A Textbook of Medical Conditions for Physiotherapists

by the same author

PHYSIOTHERAPY IN SOME SURGICAL CONDITIONS

NEUROLOGY FOR PHYSIOTHERAPISTS

CHEST, HEART AND VASCULAR DISORDERS FOR PHYSIOTHERAPISTS

A Textbook of Medical Conditions for Physiotherapists

edited by JOAN E. CASH BA, FCSP, DIP.TP

A companion volume to
Neurology for Physiotherapists
Chest, Heart and Vascular Disorders for Physiotherapists
Physiotherapy in Some Surgical Conditions

FABER AND FABER LIMITED
3 Queen Square London

First published in 1951
by Faber and Faber Limited
3 Queen Square London W.C.1
Reprinted 1951 and 1954
Second edition 1957
Reprinted 1959 and 1962
Third edition 1965
Reprinted 1968
Fourth edition 1971
Reprinted 1973 and 1975
Fifth edition 1976
Printed in Great Britain by
Butler and Tanner Ltd
Frome and London

ISBN 0 571 04894 3 (Faber Paperbacks)
ISBN 0 571 04893 5 (hard-back edition)

Foreword

by the late F. D. HOWITT CVO, MA, MD, FRCP

Physician, with charge of Physical Medicine, Middlesex Hospital
Honorary Consultant in Physical Medicine to the Army
Senior Physician to the Arthur Stanley Institute for Rheumatic Diseases

---

It gives me particular pleasure to write a short foreword to this book, partly because I have read it with great interest, and partly because I am convinced that it supplies a long-felt need.

The face of medicine in this country has changed considerably in recent years, mainly as the result of dire necessity imposed upon us by two World Wars. It has become less departmentalized, and has assumed a more purposeful character. We have come to realize that the achievement and maintenance of health, the conduct of serious disease and injury, and the rehabilitation and revocation of disabled persons are, none of them, a one-man job. Success can only be achieved by team-work, and in this team there are no two members more important than the doctor and the physiotherapist. Each has his separate function to fulfil, yet neither can fulfil it adequately unless he works in harmony with the other.

I suspect that Miss Cash had some difficulty in selecting the title for her book. It would manifestly be an impertinence for a doctor to write a textbook on physiotherapy for doctors, although there is great need for such a work. For it is most important that before prescribing the various forms of physical treatment, a medical man should be fully conversant with their uses and abuses, actions and reactions, indications and contra-indications. He should also realize the difficulties which beset the physiotherapist, when faced with an incorrect or inadequate prescription. It would be equally presumptuous for a physiotherapist to attempt to write a textbook on medicine for physiotherapists. Yet it is vital that the physiotherapist should appreciate the problems which the doctor has to face when assessing the likely value of physiotherapy in conjunction with other medical measures; its effect upon the constitutional and psychological condition of the patient; its prospects and sometimes its dangers. All physical treatments, whether preventive, corrective or remedial should be welded into a general and organized scheme. These are the points which Miss Cash has so admirably stressed from the viewpoint of the physiotherapist.

The author has aimed at simplicity, both in the general layout and in the description of the various medical conditions. The rationale for treatment has been fully explained in each instance, and there is a refreshing freedom from extravagant claims. It is up to date, and should serve equally as a work of reference for the qualified physiotherapist and for the senior student preparing for her diploma.

FRANK HOWITT

Preface to the First Edition

In writing this book the author has not attempted to teach any new material but rather to explain in detail some of the medical conditions most often seen in a department of physical medicine. It is, therefore, a book for students of physiotherapy, and it is hoped that with a better understanding of the changes occurring in these conditions the physical treatment may be carried out with a greater degree of intelligence, interest and improved efficiency.

The subject matter covers many medical conditions, but it was felt that a chapter on physical treatment in the surgical group of respiratory conditions should be included, as many chest conditions alternate between surgical and medical treatment and the physiotherapist is required to treat cases throughout both stages.

Each chapter, as well as describing medical conditions, is followed by a short outline dealing with the broad principles of treatment of these conditions by physical measures. In certain of these diseases there is little information available about the physical treatment, and so to fill in this gap a fuller account has been given.

Preface to the Fifth Edition

This edition has been completely rewritten and re-illustrated in order to bring the book up to date. The sections on neurological and respiratory disorders have been omitted because they have been more fully dealt with in separate textbooks. The section on rheumatic disorders has been considerably enlarged and it includes many new photographs. Much has been added to physiotherapy in paediatrics, including a chapter on mental subnormality, as it was felt that more information would be helpful to physiotherapy students. A revised chapter on burns has been included. Each section is followed by a bibliography.

The Editor would like to welcome the new contributors and to thank all the authors. She owes them a very deep debt of gratitude for their interest and cooperation and for giving so freely of their time.

Acknowledgments

Miss Cash would like to express her very sincere thanks and appreciation to all those who have helped her, and especially to Miss D. Caney, Principal of the School of Physiotherapy, Queen Elizabeth Hospital, Birmingham, for her advice on Part I, General Pathology and for her help and support throughout the preparation of this fifth edition. Her thanks also go to Mr G. P. Grieve of the Royal National Orthopaedic Hospital, Miss M. H. Gray of the Victoria Infirmary, Glasgow, and Miss J. Dutton of the Wrighton Hospital, Wigan, all of whom have advised and helped her.

Miss Cash owes a very deep debt of gratitude to all the contributors for their interest, co-operation and hard work. Especially she would like to thank Dr Alastair G. Mowat for his help with the editing of Part II, Rheumatic Disorders.

Miss Cash would like to thank Miss P. Jean Cunningham and Miss H. E. Potter of Faber and Faber Ltd for editing the final manuscript, and Mrs Audrey Besterman for line drawings. Her thanks also go to Miss H. Baines for typing some of the manuscript.

Mr Bannister wishes to express his gratitude to Mr J. L. Stephen, MA MCH FRCS, for the benefit of his knowledge, guidance and advice for many years, and for permission to use photographs of his patients, and to Auto-Med Ltd for the loan of their Auto-Pulse Unit with which air compression trials were carried out.

Miss Caney would like to thank Dr Ernest Fairburn, MD FRCP, Consultant Dermatologist, United Birmingham Hospitals, for his help.

Miss Graveling would like to thank the consultants of the Orthopaedic Department of the Norfolk and Norwich Hospital. She would like to express her thanks to many physiotherapists including Mrs B. Goff (Oswestry), Miss S. Kelly (Birmingham), Mr G. Grieve (for the loan of photographs) and all the physiotherapy staff at the Norfolk and Norwich Hospital. Plates 11/1–11/7 were first published in *Physiotherapy*, 1971, and are reproduced by permission of the Chartered Society of Physiotherapy. She would particularly wish to thank Mr Hugh Phillips, Consultant Orthopaedic Surgeon, for considerable help and encouragement, Mr R. Burn and staff of the photographic department, Mrs J. Tart and Miss C. Russel for typing.

Miss Kennedy would like to express her thanks to the staff and patients of the paediatric unit of St George's Hospital, and in particular to Dr Hugh Symons and Dr David Robins for their help and co-operation in the preparation of Part III, Physiotherapy for Children. She would also like to thank Miss Glennifer Hodges of the photographic department for the photographs.

Miss Marshall would like to thank Miss B. Shotton, Principal of the School of Physiotherapy, Bristol Royal Hospital (Infirmary branch), for her help in the preparation of Chapter 15, Non-articular Pain.

Dr A. G. Mowat and Mrs J. Abery wish to thank their colleagues in the medical team for advice and encouragement and they are especially grateful to Mrs Margaret Evans for typing, to Mr R. Emanuel for the photographs and to Mr G. R. Bartlett, DIPCD, for Fig. 7/1. They wish to thank the Arthritis and Rheumatism Council for the use of figures which first appeared in reports in *Rheumatic Diseases*, No. 48, on which Figs. 8/1, 8/2, 8/4, 8/5 and 8/6 are based.

Miss Wootton wishes to thank Mr T. D. Cochrane, FRCSE, Consultant Plastic Surgeon, Queen Victoria Hospital, East Grinstead, for help and encouragement he has given and the interest shown in her writing of Chapter 21, Burns.

Contributors

Joan M. Abery, MCSP
Senior Physiotherapist, Rheumatology Unit, the Nuffield Orthopaedic Centre, Oxford

C. R. Bannister, MCSP
Assistant Superintendent Physiotherapist, St Mary's Hospital, Harrow Road, London

Doreen Caney, MCSP DIP.TP
Principal, School of Physiotherapy, Queen Elizabeth Hospital, Birmingham

Joan E. Cash, BA, FCSP, DIP.TP
formerly of the Queen Elizabeth Hospital, Birmingham

B. M. Graveling, MCSP DIP.TP
Superintendent Physiotherapist, the Norfolk and Norwich Hospital, Norwich

Barbara Kennedy, MCSP
Superintendent Physiotherapist, Paediatric Department, St George's Hospital, Blackshaw Road, London

Christine M. Marshall, MCSP DIP.TP
Assistant Principal, School of Physiotherapy, Queen Elizabeth Hospital, Birmingham

Alastair G. Mowat, MB, FRCP(ED)
Clinical Lecturer in Rheumatology, University of Oxford, and Consultant Rheumatologist, the Nuffield Orthopaedic Centre, Oxford

Rosemary Wootton, MCSP
Superintendent Physiotherapist, the Queen Victoria Hospital, East Grinstead

Contents

Figures

Plates

PART I

General Pathology

JOAN E. CASH, BA, FCSP, DIP.TP

Chapter 1

Inflammation and Healing

Inflammation is the response of the body to injury. It may be defined as the reactive train of events affecting both vessels and cells which occurs in the vital tissues surrounding a site of injury. This is only true provided the injury has not been so severe as to destroy the area. It fulfils a two-fold purpose: (a) removal of the irritant, debris and dead cells; (b) preparation of the way for repair.

Causes

Any factor which damages the cells sets up the process of inflammation. Such factors may include:

(a) mechanical factors as in trauma;
(b) chemical agents such as corrosive acids and alkalis;
(c) microbiological agents;
(d) physical agents including excessive heat or cold;
(e) immunological factors as in antihistamine diseases.

THE BASIC CHANGES OF INFLAMMATION

Whatever the causes of inflammation, the reaction follows a basic pattern:

(a) changes in the calibre of the small blood vessels, arterioles, capillaries and venules;

(b) alteration in the rate of blood flow and increase in the permeability of the walls of the venules and capillaries;

(c) rearrangement of the cells in the vessels, emigration and diapedesis;

(d) transudation and exudation;

(e) changes in the lymph flow;

(f) changes in the groundwork of the surroundings of the tissues.

Changes in the calibre of the small vessels

Following a transient vasoconstriction, the arterioles, capillaries and venules dilate and capillaries not previously patent open up. This dilatation is the result of stimulation of the axon reflex and the release of chemical substances. In the early stages many substances have been thought to be responsible but there is still uncertainty as to which of these is really important. There is probably a variety of proteolytic enzymes and polypeptides concerned.

Alteration in the rate of blood flow and increase in the permeability of the vessel walls

Concurrently with vasodilatation the rate of flow increases, but within 10 to 15 minutes the flow slows and the blood may even stagnate. This is due to: (a) the increased viscosity of the blood resulting from the loss of fluid into the intercellular spaces; and (b) the increase in peripheral resistance. When the vessels are normal the blood cells occupy the centre of the stream and there is a clear zone of plasma adjacent to the walls of the vessels. This decreases the resistance to blood flow.

When the tissues are damaged the endothelial cells swell and become coated with a gelatinous substance of uncertain origin and the red cells run into rouleaux, displacing the lighter white cells into the clear zone. These cells then adhere to the sticky endothelium. The exact cause of this adherence is not yet known. Platelets also tend to adhere and little masses of white cells and platelets form and may even occlude the lumen. Thus thrombosis of small vessels is quite possible. The adherence of the white cells to the vessel walls is known as *margination.*

At the same time as the blood flow slows, the permeability of the walls of the venules and capillaries increases. This ensures that more water and protein molecules pass into the tissues and it makes the escape of white and red cells easier.

Emigration and diapedesis

Subsequent to the rearrangement of cells and adherence to the walls of the capillaries, the phagocytic cells pass out of the vessels by pushing their way between the cells and then bursting through the basement membrane. This is known as the process of *emigration.* The first cells to pass out are the neutrophils. These are followed by the larger, slower-moving monocytes, usually known when they reach the tissue spaces as macrophages. The cells move towards the damaged area. It is not certain whether this is simply a random movement or whether they are attracted by products released by the injured tissues or bacteria.

The neutrophils ingest damaged cells and bacteria, and then start the process of digestion. They have only a short life of two to three days, and any undigested particles which are liberated into the intercellular fluid on the death of these cells, together with tissue debris, are removed by the macrophages. In many cases of inflammation some red cells leave the capillaries. They follow the white cells simply by being ejected through the gaps made by these cells under the influence of the hydrostatic pressure of the blood. This process is known as *diapedesis*, a term originally applied to the passage of the white cells, but now more commonly used for the red cell ejection.

Transudation and exudation

A *transudate* is the fluid which filters through the capillary wall as a result of an increase in hydrostatic pressure. It has a low specific gravity and contains glucose, salts and other small molecules able to pass through the normal vessel wall.

An *exudate* occurs in inflammation when changes in the capillary cells allow larger molecules to pass through into the tissues. Since the fluid formed will therefore contain the larger molecules of plasma proteins, it will have a higher specific gravity.

Normally fluid with substances in solution, excluding plasma proteins, passes out into the tissues from the small vessels under the influence of hydrostatic pressure and is attracted back by the osmotic pressure exerted by the plasma proteins. When damage occurs the venules and capillaries become more permeable. It is not yet certain what produces this change. The result of this increased permeability is that more fluid, rich in plasma proteins, passes into the tissue spaces. The intercellular fluid has, therefore, a higher osmotic pressure and less fluid is attracted back into the capillaries. In addition metabolic processes in the tissues are speeded up and the consequent breakdown of large protein molecules into smaller ones further increases the osmotic pressure of the intercellular fluid. This allows the exudate to diffuse more widely so that tension does not rise so rapidly in the tissues. An immediate rise in tension would tend to prevent fluid exudation.

This exudate is important for three reasons: (a) it dilutes toxic agents; (b) it allows the passage of substances and antibodies into the affected area; (c) since the fluid has a high protein content it tends to clot. A fibrin network is formed which prevents the spread of harmful agents and provides a scaffolding for the movement of phagocytic cells and for the growth of new tissues if this is necessary.

The nature and quantity of the transudate or exudate varies with the agent causing the inflammation and its severity.

THE AGENT

Should micro-organisms be responsible for the inflammatory reaction, some, such as the streptococci, induce a thin pus which spreads easily. Others, such as the staphylococci, produce a thick pus which collects in the area of injury. The tubercle bacillus produces granulomas which consist of little masses of epitheloid cells surrounded by a circle of mononuclear leucocytes and lymphocytes. In some conditions, for example rheumatic fever, the exudate is fibrinous and fibrinoid deposits tend to occur. There may also be necrotic areas in the walls of the blood vessels.

THE SEVERITY OF THE INJURY

If the injury is slight there is usually a thin transudate which, since it has a low protein content, fails to clot and is readily re-absorbed (serous inflammation). In more severe damage the permeability of the small vessels is considerably increased, the larger fibrinogen molecules now pass out, clotting of the exudate therefore occurs, fibrin is formed and this may later be broken down by enzymes or it may eventually be organized into fibrous tissue (fibrinous inflammation). Still greater injury and tissue destruction results in larger quantities of phagocytic cells invading the area with consequent pus formation (purulent inflammation).

Changes in the lymph flow

There is an increase in the local lymph flow and the lymph contains more white cells and proteins than usual. This change causes the removal of some excess fluid and debris to the lymph nodes whose reticulo-endothelial cells deal with the debris.

Changes in the groundwork of the surrounding tissues

An early and important change is in the groundwork of the tissues. This changes from a gel to a fluid so preventing an early rise in tissue tension and allowing diffusion of the excess fluid.

RESOLUTION, CHRONICITY, SUPPURATION

Resolution

If the inflammatory agent is very mild the damaged cells and the exudate will be quickly removed and the area will rapidly return to normal. This is known as resolution. A more severe injury, provided it is not accompanied by much tissue destruction, should also resolve but the process will take a little longer, possibly up to several weeks. This return to normal occurs in the following way:

(a) *Removal of excess fluid.* Some of the fluid exudate flows back into the capillaries because, with the removal of the irritant, the vessels return to normal and the balance between hydrostatic pressure and osmotic pressure is restored. Much of the fluid is carried by the lymphatics to the regional lymph nodes.

(b) *Removal of cellular debris and damaged phagocytes.* Some debris is carried in the lymph stream to the nodes where it is dealt with by the cells lining the sinuses. Dead leucocytes are removed by the monocytes.

(c) *Undamaged polymorphs* pass back into the blood and lymph streams and macrophages wander back into the surrounding connective tissues.

Chronicity

Inflammation can fail to resolve because the irritant is not removed by the acute reaction. It then passes into the stage of chronicity characterized by proliferation of connective tissues (p. 9).

Suppuration

Pus production is the result of several factors: (a) considerable destruction of tissue either at the time of injury or by the continued action of bacteria; (b) the presence of micro-organisms which release toxic substances causing further damage to cells; (c) the stagnation of blood in the small vessels cutting down nutrition sufficiently to cause death of cells.

The destroyed tissue cannot be cleared away until it is softened and liquefied. The first step is the invasion by polymorphonuclear leucocytes followed later by lymphocytes. The normal life of the leucocytes is only a few days and in addition many will be destroyed by the micro-organisms. These dead cells together with tissue cells release protein-splitting enzymes whose function is to digest the solid debris. The resulting fluid is *pus.*

Pus is liquid containing: (a) dead and dying white cells; (b) inflammatory exudate and fibrin; (c) dead and living micro-organisms; (d) the products of tissue breakdown, nucleic acids and lipids.

The viscosity of the pus depends upon the degree to which the debris is liquefied as well as on the causative agent (p. 5). If the pus is thin and watery it tends to spread easily and a considerable area may become affected (cellulitis). If the pus is thick it tends to remain localized and the cavity in which it is contained is known as the *abscess cavity.* The pus tends to track in the line of least resistance until it reaches and breaks through a free surface. When the pus is able to discharge either this way, or preferably by surgical intervention, the cavity will heal by granulation tissue unless a chronic infection develops, in which case more pus is formed, the walls of the cavity become thickened by fibrous tissue and pus persistently discharges so that a sinus is formed. Occasionally the abscess fails to discharge and pus becomes walled off by thick fibrous tissue. Gradually fluid is absorbed and the pus thickens into a porridge-like consistency, which may become calcified.

SIGNS AND SYMPTOMS

Inflammation is characterized by redness, heat, pain, swelling and loss of function. There may also be rise of temperature, respiration and pulse rate, together with other signs of fever. The presence and severity of these signs depend upon the degree of the injury done to the tissues and the efficacy of the body's defence mechanism in that area.

Redness

This is due to the vascular dilatation and consequent hyperaemia. Dilatation of the capillaries produces a dull red area, dilatation of arterioles a brighter red flare. This can be seen if the skin is firmly stroked with a hard object. The immediate response is a white line caused by temporary vasoconstriction. This is followed by a dull red line which is rapidly surrounded by a bright red flare. The dull red area then swells and a wheal may appear due to the exudate causing the red line to become paler. This is the triple response of the skin to injury, described by Lewis.

Heat

Dilatation of arterioles increases the blood supply to the part. If the temperature of the affected area is lower than that of the blood because the area is in contact with the external environment, the increased blood flow will raise its temperature. Heat is not felt in deeper tissues for this reason and because the organs do not have heat-sensitive nerve endings.

Pain

This is at least partly due to tension created in the tissues by the exudate. It will, therefore, be greatest if there is little room for swelling, resulting in greater pressure on pain-sensitive nerve endings. It may be that pain is also the result of concentration of hydrogen ions in an inflamed area or due to chemical substances liberated by damaged tissues.

Swelling

Inflammatory exudate accumulating in the affected area produces swelling, the amount depending on the severity of the inflammatory changes, the tension of the particular tissues and the extent to which the fluid can diffuse away. It may also be due to increased activity of special secreting cells involved in the injury. Thus if a synovial membrane is inflamed there will be inflammatory exudate causing swelling of the membrane and increased synovial fluid producing an effusion into the joint cavity.

Loss of function

Inflammation will upset the functions of the tissues. For example, if a joint is inflamed it is painful and there will be reflex inhibition of the muscles acting on the joint. Swelling would also make movement difficult.

CHRONIC INFLAMMATION

This type of inflammation is characterized by the formation of fibrous tissue, causing thickening, loss of elasticity and pliability of the tissues and disturbance of function.

It is due to:

(a) The persistence of the agent which initiates acute inflammation because: (i) the body's defensive mechanism to a particular micro-organism such as the tubercle bacillus may be low; (ii) the factors which delay healing may be present; (iii) a foreign body may not have been removed by the acute reaction.

(b) The agent has caused so mild a reaction that it has not been recognized by the body. Pneumoconiosis is an example of this. Asbestos workers inhale particles of asbestos. These particles are too large to be removed by the macrophages so they remain in the alveoli and stimulate a mild reaction which is followed by extensive fibrosis of the lung. Certain micro-organisms produce only a fleeting acute reaction but tend to remain in the tissues, causing chronic irritation.

Two types of chronic inflammation are found: (a) that which follows acute inflammation; (b) that in which there has been no appreciable acute reaction.

There is little difference between the changes which occur in the two types, so they will be considered together.

Changes

The changes are a mixture of the vascular and proliferative changes of acute inflammation – the attempt to clear the debris and the micro-organisms and the processes of healing. This is the state in which inflammation and healing are going on at the same time.

In many cases of chronic inflammation there is extensive exudation of protein-rich fluid leading to the production of considerable quantities of fibrin. This is particularly seen in chronic, suppurative inflammation and inflammation of serous sacs. Many cells are present in the area including large quantities of macrophages which may have fused to form giant cells. These cells soften and remove the dead cells and debris.

Lymphocytes and plasma cells are also found in great numbers. The function of the latter cells is uncertain but they are a feature of the granulation tissue in chronic inflammation. Endothelial cells are also present forming new capillaries. These are especially noticeable in the lining of chronic abscess cavities and they break down readily leading to haemorrhage.

Fibroblasts are present in large numbers and lay down the collagen which produces a large quantity of fibrous tissue. If the cells of the chronically inflamed tissue can divide, then regeneration occurs. Quite often there is excessive production of new cells, which is particularly noticeable in epithelial tissues.

Signs and symptoms

These depend on the area involved. Fibrous tissue replacing specialized tissue cannot carry out the functions of the tissue in which it is formed. It may, for example, form adhesions binding the lung to the chest wall and interfering with expansion; it may 'stick' ligaments to the bones over which they pass, limiting movement; it may bind tendons in their sheaths and interfere with the work of muscles. It can reduce the elasticity of tubes as in chronic bronchitis and if it replaces glandular tissue reduce secretions.

Chronic suppurative inflammation may give rise to haemorrhage, as in stomach ulcers, and it always gives rise to general symptoms of loss of appetite, loss of weight, anaemia, headache and tiredness.

HEALING

In the floor of any open and healing wound tiny raised red dots can be clearly seen. To this tissue the term *granulation tissue* has been applied. The name originates from the Latin *granum*—a seed or granule. Each dot or granule consists of new blood vessels, macrophages, fibroblasts and other cells.

No matter what body tissue is damaged, healing begins with the formation of granulation tissue. The final result may differ depending upon whether the parenchymal cells are capable of mitotic division or not. The cells of some tissues such as epithelium, bone marrow, lymph glands and the spleen continue to divide throughout life. Such tissues have great powers of regeneration. Some cells, for example the cells of the liver, have the power to divide but only do so if the need arises. On the other hand nerve and muscle cells have no power to reproduce themselves and in this case granulation tissue will eventually be converted into scar tissue.

Regeneration is the replacement of lost tissue by similar tissue. *Repair* is replacement by scar tissue when the cells of the damaged organ or tissue are unable to divide.

Repair

The process of repair is best understood in the healing of open wounds but the same changes will occur in all other areas of the body where the parenchymal cells are not capable of reproducing the original tissue.

Healing of skin wounds

If there is little tissue loss and no infection, such wounds heal by first intention (primary union). With more destruction healing occurs by second intention (secondary union).

HEALING BY FIRST INTENTION

This should occur following a clean cut or surgical incision and follows a basic pattern:

(a) *Blood clot.* This fills the small gap and the crust on the surface seals the wound. The fibrin of the clot serves the purpose of providing a scaffold along which the epithelial cells and fibroblasts can grow into the gap.

(b) *Inflammatory reaction.* This occurs in the edges of the wound and is characterized by fluid and cellular exudate.

(c) *Invasion of the clot by phagocytic cells.* These begin the work of liquefying the fibrin (formed in the process of clotting) and any debris caused by the injury. This starts within the first 24 hours.

(d) *Proliferation of cells.*

(i) The *endothelial cells* of both blood and lymph capillaries multiply and form buds which grow out into the fibrinous scaffolding. These buds rapidly develop a lumen and form loops through which the blood flows (granulation tissue). The loops anastomose with each other and a network of new capillaries develops. At first the new blood vessels are all capillaries but gradually some acquire a muscular coat to form arterioles, while others enlarge to form venules.

(ii) *Fibroblasts* grow out from the margins of the wound with the capillaries into the fibrinous scaffolding and gradually fibres form around them. It is not certain how these fibres form but they only do so in the presence of fibroblasts. Within four to five days some collagen is present and this increases over the next two to three weeks. The fibroblasts are also thought to be responsible for the production of the groundwork substance of the new tissue.

(iii) *Epithelial cells* from the margins of the wound multiply and migrate over the surface of the wound and fuse at the centre. At first just a single layer of cells covers the wound, which therefore looks bluish in appearance, but quickly these cells divide and differentiate until normal skin is formed devoid only of hair follicles, sweat and sebaceous glands, which, if destroyed, cannot reproduce themselves.

With a minute gap the wound is healed within a few days though as more collagen forms its strength increases over several weeks.

HEALING BY SECOND INTENTION

There is no real difference in the healing process except that there is necrotic tissue and debris to be removed and a gap to be filled. The process of healing therefore takes longer. More granulation tissue is formed and more scar tissue results. The gap is filled by clotted exudate and blood. Phagocytic cells invade the clot. Capillaries and fibroblasts grow in from the sides and floor of the wound, filling it with granulation tissue.

If the cells of the damaged tissue can divide, new cells infiltrate the granulation tissue, but if they cannot, the tissue becomes increasingly fibrous. The collagen fibres thicken and new layers are laid down at right angles to each other, so that eventually a tough bundle or membrane of collagen fibre is formed. Tension on these fibres seems to determine the direction in which they lie.

Epithelial cells at the edges of the wound multiply and migrate down the sides into the wound between the connective tissue and the clot, forcing the latter up. As the granulation tissue grows up from the floor and sides, the tongues of epithelial cells growing down on the edges of the gap are forced up until they cover the surface. Should there be much loss of epithelium, cells are obtained from the bases of the hair follicles and sweat glands.

While all this is going on some of the new blood vessels begin to atrophy while others show such proliferation of the endothelium that their lumen is obliterated. As devascularization and thickening increase, pale avascular scar tissue is formed. This has a great tendency to contract, thereby deforming the surrounding tissues.

Rate of healing

A rough guide to the times taken for the various stages of healing in a clean incised wound is as follows:

(a) The clotting of the blood and the formation of the scab which seals the wound occurs within the first few hours.

(b) The migration and proliferation of epithelial cells to form new skin, of endothelial cells to form new blood vessels, and fibroblasts to form collagen and groundwork substances begins within the first 24 hours. Fine fibrils appear two days after injury. These thicken to form collagen fibres by about the fourth day. Collagen formation then increases rapidly for three to four weeks and as this increases devascularization also occurs. The tensile strength of the healing area is good by four weeks and is back to normal by about six to eight weeks.

Wounds which heal by second intention pass through the same stages but make a slower start since debris and destroyed tissue have to be removed first. The gap requires filling and epithelization cannot occur until there is a good base over which epithelial cells can migrate.

The actual rate of healing is influenced by both local and general factors.

LOCAL FACTORS

One of the most important of these is the vascularity of the damaged tissue. A *good blood supply* is necessary both for an inflammatory reaction and to support the processes of repair. Circulation varies in different tissues. Some, such as bone and muscle, are highly vascular; others, such as cartilage and ligaments, have very poor nutrition and heal less readily. When the circulation is impaired by disease, healing can be seriously affected, as can be readily seen in peripheral vascular disease. The blood supply can also be reduced by: (a) prolonged pressure; (b) oedema; (c) chronic inflammation since this is accompanied by thickening of the intima and obliteration of the lumen of the blood vessels.

Infection will delay healing since the toxins produced by micro-organisms destroy tissue.

Persistent irritation will cause healing to be slowed, e.g. the presence of foreign bodies.

Continual breakdown of granulation tissue due to rough handling will delay healing. Repeated dressing of a wound will have a similar effect.

Too early movement will sometimes delay healing if it causes further damage or destruction of granulation tissue.

The speed of healing is increased by physical measures which stimulate the circulation. Thus heat, ultraviolet light and moderate exercise may all help the healing process if applied correctly.

Healing of other soft tissues

Healing of damaged tendons takes place in an identical way to that of other soft tissues except that tendon cells are found in the granulation tissue and very slowly regeneration will occur. If the ends of the tendon are not joined, however, union will be by fibrous tissue and the danger is then that repeated stretching due to movement will elongate the fibrous tissue, lengthening the tendon and reducing power.

In a minor injury of a muscle with rupture of individual fibres, regeneration can occur but in more severe injuries scar tissue forms. Cardiac muscle fibres have no ability to divide, consequently damage to the heart muscle is healed by fibrous tissue – an infarct is converted into fibrous tissue.

Nerve tissue within the brain and spinal cord has no power of regeneration since nerve cells cannot reproduce, and axons can only grow if there is a neurilemma. Nerve fibres in the central nervous system do not have a neurilemmal sheath. Peripheral nerves on the other hand can regenerate if the cells of origin of the axons are still intact.

Healing of bone

Again the fundamental basis of repair of bone is by the formation of granulation tissue.

The final result is, however, different for two main reasons. In the first place, bone-forming cells are available in the periosteum, endosteum and bone marrow, and in the second place, when there is hyperaemia round bone, calcium is absorbed from the bone and is in high concentration in the surrounding fluid. Thus two main essentials for bone formation – bone-forming cells and calcium, are available. (For full details of repair, see *Physiotherapy in Some Surgical Conditions* edited by J. E. Cash.)

REFERENCE

Lewis, Sir Thomas. *Vascular Disorders of the Limbs.* Macmillan 1949.

For Bibliography see p. 35.

Chapter 2

Oedema

Oedema may be defined as the accumulation of fluid in the intercellular tissue spaces and/or the body cavities. At first excess fluid is absorbed into the cells and fibres, rendering the area firmer and heavier. When the fluid can no longer be absorbed it collects in the spaces and cavities.

Oedema can be either general or local. When excess fluid is formed in the body cavities it is sometimes specially named according to the serous cavity in which it is formed, e.g. hydrothorax, hydroperitoneum, hydropericardium.

NORMAL FORMATION AND DRAINAGE OF TISSUE FLUID

Formation

Tissue fluid is formed under the influence of three main factors: (i) hydrostatic pressure; (ii) osmotic pressure; (iii) the permeability of the capillary walls.

HYDROSTATIC PRESSURE

The blood pressure in the capillaries is higher than the pressure of the tissue fluid, consequently water and dissolved substances diffuse through the capillary wall into the tissues.

OSMOTIC PRESSURE

The osmotic pressure of the blood is largely dependent upon the plasma proteins, particularly upon the serum albumin. The capillary wall is not normally permeable, to any extent, to the larger molecules of these proteins, though a very small amount does pass through. As a result the osmotic pressure of the capillary blood is greater than that of the tissue fluid. An attractive force is therefore exerted to withdraw the fluid from the tissue space.

PERMEABILITY OF THE CAPILLARY WALL

The capillary endothelium is permeable to certain substances and not to others. Water, glucose and salts may all pass through, provided they are in greater concentration on one side of the membrane than the other. The larger molecules of the plasma proteins cannot normally diffuse, to any extent, through the endothelial cells.

Permeability can be altered. Any factor which brings about dilatation of the capillary will also increase the capillary pore size and under these circumstances the plasma proteins may enter the tissue fluid, raising its osmotic pressure and lowering that of the blood.

Drainage

Absorption of tissue fluid occurs into the blood and lymph capillaries. Since the osmotic pressure of the blood in the capillaries is greater than that of the tissue fluid, fluid is attracted back into the capillaries. At the same time the hydrostatic pressure of the tissue fluid is greater than that within the lymph capillaries, consequently fluid flows from the intercellular spaces into the lymph vessels. The small quantities of proteins in the tissue fluid will pass into the lymph vessels since these are more permeable than the blood capillaries. This ensures that the osmotic pressure of the tissue fluid remains low.

A balance is kept between the fluid which is formed and that which is absorbed. Thus fluid passes into the tissues and from here into the lymph vessels and so to the lymphatic glands under the influence of hydrostatic pressure and it passes back into the blood vessels under the influence of the attractive force of the osmotic pressure of the blood.

The quantity of fluid varies with rest and exercise. Activity of the muscles brings about vasodilatation and increased formation of metabolites. Vasodilatation causes increased formation of tissue fluid, while increased metabolites may raise the osmotic pressure of the tissue fluid, so that the attractive force of the capillary blood is lessened. The stiffness which follows strenuous exercise is the result of increased fluid in the tissue spaces.

FACTORS RESPONSIBLE FOR OEDEMA

Oedema may be the result of the following changes: (i) increase in hydrostatic pressure of the blood; (ii) fall in osmotic pressure of the blood; (iii) increased capillary permeability; (iv) lymphatic obstruction; (v) venous obstruction; (vi) slowed rate of flow of blood and lymph.

Increase in hydrostatic pressure

This will, if it is sufficiently prolonged, cause oedema. It is not the only cause, since a rise in hydrostatic pressure in the capillaries means a disturbance of the circulation with change in the endothelium and increased permeability.

A rise in hydrostatic pressure may be the result of general or local factors. If the heart fails to maintain a normal circulation, there will be congestion in the veins and hydrostatic pressure will rise in the capillaries. Increased filtration will therefore occur. An obstruction in a large vein will have exactly the same effect, though it will be localized to the area which is drained by that vein.

Fall in osmotic pressure

This will lessen the attracting force exerted by the blood, and fluid will tend to accumulate in the tissues. Locally it may arise because the permeability of the capillary wall is increased and plasma proteins pass into the intercellular fluid. This occurs in inflammation. A fall in the general osmotic pressure may be the effect of one type of kidney disease in which a greater quantity of plasma proteins is lost through the kidney.

The plasma proteins may also be deficient due to starvation, and in this case a nutritional oedema may develop.

Increased capillary permeability

Trauma or nutritional disturbances may alter the permeability of the endothelium. A capillary reacts to irritation not only by dilating but also by changes in the endothelial cells which form the vessel. A great quantity of fluid may enter the tissues as a result of this factor, both in severe lacerations and in burns.

Any factor which disturbs the nutrition of the cells will also increase their permeability. If the blood is circulating unduly slowly, it loses oxygen and gains more than the normal amount of carbon dioxide. This disturbs the physical state of the endothelium and tissue fluid increases. Oedema will therefore occur, not only following trauma but also in all cases of venous congestion.

Lymphatic obstruction

Tissue fluid may be formed normally but its drainage may be impaired because the lymph channels are blocked or because they have been removed surgically. Blocking may be due to one of the following:

(i) The action of parasites such as the worm producing filariasis. This worm causes fibrosis in the vessels and glands. The oedema can be so severe in the legs and external genitalia that the name elephantiasis has been given to the condition.

(ii) Inflammation of the vessels and lymph glands.

(iii) Pressure of tumours or scar tissue.

Venous obstruction

Obstruction to the return of venous blood to the heart will cause oedema. This can be due to right-sided heart failure, or to local obstruction arising from deep vein thrombosis or massive scar tissue formation. Overloading of the veins results in a rise in hydrostatic pressure in the venules and capillaries.

Slowed flow of blood and lymph

Weak or paralysed muscles, stiff joints and poor action of the diaphragm will all reduce the venous and lymphatic return so that tissue drainage is impaired.

EFFECTS OF OEDEMA

The presence of extensive oedema is liable to set up an arterial spasm and so cause an anaemic condition of the area. Even if it fails to cause spasm it causes anaemia because, as the hydrostatic pressure of the tissue fluid rises, pressure is exerted on the capillaries and arterial inflow is retarded.

Persistent fluid in the tissue spaces interferes with the nutrition of the cells since fresh nutrient substances and gases are not available and waste products are not removed; metabolism is therefore seriously impaired and the function of the area diminished.

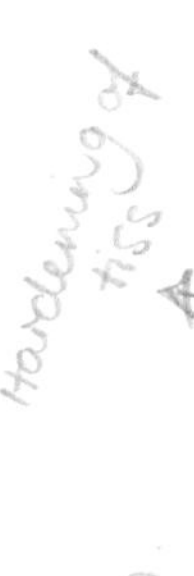

In the course of time, the fluid will tend to organize into fibrous tissue and the area becomes indurated. The speed with which this occurs depends upon the characteristics of the oedema fluid. If it contains a high percentage of protein it will clot readily. This condition exists when the fluid is largely the result of increased capillary permeability, and is less likely when the major factor in its formation is either raised hydrostatic pressure or low osmotic pressure. Should the fluid clot, it forms a mass foreign to the tissues and they will react by proliferation. Cells and blood vessels invade the clotted fluid and it gradually becomes converted into fibrous tissue. This may have serious effects because the fibrous tissue tends to shrink. As it shrinks it may obliterate blood vessels, so causing anaemia and gross disturbance in local nutrition. It may, if it has occurred in the periarticular structures, cause limitation of movement in joints. Should the fluid have invaded muscles, elasticity and extensibility will be impaired. Muscular contraction may be seriously hampered by the presence of scar tissue. Should oedema occur in serous membranes, adhesions may form, causing interference with the movements of the underlying organs.

In addition to all these ill-effects, the presence of fluid distending the tissue spaces is a source of permanent discomfort and annoyance to the patient.

TYPES OF OEDEMA

Oedema occurs in many different conditions. Often therefore a special name is used to indicate the type

General oedema: (i) cardiac
(ii) renal
(iii) starvation
Local oedema: (iv) traumatic
(v) obstructive
(vi) paralytic
(vii) oedema due to poor muscle tone and laxity of the fascia.

Cardiac oedema

This is seen in right ventricular failure when the ventricle fails to pump out the venous blood adequately. This leads to back-pressure and congestion in the veins. If the patient is up and about, it is most marked in the lower extremities where the hydrostatic pressure is normally highest. If the patient is confined to bed it occurs in the sacral region. The oedema is worst at night when the heart is tired, and is least in the morning. Since it is mainly due to the rise in pressure in the venules and capillaries it has a low protein content and does not clot readily. If a finger is pressed over the area and then removed a depression will be left which will slowly fill as the fluid is pressed out of the tissues under the finger and then is formed again. This is known as 'pitting on pressure'.

Renal oedema

This is most usually the result of a drop of osmotic pressure arising from increased permeability of the glomeruli to plasma proteins. The oedema is widespread and, having a low protein content, pits on pressure. It is often noticeable in the face, particularly in the lax tissues around the eyes, and is worse in the morning, tending to be dispersed by muscular action during the day.

Starvation oedema

This is probably partly due to a drop in the osmotic pressure of the blood as a result of a deficiency of proteins, partly due to nutritional disturbances with loss of fat and laxity of the tissues, and partly due to decreased heart action and slowing of the circulation.

Traumatic oedema

One of the most serious effects of extensive burns is the great loss of fluid into the tissues. This is also seen to a lesser degree in injuries such as extensive laceration, fractures and dislocations. Various factors enter into this type of oedema.

(i) Rise of local hydrostatic pressure due to the irritation of the sensory nerve endings and the release of a histamine-like substance, bringing about extensive vasodilatation and hyperaemia.

(ii) Increase in the permeability of the dilated capillaries caused by the injury.

(iii) Injury and possibly thrombosis of the lymphatic vessels and veins with interference to the drainage of tissue fluid.

(iv) Diminished function reducing the pumping effect of muscle action and joint movement on the soft-walled vessels.

The fluid formed has a very high protein content and clots and organizes readily. For this reason the final effects on the area may be serious if care is not taken.

Obstructive oedema

This type of oedema is non-inflammatory in origin. It develops if either veins or lymphatics are obstructed. This may be the result of: (i) deep venous thrombosis; (ii) filariasis; (iii) pressure of scars or tumours; (iv) removal of lymph glands and vessels.

In a condition such as phlegmasia alba dolens (white leg), femoral thrombosis and chronic inflammation of the lymph vessels are probably both responsible. The oedema which occasionally follows radical mastectomy is an illustration of obstructive oedema which may be due to removal of lymph glands or to pressure of axillary scar tissue. The presence of fluid is mainly due to a rise in hydrostatic pressure and the fluid will have a low protein content and will clot only slowly. Nevertheless in the course of time it will organize.

Paralytic oedema

Oedema tends to develop in the presence of extensive muscular paralysis. It is due either to paralysis of the vasoconstrictors causing widespread vasodilatation, congestion and increased filtration, or to decreased function and loss of the pumping effect normally exerted on the veins and lymphatics. If the circulation is slowed as a result of either or both of these factors, the oxygen tension of the blood will fall and the capillaries will therefore become more permeable. The fluid is likely to have a high protein content and will readily organize.

Oedema due to poor muscle tone and laxity of fascia

In the erect position, venous blood from the legs and abdomen has to return to the heart against the force of gravity. It would therefore have a tendency to stagnate in these regions if it were not for certain factors.

(i) The deep fascia of the lower extremity is particularly strong and extensive and acts as a kind of elastic stocking to support the veins. Many of the muscles either insert directly into this fascia or send expansions to reinforce it. The fascia is affected either by prolonged recumbency or by immobilization of the limb in a rigid support since the muscles inserting into it will become weaker and hypotonic and the fascia will become less tense.

(ii) The tone of the muscles of the legs and abdominal wall plays a very important part in the prevention of 'pooling' of blood, thus any factor which causes decrease in tone may lead to venous congestion.

(iii) The vasomotor mechanism causes an increase in the tone of the veins when the posture is changed from lying to standing, but if this mechanism has not been fully in use for a period of time, then when it is required it does not act as effectively as it should.

Oedema therefore tends to occur when a patient first gets up after a long period in bed, particularly if the illness has been one such as rheumatoid arthritis, in which the muscles have been directly affected and their strength and tone reduced. It will also develop when a plaster splint is removed after a prolonged period of immobilization. In each case the inadequately constricted or supported vessels tend to dilate, venous congestion develops and excess tissue fluid is formed, partly under the influence of a raised hydrostatic pressure and partly as a result of increased capillary permeability. The fluid will have a high protein content and will clot readily.

Idiopathic oedema

There are a few people in whom oedema tends to develop without known cause. This is an hereditary oedema which has certain peculiar features. It affects women mainly and may involve one or both legs. No treatment appears to be effective. It causes no outstanding symptoms, but it brings about an unsightly thickening of the legs.

TREATMENT BY PHYSIOTHERAPY

The treatment of oedema depends upon the type.

GENERAL OEDEMA

This is rarely treated by physical measures. In these cases the treatment is medical, and if the heart lesion or the kidney disease can be alleviated, oedema is likely to disappear. Occasionally a case of cardiac oedema is met by the physiotherapist, when the main object is to hasten the absorption of fluid by the lymphatic vessels and so give the patient temporary relief from discomfort until such time as the production of excessive fluid ceases. This oedema will be treated on the same lines as obstructive oedema but with particular precautions owing to the cardiac condition.

Local oedema

This type more commonly presents itself for physical treatment and a careful consideration of its cause must first be made.

TRAUMATIC OEDEMA

When trauma is extensive some oedema is almost inevitable. The main principle of treatment is the prevention of organization into fibrous tissue. Efforts must be made to:

(i) Decrease the formation of the tissue fluid by rest and firm support.

(ii) Speed its absorption by encouraging its movement into areas in which the veins and lymphatics have not been damaged, and speed the flow of venous blood and lymph in these regions. Such measures as superficial heat and massage to the region proximal to the injury will assist.

(iii) Keep the fluid moving so that it cannot clot, by elevation of the limb and rhythmic muscle contractions to press the fluid out of the tissue spaces. If muscle contractions are difficult to obtain, minimal faradic contractions may be used temporarily.

In nearly every case functional use of the limb can be encouraged early, so stimulating the tissue drainage and preventing organization.

OBSTRUCTIVE OEDEMA

The excess fluid in this case is the result of obstruction in the venous or lymph drainage or in both. Whether the oedema will subside will depend upon how well the unobstructed vessels will dilate to do the work of the obstructed ones. The principle underlying the use of physical means is the attempt to encourage the development of a good collateral circulation. Any measures which press the fluid out of the tissue spaces and force it proximally are likely to assist, e.g.

(i) Faradism under pressure.

(ii) Strong muscle contractions followed by relaxation.

(iii) With the limb elevated the fluid should be mechanically pushed on by slow, deep effleurage and vigorous active movements which press the fluid on in the veins and lymphatics.

(iv) A firm support to prevent accumulation of fluid. A one-way stretch elastic bandage must be worn and it is the physiotherapist's duty to teach the patient how and when to apply it and to give instructions about washing the bandage and its replacement when necessary.

In these cases of obstructive oedema the condition is sometimes a long-standing one and some of the tissue fluid may have organized into firm fibrous tissue which by pressure has further impeded the circulation. If these areas of induration are localized (such as may be seen around gravitational ulcers, Chapter 20) an attempt may be made to soften the fibrous tissue by the use of ultrasound and deep finger kneadings.

The most important part of the physical treatment is to teach the patient that the best way to reduce and prevent recurrence of swelling is active use of the limb while wearing a firm support. Thus walking and active exercises in the support are essential, but standing and sitting with the limb dependent are to be avoided.

PARALYTIC OEDEMA

Since the excess fluid is the result of vasodilatation and lack of use, it is difficult to prevent its formation. Continual dispersal of the fluid and movement to prevent clotting are therefore essential. Unlike traumatic oedema this cannot be carried out by the use of rhythmic contractions and active movements. Passive means must be used:

(i) Elevation of the part.

(ii) Passive movements of joints.

(iii) Artificial exercise of the paralysed muscles by means of the interrupted direct current will exert a pumping effect on the veins and lymphatics and will keep the tissue fluid moving.

(iv) Light massage is sometimes effective in dispersing the fluid into regions not affected by the paralysis, but care must be taken not to increase the paralytic vasodilatation nor to bruise or stretch the atonic muscle fibres.

OEDEMA DUE TO POOR MUSCLE TONE AND LAXITY OF THE FASCIA

Since the oedema is the result of lack of muscle tone and poor condition of fascia, the principle of treatment by physiotherapy is to bring back to normal the strength and tone of the musculature. This can be carried out by the use of maximal resisted exercises. While this is being done, constant seeping of fluid into the tissues should be lessened by repeated elevation of the limb and by firm pressure using elastic bandages. Any fluid which forms must not be allowed to organize, and measures such as those used in obstructive oedema (p. 22) are of value.

In all cases of oedema it is worth noting that the vessels in the region of the oedema should not be encouraged to dilate since this results in increased filtration of fluid. Dilatation of vessels which are not always patent is, however, desirable in areas proximal to the oedema. For this reason it is wiser to avoid the use of heat directly over the area. The immersion of an oedematous hand or foot in hot paraffin wax usually increases the tension in the tissues. If, due to oedema and arterial spasm, the limb is cold and blue, heat can be given to the trunk. The limb is then indirectly warmed without increasing the oedema.

For Bibliography, see p. 35.

Chapter 3

Thrombosis and Embolism

THROMBOSIS

A thrombus is a solid body formed in the cardiovascular system from the constituents of blood. Blood platelets adhere to the lining of the vessel, thromboplastin is liberated, and fibrin is formed and deposited on the little mass of platelets. More platelets then adhere and some white and red cells are trapped in the fibrinous network. The thrombus may then build up slowly, if the blood flow is normal, or quickly if the flow is slow. If the mass forms in the heart or aorta it rarely occludes the cavity but adheres to the wall, when it is known as a *mural thrombus*. If it forms in smaller arteries or in veins or capillaries it may completely block the vessel, and is sometimes known as an *occlusive thrombus*.

If a vein is involved, stasis then occurs proximal to the thrombus and the blood therefore clots to the point at which the next tributary vein joins the affected vein. Propagation of the clot may then occur because the proximal end of the clot may present a rough surface and platelets from the incoming blood start to adhere. Clotting then develops proximally to the entry of the next tributary. Eventually a clot one or two feet long may form.

If the thrombus does not dissolve, its presence causes an inflammatory reaction in the walls of the vessel. Capillary buds and fibroblasts grow into the solid mass from the deeper layers of the vessel wall while phagocytic cells remove the cellular content. Thus the thrombus becomes firmly adherent to the vessel. At this point it is unlikely to be displaced, though the proximal clot is not thus organized and can break off.

Canalization of the thrombus gradually occurs. Endothelial cells multiply and grow into the mass between the strands of fibrin, forming new capillaries. These may join up to form channels permeating the thrombus so that the circulation in the area is re-established.

Causes

The deposit of platelets is the main feature in thrombosis and this may occur in three circumstances: (a) local injury to the endocardium or endothelium; (b) stasis and turbulence of blood flow; (c) alteration in the coagulability of the blood.

LOCAL INJURY TO THE ENDOCARDIUM OR ENDOTHELIUM

This causes some change, whose effect is the adherence of blood platelets. The injury may be due to:

(i) disease such as occurs in atherosclerosis;

(ii) surgery and accidents;

(iii) anoxia;

(iv) pressure on vessels (such as may occur on the veins of the calf of the leg when a patient is unconscious);

(v) chemical irritants (accounting for the inflammation and thrombosis seen in the 'drip' leg);

(vi) rheumatic heart disease in which the valves become inflamed and platelets are deposited along the edges of the cusps;

(vii) coronary heart disease – damage to the endocardium close to the myocardial infarct results in the formation of a mural thrombus.

STASIS AND TURBULENCE

At normal speed of the blood flow the cellular content of the blood travels at the centre of the stream, leaving a clear zone of plasma near the walls of the vessel. With slowing of the flow and turbulence, the platelets and white cells fall out into the clear zone and are therefore more likely to adhere to the endothelium. Slowing of flow may occur in the following circumstances:

(a) If a patient is confined to bed for any length of time or if a limb has to undergo prolonged immobilization.

(b) Congestive cardiac failure.

(c) Abnormal dilatation of arteries (as in aneurysm) or of veins (as in varicose veins), such dilatations giving rise to the slowing in blood flow and turbulence.

(d) An increase in the number of red blood cells. This tends to occur in congenital cyanotic heart disease and causes increase in the viscosity of the blood.

ALTERATION IN THE COAGULABILITY OF THE BLOOD

It is known that about the tenth day after childbirth or surgery (the time at which thrombosis seems to occur most frequently) there is a rise in the number of platelets in the bloodstream. These young platelets have a greater adhesiveness.

Site

While thrombosis can occur in any part of the cardiovascular system, the commonest site is in the veins where it is associated with congestive heart failure, immobilization and varicose veins. It also appears to be a complication of advanced cancer and it is suggested that it is then due to the release of tissue factors from necrotic tumours (Robbins and Angell), which affect the coagulability of the blood. Some authorities believe that the incidence of venous thrombosis is increased by the use of oral contraceptives.

Venous thrombosis tends to complicate surgery and childbirth because several agents are then present together. These include a rise in the number of platelets and amount of thromboplastin (the latter released from damaged tissue); slowing of blood flow due to inactivity and (in the case of high abdominal or thoracic surgery), reduced respiratory excursion. Minor damage to the endothelium of blood vessels may well occur due to pressure on the calves when the patient is unconscious.

Effects of thrombosis

The effects of thrombosis will depend upon the vessel affected, the degree to which the mass occludes the lumen, and the state of the collateral vessels:

(a) Some thrombi are dissolved, probably the results of a plasminogen activator in the endothelium.

(b) Some thrombi shrink and become canalized.

(c) Some may become detached and form emboli and the effects then depend upon where the embolus becomes impacted.

If collateral circulation is not rapidly established in arterial thrombosis, death of tissue occurs, the dead tissue is gradually softened by autolysins and protein-splitting enzymes, and replaced by granulation tissue from the surrounding unaffected tissue. The granulation tissue changes into fibrous tissue. Such an area is known as an *infarct* and its seriousness depends upon the ability of the undamaged tissue to do the work of the destroyed tissue.

For details see *Chest, Heart and Vascular Disorders for Physiotherapists*, edited by J. E. Cash.

EMBOLISM

An embolus is a foreign body circulating in the bloodstream. When it enters a vessel too small to allow it to pass, it becomes impacted and completely blocks the vessel, producing a state of anaemia.

Though the embolus is nearly always part or the whole of a detached thrombus, it can be a globule of fat derived from ruptured fat cells or it can be air. In the former case it is a complication of fractures in which the fat, in a liquid form, is released from the ruptured fat cells of the bone marrow and passes into the veins of the cancellous spaces. In the latter case air may enter the bloodstream and so reach the heart, where it becomes churned up with the blood, forming a frothy mass which interferes with the passage of blood through the heart.

Emboli derived from a thrombus most often enter the venous circulation and so reach the right side of the heart to become impacted in the pulmonary vessels. Emboli formed in the left side of the heart may block the coronary or cerebral vessels.

EFFECT OF EMBOLISM

Both thrombi and emboli block the vessels, but the former usually produce a gradual blocking with a state of chronic anaemia. The effect of the latter is sudden, no time having been allowed for the dilatation of collateral vessels supplying the same area. In this case the result depends upon the presence of collateral vessels and the speed with which they open up. If the embolus impacts in a small vessel with many anastomosing branches, no ill effect may occur. If it obstructs a large vessel, such as the axillary artery, the limb would rapidly become cold, pulseless, cyanotic and oedematous. But warmth and colour would gradually return since blood can reach the limb through the branches of the subclavian artery, and provided these are healthy, they will rapidly dilate. There may be some residual effects, but the health of the limb will be maintained.

Should the obstruction occur in one of the main cerebral or coronary arteries which are entirely responsible for the nutrition of one area of the brain or heart, that area of tissue must inevitably undergo necrosis and infarction occurs.

REFERENCE

Robbins and Angell. See Bibliography, p. 35.

Chapter 4

Atrophy and Hypertrophy; Hypoplasia and Hyperplasia; Neoplasia

Alteration in the size of individual cells and fibres or of an organ as a whole is not uncommonly seen. Such alteration in size is invariably accompanied by alterations in function and in many cases, though not in all, is the result of disturbances of nutrition. For any cell or fibre to maintain its normal size once it reaches full development, it must carry out its normal function, its metabolism must continue undisturbed and its nervous connections must remain intact. It follows that disturbance of any one of these factors may cause increase or decrease in size. In addition such factors as the influence of toxins, the effect of the secretion of ductless glands and interference with the blood supply must all be considered.

ATROPHY

This is diminution in the size of tissues. If the term is applied to muscles or organs it refers to the specialized elements and not the supporting framework, although in certain cases the connective tissue may increase at the same rate or even faster than the atrophy of the special cells. This increase of interstitial structures may be explained by the fact that the atrophied cells and fibres are probably receiving and using less nutrient products and oxygen, and more are therefore available for the less specialized tissues.

Common causes of atrophy

(i) One of the commonest causes of atrophy is *diminished function.* It is often seen in limbs which have been immobilized for a period of time. This is due to impaired metabolism since decreased metabolic processes mean decreased anabolism and therefore decrease in size. Disuse atrophy, as this type is called, is seen not only in muscles but also in other tissues which have lost their function, such as the ovaries after the menopause.

(ii) *Injuries and disease of joints* are almost invariably accompanied by rapid and severe atrophy of the muscles acting on the affected joints. Such atrophy is often much more profound than could possibly be accounted for by disuse. The probable explanation is that either sympathetic fibres are disturbed and nutrition consequently impaired, or that reflex atrophy is the result of irritation of sensory nerve endings, and so messages pass to the spinal cord and thus to the lateral and anterior horns of grey matter, causing inhibition of activity of the cells.

(iii) Atrophy is seen in *circulatory disturbances*. A slow progressive diminution in the lumen of the main vessels of a limb means gradual cutting down of the nutrition to all the tissues of that part and all specialized cells and fibres consequently shrink in size. Involvement of skin, muscles, joint structures and bone is seen in advanced arteriosclerosis and Buerger's disease.

(iv) *Continuous pressure* is responsible for atrophy, partly because it reduces the blood supply to the part and partly because it impairs function and so catabolism. The presence of a tumour is liable to lead to atrophy of the tissues on which it grows.

(v) In *disease of the lower motor neurones*, atrophy will be present in all structures supplied either by the damaged neurones or by any other nerve fibres running with them. Several explanations arise for this:

(a) Since no nerve impulses can reach the motor end-plates there can be no muscle tone or power of contraction and the result is abolition of catabolic processes with atrophy of muscle fibres.

(b) The vasoconstrictor fibres running with the motor fibres are also liable to be involved and if this occurs, paralytic vasodilatation results in circulatory stasis and impairment of nutrition to all the structures in the region. Such atrophy is serious because it is likely to continue over a long period and will therefore be followed by degeneration of the tissues and permanent impairment of function.

Most cases of atrophy are local but a generalized atrophy is seen in chronic starvation and in fevers. In the latter case the toxins stimulate protein metabolism and a rapid wasting takes place, particularly in the muscles. It is probably also partly due to impaired digestion and absorption.

Effects of atrophy

The primary effect is decreased function. In the case of muscular tissue power depends on the number and size of the fibres. While atrophy does not normally affect the number it does affect size, and muscle power is therefore markedly reduced. In addition atrophy may mean loss of elasticity. This is seen in the skin and may lead to limitation of function.

HYPERTROPHY

This is an increase in the size of the specialized elements of a tissue. Increase in the quantity of the connective tissues, such as in some types of muscular dystrophy, is not true hypertrophy. The change in size is due to increased functional demands or overactivity of the ductless glands.

Hypertrophy may be physiological or pathological. *Physiological hypertrophy* is not associated with disease. It is well illustrated in the case of the pregnant uterus or in the muscles of the athlete. Muscles in either case are called upon to do extra work and the effect is hypertrophy.

Pathological hypertrophy, as its name implies, is associated with disease. An example of such an occurrence is hypertrophy of the heart – stenosis of the mitral valve hinders the flow of blood from the left atrium and the effect is an increase in the breadth and length of the muscle fibres of the atrium. A similar hypertrophy may be seen in the involuntary muscular coat of the stomach when there is stenosis of the pyloric sphincter.

There is a limit to the amount to which any cell can hypertrophy and when this point is reached there is either hyperplasia or the functional demand fails to be met.

Pathological hypertrophy is sometimes compensatory. One group of cells and fibres enlarges to take over the work which should be done by damaged or lost tissue. This may be seen in one lobe of a lung when the other lobes have been removed, or in one kidney when the other becomes diseased and fails to function.

Hyperfunction of the pituitary gland in the adult leads to hypertrophy in the form of enlargement of the girth of the bones and thickening of the connective tissues throughout the body.

Effects of hypertrophy

With the exception of the last-mentioned type of hypertrophy, increased size means greater function. Hypertrophied muscles have always greater power than normal muscles, provided that it is the whole muscle which is hypertrophied and not only a few groups of its fibres.

HYPOPLASIA AND HYPERPLASIA

These should not be confused with atrophy and hypertrophy. The latter terms invariably refer to size, the former to number. Hypoplasia and hyperplasia most commonly occur before the tissues have reached maturity and are then developmental defects, often of unknown origin.

Hypoplasia means a decreased number of cells or fibres and may be the result of disturbance of the ductless glands controlling growth and development, such as in pituitary dwarfism.

Hyperplasia is an increase in the number of cells and fibres, either as a result of increased activity of ductless glands during the period of growth, or due to greater functional demands which cannot be entirely met by hypertrophy. Hyperplasia of bone marrow very readily occurs on a demand for increased blood; division of liver cells may cause hyperplasia of the liver if a section of that organ is surgically removed; hyperplasia of the glandular tissue of the breast occurs in puberty and pregnancy. It is possible that some hyperplasia of cardiac muscle may take place but it is not a feature of voluntary muscle cells.

NEOPLASIA

This is too vast a subject to be dealt with fully in a textbook of this type, but since the physiotherapist has to treat patients suffering from tumours, a brief description of some of the features of neoplasia has been included.

The term 'neoplasia' means new growth and the mass of cells comprising the tumour is known as a 'neoplasm'.

Most cells in the human body can proliferate, but their proliferation is under control and when it is no longer needed it ceases. In neoplasia, cell increase appears not to be under any control. The multiplication occurs spontaneously or as a result of some abnormal stimulus, and once started it continues even though the stimulus has ceased.

The new cells have certain characteristics: (i) there are usually differences in the structure and relationship of the cells to one another; (ii) they lose the specialized functions of the cells from which they originated and appear to be mainly concerned with proliferation; and (iii) they have the power to multiply and form new masses at sites distal to their origin if they are carried away in the blood or lymph stream.

As the cells multiply they may form masses supported by connective tissue, the stroma, and blood vessels, producing a tumour, or they may spread rapidly into the surrounding tissues when no mass may form, or both may happen at the same time.

A peculiar feature of the tumour is its ability to divert to itself a large proportion of nutritive substances, so that the rest of the tissues of the body suffer. Thus a tumour may grow to large proportions while the rest of the body wastes.

Tumours are often divided into benign and malignant, though rarely there may be no clear distinction between the two and a benign tumour may suddenly begin to become malignant.

Benign tumours

This type grows slowly, it usually possesses a capsule and its cells do not invade the surrounding tissue or spread to distant sites. The arrangement of its cells closely resembles that of the organ or tissue on which it grows.

While not normally affecting the general health of the patient, it can have serious effects by blocking tubes or, if it is growing in glandular tissue, it can cause irritation and so increased secretion.

A benign epithelial tumour of surface epithelium is known as a papilloma, of glandular tissue as an adenoma. Benign connective tissue tumours are usually named according to the tissue on which they grow: fibroma; osteoma; chondroma; lipoma; haemangioma; meningioma.

Malignant tumours

These usually grow much more quickly than benign tumours, though different types have different growth rates. They do not often develop a capsule and the cells invade the surrounding tissues, following the tissue planes in the line of least resistance. Fascial sheaths tend to confine them and cartilage to resist them. The thin walls of lymphatics, veins and capillaries are particularly liable to be penetrated and the lymph vessels and veins form the most common way in which malignant cells spread to form metastases (secondary deposits) at a distance from the primary site. Little groups of cells may form emboli and are carried round in the lymphatic and blood circulation until they become impacted in the capillary network. Here they multiply and secondary deposits are formed. If such emboli are travelling in the venous circulation or enter the venous stream via the thoracic or lymphatic ducts, the first capillary network will be in the lungs. Secondary growths in the lungs are therefore common. Emboli in the portal circulation will impact in the liver and cause metastasis here.

Malignant tumours produce many ill-effects. They cause pressure and obstruction; they cause cachexia (progressive weakness, weight loss and wasting), they destroy tissue and may undergo secondary infection. Anaemia is a frequent feature and if surface epithelium is involved haemorrhage often occurs. Pain is a common feature with its effect on general health.

A malignant tumour of surface or glandular epithelium is known as a carcinoma, while if connective tissue is involved the term sarcoma is applied; thus we hear of liposarcoma, fibrosarcoma, osteogenic sarcoma. Various terms have been used for malignant tumours of lymphoid tissue, of which lymphatic leukaemia is one. All malignant tumours are cancers, this classification being used because of their characteristic spread into surrounding tissues.

Though some malignant tumours can occur at any age, most tend to develop after the age of fifty and they seem to be slightly more common in men than in women, though some are peculiar to women and some to men.

Causes

The cause is not yet certain but some points are becoming clearer. Some types of tumours are common in certain occupations, and certain agents appear to predispose a whole area of tissue to neoplasia. These agents are carcinogenic and may be chemical or physical. *Chemical agents* may be derived from coal tar and mineral oils. Workers using arsenic seem liable to develop cancer of the skin of the limbs and face. Carcinoma of the lungs is more common in those whose occupation brings them in contact with hot tar fumes, nickel and asbestos, or in those who are heavy smokers. *Physical agents* which appear to predispose the tissues are radioactive elements, X-rays and strong ultraviolet radiations.

While chronic irritants probably do not themselves produce cancer, they may promote neoplasia in a tissue already predisposed by a carcinogenic agent.

Hormones appear to have some influence on the growth of tumours. Some breast tumours appear to depend for their growth on oestrogen, progesterone and prolactin, and ovariectomy and bilateral adrenalectomy sometimes causes a temporary regression in such cancers. In recent years some lesions of epithelial surfaces have been recognized in which the cells show changes, but in which there is not true malignancy or invasion of surrounding tissues. If such lesions can be detected treatment can be instituted which may prevent development of neoplasia and loss of life. In this, for example, lies the importance of the taking of cervical smears, since such changed cells are shed, and trapped in the mucus of the cervix.

Physiotherapy in relation to tumours

Physical measures may be needed to help to relieve the effects of tumours. Again they may help in the treatment of neoplasia by surgery. For example, a tumour may be causing obstruction of a bronchus giving rise to accumulation of secretion and collapse of an area of lung, and postural drainage and coughing may be essential. A bilateral adrenalectomy or a radical mastectomy will require routine pre- and postoperative physiotherapy. Exercises may be needed to strengthen muscles and improve posture following surgery to remove lymph nodes and soft tissues in the region of tumours, as in block neck resection in laryngopharyngectomy. The fact that the patient is or has been suffering from a tumour does not affect physiotherapy in such cases.

BIBLIOGRAPHY

Boyd, W. *A Textbook of Pathology*. Kimpton, 8th ed. 1970.

Dible, J. H. and Davie, T. B. *Pathology*. Churchill Livingstone (out of print).

Florey, Sir H. (ed.) *General Pathology*. Lloyd-Luke, 4th ed. 1970.

Martin, P., Lynn, R. B., Dible, J. H. and Aird, I. *Peripheral Vascular Disorders*. Churchill Livingstone, 1956.

Robbins, S. L. and Angell, L. M. *Basic Pathology*. W. B. Saunders Co. 1971.

Walter, J. B. and Israel, M. S. *General Pathology*. Churchill Livingstone, 3rd ed. 1970.

Wright, G. P. *An Introduction to Pathology*. Churchill Livingstone, 3rd ed. 1964.

PART II

Rheumatic Disorders

Chapters 5 to 14 inclusive are edited by ALASTAIR G. MOWAT, MB, FRCP(ED)

Chapter 5

Polyarthritis of Unknown Cause – I

including rheumatoid arthritis and juvenile rheumatoid arthritis

by ALASTAIR G. MOWAT, MB, FRCP(ED)
and JOAN M. ABERY, MCSP

Introduction

Arthritis affects as many as 5 million people in the United Kingdom, a very large majority of whom are afflicted by two quite separate diseases. Approximately 1.5 million people have rheumatoid arthritis, although fortunately only a small proportion have serious disease or disability, while approximately 3.5 million people suffer from various forms of degenerative arthritis, osteoarthrosis. Although many patients with degenerative arthritis have ceased to be wage-earners, it has been estimated that the combined cost of lost production and sickness payments attributable to arthritis exceeds £300 million per annum. This far exceeds the annual cost to the nation of all strikes and places arthritis second only to chronic bronchitis in this unattractive 'league'. These figures, although important, fail to emphasize the real problem of arthritis, which is that the quality of the lives of these patients is impaired by pain and disability.

Fortunately, there is a growing interest in and concern for these patients. This is reflected in a growing public awareness of the problems of the disabled and in action by the Department of Health and Social Security to increase the number of doctors in the field of arthritis and to develop Demonstration Centres for the treatment of the disabled. At the same time, increasing financial support for research into the causes and treatment of these diseases has begun to show important results, with the availability of new drugs, the use of better programmes of management and the development of an exciting range of new orthopaedic prostheses and appliances.

The following chapters describe the common forms of joint disease. In Chapter 5 the most common inflammatory joint disease, *rheumatoid arthritis*, is described together with its variant juvenile rheumatoid arthritis. The more common of the other inflammatory joint diseases are described in Chapters 6 and 7. There are very large numbers of such conditions and the therapist is referred to larger textbooks for details of those not described. (See Bibliography, p. 104.)

Chapter 8 describes the general principles of management of joint disease, the management and reduction of disability by a variety of physical means, ranging from splints, through walking aids to wheelchairs and various aids to daily living; while Chapters 9 and 14 describe the role of orthopaedic surgery in the treatment of arthritis and the commonly used drugs. It must, however, be emphasized from the outset that there are no general rules for the management of patients with arthritis and that an individual programme of treatment has to be planned for each patient after careful assessment of his or her problems. These chapters contain sufficient information for sensible programmes of management to be planned. Such management will reduce disability and improve the quality of the arthritic's life.

CLASSIFICATION OF JOINT DISEASE

POLYARTHRITIS OF UNKNOWN CAUSE: (Chapter 5)

Rheumatoid arthritis
Juvenile rheumatoid arthritis

POLYARTHRITIS OF UNKNOWN CAUSE: (Chapter 6)

Ankylosing spondylitis
Reiter's disease
Psoriatic arthropathy
Arthropathy of ulcerative bowel disease

A common thread of genetic influence, familial aggregation and spinal involvement runs through this group of sero-negative polyarthritides.

ARTHRITIS DUE TO INFECTION: (Chapter 7)

Rheumatic fever
Septic arthritis
Gonococcal arthritis
Brucellosis
Tuberculosis
Viral arthritis
Erythema nodosum

Although the pattern of arthritis differs widely, infection or an allergic process secondary to infection is important in all the diseases in this group.

CONNECTIVE TISSUE DISEASES: (Chapter 7)

Disseminated lupus erythematosus
Dermatomyositis
Scleroderma
Sjögren's syndrome
Polyarteritis nodosa
Polymyalgia rheumatica

These connective tissue diseases, most of which are rare, have an inflammatory reaction in arterioles as a common pathological basis. Important immunological abnormalities are often present. Although multisystem disease is the rule, there are prominent and often early symptoms and signs in the musculoskeletal system and the involvement of the joints may resemble that found in rheumatoid arthritis. Most carry a poor prognosis.

CRYSTAL ARTHRITIS: (Chapter 7)

Gout
Pyrophosphate arthropathy (pseudo-gout)

OTHERS:

Arthritis associated with malignant disease
Arthritis associated with haemophilia
Arthritis associated with neurological disease

DEGENERATIVE ARTHRITIS: (Chapters 10–13)

Osteoarthrosis
Spondylosis and intervertebral disc disease

NON-ARTICULAR PAIN: (Chapter 15)

RHEUMATOID ARTHRITIS

Rheumatoid arthritis is a common inflammatory disease of joints, characterized by symmetrical, peripheral polyarthritis often associated with systemic features. The name rheumatoid disease may be preferred since it directs attention to the whole patient.

INCIDENCE

Rheumatoid arthritis affects some three per cent of the population of Great Britain. Although it was once thought only to affect populations living in temperate climates, it is now clear that the incidence of the disease is much the same the world over, but causes less disability amongst those living in warmer climates. Two-thirds of cases begin before the age of 50 but no age group is exempt. An acute onset in the eighth or ninth decade is well documented, although the disease tends to be more benign and spontaneous remissions are more common. The disease affects females to males in a ratio of 3:1.

Clearly the disease afflicts young people at the most important time of their lives, when wage-earning is at a peak and when housewives have young children to look after. It is these reasons, together with the chronicity of the disease, which necessitate the total management of the patient and not just of the joint disease.

Clinical features

The disease is characteristically polyarticular and although the onset may be monarticular the spread to involve other joints, usually producing symmetrical disease, is often rapid. The small joints of the hands and feet are first affected in 70 per cent of patients, although in older patients the shoulder joint is commonly involved first. The onset is acute, with fever and constitutional symptoms in 20 per cent of patients.

The patients complain of loss of function, pain and stiffness, most characteristically in the morning. The joints and the surrounding periarticular structures, tendons, ligaments and joint capsules are tender and swollen (Plate 5/1). Synovial proliferation and joint effusions may be marked. There is limitation of joint movement and correctable flexion deformities may follow at many joints. These flexion deformities accommodate the swollen and proliferating tissues with a reduction in pain (Plate 5/2). If the inflammatory process is unchecked further deformity and disability will result due to the progressive damage to joint cartilage, subchondral bone and periarticular structures and to the associated muscle spasm. Flexion contracture is the common deformity in a large joint. *In the hands* more characteristic deformities such as ulnar deviation, swan neck (hyperextension at the proximal interphalangeal and flexion at the distal interphalangeal joints) and boutonnière deformities (flexion at proximal interphalangeal and hyperextension at distal interphalangeal joints) of the fingers may develop. *In the feet*, broadening of the forefoot, clawing of the toes and plantar callosities may develop. These changes are due to alterations in the intricate mechanical arrangements of the tendons, ligaments and joints.

Any synovial joint may be affected, but involvement of the sacro-iliac joints and the spinal joints (except those in the cervical spine) is uncommon. Progressive disease causes further loss of cartilage and bone with subluxation of joints. The end result is ankylosis.

However, it must be appreciated that the progress of the disease and the ultimate damage produced by the disease varies considerably. A large proportion of patients have very mild disease which causes little or no disability or deformity and may not necessitate advice from their family doctor, let alone a hospital specialist. Others may have disease of acute onset which causes considerable pain and disability for several weeks or months but which is subsequently well-controlled by appropriate therapy and then causes little trouble. Yet others may have disease with a gradual onset which causes progressive, severe damage despite all attempts at control. Certainly natural variations in the intensity and activity of the disease are common and these tend to produce remissions or relapses lasting many months. The variability in the natural history of the disease makes a uniform description impossible and makes discussion and management of individual cases difficult.

Extra-articular features

Rheumatoid arthritis is a *systemic disease*. Loss of appetite and weight, general malaise and depression are common. A low-grade fever may be present. Generalized osteoporosis with more marked juxta-articular osteoporosis occurs and muscle wasting is prominent, around both involved and uninvolved joints. Lymph node and splenic enlargement is common. Almost all patients have some degree of anaemia due to abnormalities in iron metabolism. Oral iron therapy is of no value. The anaemia can be improved by controlling the disease or by parenteral iron therapy.

Tendons, in synovial sheaths, and *bursae* become involved in the same pathological process as affects the joint synovium. Tendon involvement may impair function, and stretching or rupture of tendons, particularly the extensors of the fingers, may occur.

Thinning of the *skin* due to loss of the subcutaneous fat and connective tissues is common. Shearing stresses on the skin tend to cause bruising since the small vessels are poorly supported and patients may need to protect skin overlying bone such as the shin. Fortunately wound healing after surgical procedures is normal.

Many of the complications of rheumatoid disease can be attributed to inflammatory changes in small arteries and arterioles. These can cause small necrotic lesions at the periphery, particularly around the nail folds, and may even lead to small areas of gangrene. Such vascular changes form the basis of the neurological and pleural lesions to be described and are the cause of the rheumatoid nodule. They occur only in those with positive serological tests for rheumatoid factor. Characteristic *subcutaneous nodules*, present in 20 per cent of patients, develop over any pressure areas, particularly the extensor surfaces of the forearms. Their removal, unless they become infected or for mechanical reasons, is probably unwise since they frequently recur.

Nerve involvement includes *mono-neuritis multiplex* with involvement of one or more major nerves producing such signs as foot drop and the very serious symmetrical, *peripheral neuropathy* producing motor weakness and stocking and glove sensory loss, both of which are due to vasculitis of the vasa nervorum. *Entrapment neuropathies* are a common feature of rheumatoid disease and may be the presenting complaint. Carpal and tarsal tunnel compression and entrapment of the ulnar nerve at the elbow and the lateral popliteal nerve at the head of the fibula are well documented. Proliferation of tendon sheath or joint synovial tissue in a limited space is responsible. Carpal tunnel compression occurs in 60 per cent of patients at some time. Surgical decompression of nerves may be required.

Spinal cord compression may occur. Instability of the atlanto-axial joint with subluxation of the atlas on neck flexion is a radiological finding in 25 per cent of patients (Plates 5/3, 5/4). They complain of pain, particularly with jolting movement, C1–2 root compression symptoms and occasionally demonstrate signs due to spinal cord compression. Although symptoms and signs are less common than the radiological findings would suggest, sudden death due to cord compression has been recorded and the anaesthetist should be warned if surgery is planned so that appropriate protective measures can be taken. Management of pain and root compression is by the use of cervical collars, but the presence of persistent symptoms or cord compression demands surgical fixation.

In the chest, rheumatoid *nodules* may develop in the lower lung fields and be confused with a tumour. *Pleurisy* and pleural *effusion* occur but the most serious lesion is the untreatable diffuse interstitial fibrosis which leads to progressive shortness of breath.

Various inflammatory changes in the eye may impair vision and further disable the patient.

COMPLICATIONS

Amyloidosis, the term given to the deposition in tissues of an abnormal protein, is found post mortem in 20 per cent of patients with rheumatoid arthritis. It may present as renal damage with proteinuria progressing to nephrosis but comparatively few patients show any signs of amyloidosis during life. *Septic arthritis* superimposed upon rheumatoid arthritis will occur in 3 per cent of patients. Although the septic process, which is usually due to *Staphylococcus aureus*, may be silent, the apparent flare-up of rheumatoid arthritis in only one joint should be considered as septic arthritis until proved otherwise.

Aetiology

The cause remains unknown. It seems likely that there may be several initiating factors which are distinct from a perpetuating mechanism about which there is more general agreement. Thus there is evidence of abnormal protein production, probably in the form of an antibody to altered tissues or proteins, which can produce a series of inflammatory reactions ending in the production of synovitis. The mechanism provid-

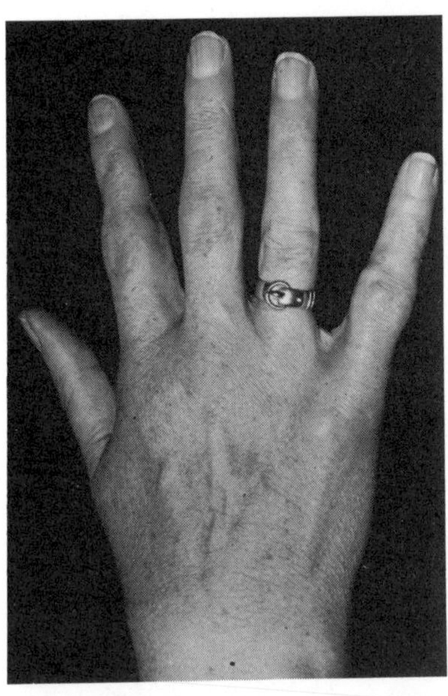

Plate 5/1 Rheumatoid arthritis. Swelling in metacarpophalangeal and proximal interphalangeal joints of 2nd, 3rd and 5th fingers (*see p. 42*)

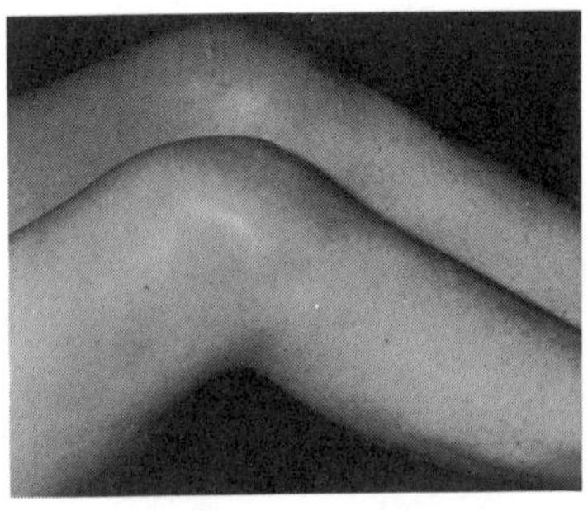

Plate 5/2 Rheumatoid arthritis. Gross flexion deformity at knee-joint (*see p. 42*)

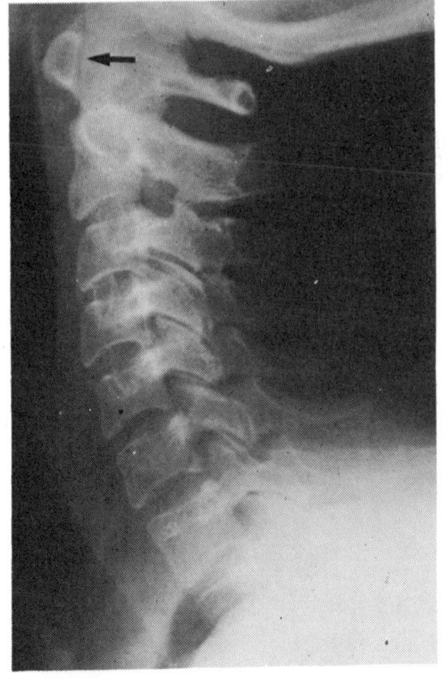

Plate 5/3 Lateral radiograph of rheumatoid neck in extension. Arch of atlas is close to odontoid process (*see p. 44*)

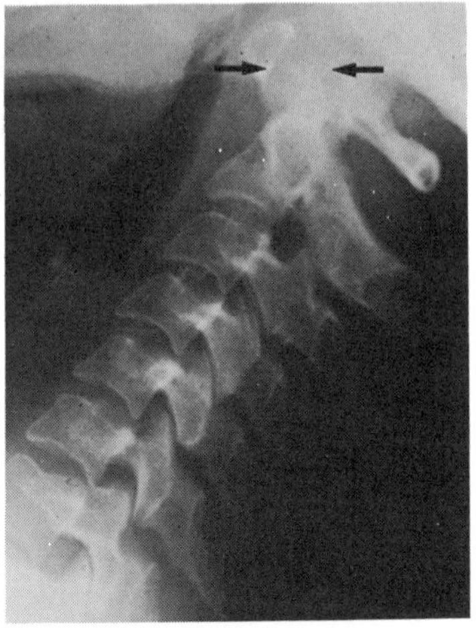

Plate 5/4 Lateral radiograph of the same neck in flexion, showing large gap between anterior arch of atlas and odontoid process (normal gap 2–3 mm)

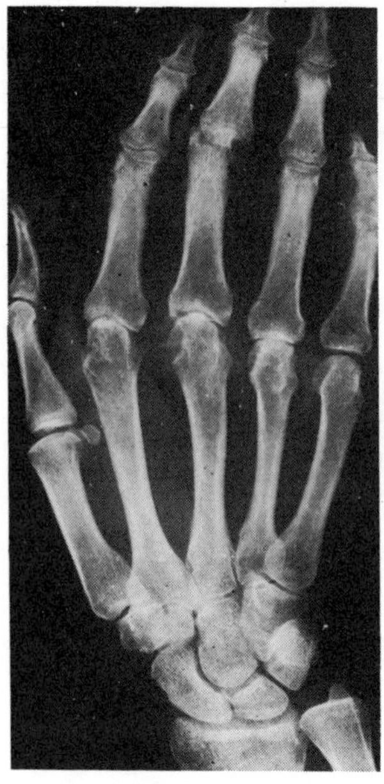

Plate 5/5 Rheumatoid arthritis. Hand radiograph showing osteoporosis, cartilage and bone damage, especially in 2–4 metacarpophalangeal joints and 3rd proximal interphalangeal joint

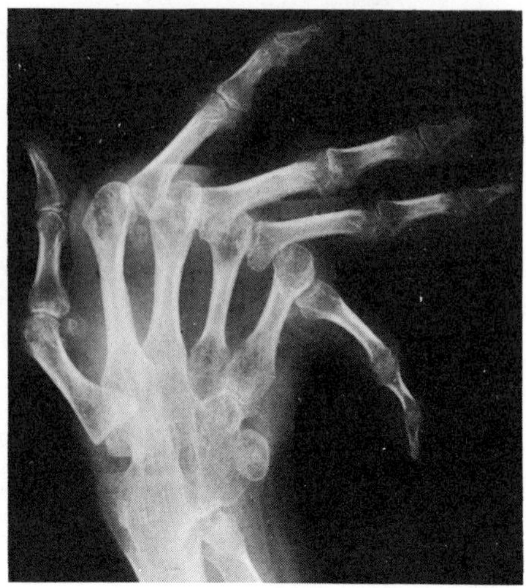

Plate 5/6 More advanced changes in rheumatoid arthritis, with subluxation at metacarpophalangeal joints and bony ankylosis at wrist with disappearance of individual carpal bones (*see p. 48*)

ing the stimulus to this antibody production is unknown but the following factors have been suggested:

A GENETIC INFLUENCE

There is a slight tendency for the disease to be aggregated in families.

TRAUMA

Many patients have mentioned traumatic incidents as a precipitating cause.

PSYCHOLOGICAL STRESS

Patients frequently suggest this reason but this reflects their natural desire to find an explanation for a disease which has no clear cause. It has been difficult to support this entity by statistical means except in some cases of identical twins in whom rheumatoid arthritis affected only the twin under stress.

INFECTIOUS AGENTS

Renewed interest has resulted in a claimed isolation of a variety of organisms from synovial tissue, synovial fluid and blood. These include diphtheroid bacilli, mycoplasma and viruses.

VASCULAR CHANGES

Alteration in the normal peripheral vascular bed, perhaps by the sympathetic nervous system, has been suggested as the primary abnormality and has been implicated to explain the striking symmetry of the arthritis in many patients.

Diagnosis

Although rheumatoid arthritis is much the commonest form of inflammatory joint disease, it is important that the diagnosis is made soundly so that appropriate treatment can be started and the implications of the disease can be explained to the patient. The American Rheumatism Association has laid down certain criteria for the diagnosis of rheumatoid arthritis:

(1) Morning stiffness.
(2) Pain on motion or tenderness in at least one joint.
(3) Swelling of at least one joint.
(4) Swelling of another joint within three months.
(5) Simultaneous involvement of the same joint bilaterally but excluding the distal interphalangeal joints of the fingers.
(6) Subcutaneous nodules.
(7) X-ray changes typical of rheumatoid arthritis.
(8) A positive test for rheumatoid factor.
(9) A poor mucin clot of the synovial fluid.
(10) Characteristic histology of the synovial membrane.
(11) Characteristic histology of the nodules.

Criteria 1–5 must be present for six weeks. When twenty other causes of polyarthritis listed by the American Rheumatism Association have been excluded the diagnosis of rheumatoid arthritis can be considered. Classical rheumatoid arthritis requires seven and definite rheumatoid arthritis five criteria. It should be stressed that the diagnosis can be made on a clinical basis by using criteria 1–5 and that the finding of a positive test for rheumatoid factor is relatively unimportant using this list of unweighted criteria.

Laboratory findings

Anaemia with a haemoglobin value of 11 g per cent is common. The white cell count is usually normal but a rise to $10–15 \times 10^9/l$ occurs with steroid therapy and superimposed bacterial infection. The *ESR* may be markedly elevated and in some patients with long-standing disease may never return to normal value. *The tests for rheumatoid factor* are positive in 70 per cent of cases. Positive tests are less common in those with onset of the disease late in life. It must be remembered that positive tests occur with increasing frequency in the normal population with age. Positive tests also occur in the other connective tissue diseases and in diseases in which marked changes in the serum globulins occur such as multiple myeloma, macroglobulinaemia, chronic infections and liver disease. Unaffected relatives of patients have a higher than expected incidence of positive tests.

RADIOLOGY (Plates 5/5, 5/6)

The sequence of radiological signs of rheumatoid arthritis are:

(1) Soft tissue changes around a joint due to synovitis and effusion.

(2) Osteoporosis.

(3) Periosteal reaction with new bone formation along the shaft adjacent to capsule attachments.

(4) Subchondral cyst formation.

(5) Narrowing of joint spaces due to cartilage loss.

(6) Loss of bone substance by erosion along the marginal areas of the joint.

(7) Subluxation and deformity.

(8) Bony ankylosis.

PATHOLOGY

Inflammation of synovial tissue in joints, tendons and bursae is the essential pathological change. The thickened, oedematous, inflamed tissue produces erosions of the cartilage surface and erodes into the subchondral bone. These erosions may become large and cystic and lead to joint destruction. Reparative changes are rarely found and the disease progresses to fibrous and occasionally bony ankylosis. Microscopically the synovium is vascular and infiltrated with lymphocytes and plasma cells which are clumped together in follicles. It must be emphasized that present pathological techniques do not allow a firm diagnosis of rheumatoid arthritis when biopsy material is examined. Very similar changes are found in many types of inflammatory joint disease.

Prognosis

One of the greatest problems arises from the *variable nature* of the disease and it is very difficult to give an accurate prognosis in individual cases. However, the general prognosis is better than many expect, especially when it is appreciated that follow-up studies have only been done on patients attending hospitals and special units, who inevitably have more severe disease. *Follow-up studies* on large numbers of patients treated by simple methods show that after 10 years 50 per cent will have improved and 50 per cent deteriorated. This important fact, which underlines the known tendency for the disease to remit and relapse, must be remembered when any form of therapy is being evaluated. Grading of such patients according to their disability shows that approximately 20 per cent have no disability; 40 per cent have moderate disability; 30 per cent have more severe disability but remain independent in the home and usefully employed; and 10 per cent are dependent upon others. The disease is inactive in 25 per cent of patients. Thus the concepts that large numbers of patients become crippled and that the disease becomes 'burnt-out' are erroneous.

Factors that suggest a poor prognosis include insidious onset, unremitting disease, the presence of nodules and other vasculitic phenomena, severe systemic involvement with a high ESR and anaemia, and the presence in the serum of rheumatoid factor in large amounts. Although *few patients die from rheumatoid arthritis* per se, the disease reduces life expectancy by five to eight years. Death from bacterial infection and renal disease is commoner than in the general population.

MANAGEMENT

The basic principles, the use of rest, exercise, splints and walking aids and domestic and occupational factors are discussed in Chapter 8. Surgical treatment is discussed in Chapter 9 and drug therapy in Chapter 14.

JUVENILE RHEUMATOID ARTHRITIS

This disease differs in a number of important respects from rheumatoid arthritis in adults and it is probably a different disease. For this reason some people prefer the eponym *Still's disease*, although this description was originally used for only one group of patients with chronic inflammatory polyarthritis and systemic symptoms.

The peak age of onset is between two and four years with a second peak around puberty. The disease may be entirely confined to the joints or there may be a systemic illness. Monarticular arthritis, commonly involving the knee, is the usual presentation. The disease may remain monarticular but in the majority becomes polyarticular with involvement of the knees, hands, wrists and feet. Early involvement of the hips, sacro-iliac joints and cervical spine is common. Although the increased thickness of the articular cartilage seems to retard the appearance of erosions, unremitting disease leads to joint damage often with bony ankylosis. Increases in periarticular vascularity, the presence of systemic disease and the use of corticosteroids may cause a variety of skeletal growth abnormalities. The small chin is one such striking abnormality.

Although general malaise, loss of appetite and weight may occur in any case, more characteristic systemic signs are found in some children with polyarthritis. These are: fever; lymphadenopathy; splenomegaly; rash – a dusky pink eruption, the distribution of which may vary from hour to hour; anaemia; white cell counts up to $20 \times 10^9/l$; pericarditis; iritis – occurs in 8 per cent of cases and is most common in the monarticular group; the ESR is elevated. Tests for rheumatoid factor are negative except in a small group of children with late onset of disease.

About 5 per cent of children carry the disease into adult life when it follows the chronic, unpredictable course of adult rheumatoid arthritis. However, involvement of the neck, sacro-iliac and hip joint is commoner, the serological tests for rheumatoid factor remain negative and the systemic symptoms disappear. Of those in whom the disease remits, 50 per cent will have no residual damage, 45 per cent will have moderate deformity and disability and 5 per cent will be severely incapacitated. A better prognosis is enjoyed by those whose disease starts in early childhood, is treated within a year of onset and whose involvement is monarticular. Juvenile rheumatoid arthritis must be differentiated from rheumatic fever, viral and septic arthritis, the connective tissue diseases and the leukaemias.

Treatment

Treatment chiefly involves the proper management of the patient as a child with the provision of the necessary hospital, home and educational facilities to achieve this end. It must be realized that many of these children will eventually earn their living by 'brain' and not by 'brawn', and that in consequence the maintenance of their education, even when in hospital, is vital.

Prevention of deformity in a disease with a high remission rate is crucial. All the methods described for adult rheumatoid arthritis are of value except that sustained immobilization in splints is inadvisable because of the tendency of joints to ankylose. Drug therapy in appropriate dosage follows similar lines. Corticosteroid therapy must be used with care because of the effect on growth. ACTH and alternate day oral steroids reduce these effects.

Surgical treatment is largely confined to reconstructive procedures. These may be carefully timed with examinations in teenagers to maintain mobility, or delayed until early adult life when the disease has remitted. Although there have been reports of the satisfactory results of synovectomy, especially in the knees, on both the local and the general disease states, the operation is not widely used. Surgical procedures are best avoided in children under the age of six years whose co-operation may be difficult to obtain.

For Bibliography see end of Chapter 9, p. 104.

Chapter 6

Polyarthritis of Unknown Cause – II

including ankylosing spondylitis, Reiter's disease, psoriatic arthropathy and arthropathy of ulcerative bowel disease

by ALASTAIR G. MOWAT, MB, FRCP(ED)
and JOAN M. ABERY, MCSP

ANKYLOSING SPONDYLITIS

Ankylosing spondylitis is a chronic inflammatory disease involving chiefly the synovial diarthrodial and cartilaginous joints of the spine. The disease occurs in one per thousand of the population, with an equal sex incidence, but males have more severe disease.

Pathology

The essential abnormality is an inflammatory reaction originating in the attachment of ligaments to bone (an enthesopathy). The inflammatory reaction, consisting of a lymphocytic and plasma cell infiltrate and increased vascularity and fibrosis, extends to involve spinal ligaments, the outer layers of the intervertebral disc and posterior apophyseal joints. Sacro-iliac joint involvement always occurs and peripheral synovial joints may also be affected, the synovial reaction resembling that found in rheumatoid arthritis. Continuing inflammation results in ossification of ligaments and the ankylosis of joints.

Clinical features

The disease usually begins between the ages of 16 and 40 years. The onset is gradual and initial complaints of lumbar backache and discomfort after rest may be ignored. Some patients may progress to serious deformity and ankylosis before seeking advice. However, most patients complain of backache and marked stiffness especially after rest and for an hour or more each morning.

Any part of the spine may be involved, although the disease usually starts in the lumbar spine and proceeds upwards. Loss of the lumbar spinal curve and progressive kyphosis of the remainder of the spine is usual (Plate 6/1). The involvement of synovial costo-vertebral joints leads to progressive reduction in chest expansion. In severe cases respiration may be entirely diaphragmatic, leading to abdominal ballooning. Any involved joint or bony prominence may be tender and pain may be elicited by forced movement of the sacro-iliac joints.

Although involvement of *peripheral joints* (most commonly the hip and shoulder) may occur in 50 per cent of patients at some time, in 10 per cent of cases synovitis of a peripheral joint or tendinitis (achilles tendinitis, plantar fasciitis) is the presenting feature and may lead to diagnostic difficulties. Many patients will have *systemic signs* of the disease such as low-grade fever, anaemia and weight loss. The ESR is usually elevated but the rheumatoid factor tests are negative.

Careful measurements of all planes of spinal movement and chest expansion are valuable in the assessment and management of ankylosing spondylitis, although such measurements are now considered less valuable in the diagnosis since these movements vary widely in the normal population and decrease with age. It is important to remember that the patient may compensate for spinal rigidity by increased hip flexion and so still be able to touch his toes. (Examination of the undressed patient avoids such errors.) Further, limitation of movement may be reversible if due to pain and muscle spasm.

Complications

Recurrent iritis, a painful inflammatory process in the eye, occurs in 20 per cent of cases and may occasionally be the presenting feature. Energetic treatment with local corticosteroids is required to avoid permanent visual impairment.

Atlanto-axial subluxation (see p. 44) is common, and hence spinal cord damage may occur especially if the remainder of the spine is rigid or the neck of the unconscious or anaesthetised patient is handled carelessly. Fracture of the rigid but brittle spine occasionally occurs.

Radiology

The diagnosis of ankylosing spondylitis cannot be considered unless there is evidence of bilateral sacro-iliitis. However in very early cases and in teenage patients the interpretation of the X-rays may be difficult. The sequential appearances in the posterior–anterior films are of erosive arthritis, marginal sclerosis and finally bony fusion with disappearance of the sclerosis (Plate 6/2). Spinal radiographs may show ligamentous ossification, ankylosis in apophyseal joints, the typical spinal deformity with squaring of the vertebral bodies and 'a bamboo spine'; an appearance due to new bone growth between adjacent vertebrae resulting from the changes in the intervertebral disc (Plate 6/3).

Differential diagnosis and aetiology

The diagnosis of ankylosing spondylitis is based upon the presentation of: (1) thoraco-lumbar pain and stiffness; (2) limited spinal and chest movement; (3) radiographic evidence of sacro-iliitis; (4) an elevated ESR in 75 per cent of cases. Similar findings may occur in Reiter's disease, juvenile rheumatoid arthritis, psoriatic arthropathy and in the arthritis associated with ulcerative colitis and Crohn's disease, although additional features in each of these diseases usually allows the correct diagnosis to be made. All these diseases may be associated with iritis, and the nature of this curious link between sacro-iliac joint disease and the eye is unexplained. These diseases are further linked by the finding of an increased familial aggregation and the fact that the tests for rheumatoid factor are negative. Genetic rather than environmental factors are likely to be important in these diseases. A tenfold increase in the incidence of ankylosing spondylitis among relatives of patients with this disease has been reported, but genetic counselling is unnecessary.

Management

The aims of management are: maintenance of spinal mobility; prevention and correction of spinal deformity; relief of pain and stiffness.

MAINTENANCE OF SPINAL MOBILITY

The importance of physiotherapy cannot be overstated. However, since the patient may require to perform exercises for many years or even the rest of his life, it is vital that he be properly taught a simple programme of exercises. Further, the purpose of spinal and chest mobilizing exercises must be explained and the patient frequently encouraged by doctor and therapist. Exercises may also be required for peripheral joints. Heat and other physical therapies have little value. Immobilization in bed or spinal supports must be avoided.

PREVENTION AND CORRECTION OF SPINAL DEFORMITY

A firm bed, the use of one pillow, and a daily period of prone lying are essential. Further, the posture adopted at work or in the home is vital. The patient must always be conscious of his spinal posture and adapt his life, chairs and work situations accordingly. The occupational therapist and physiotherapist can implement this advice.

RELIEF OF PAIN AND STIFFNESS

One of the analgesic/anti-inflammatory drugs listed on pages 159–60 should be used. Phenylbutazone and indomethacin are popular and bed-time doses relieve morning stiffness. For severe cases corticosteroids may be required. A short course of these drugs or ACTH may reduce pain and stiffness and muscle spasm and result in considerable increase in movement which the well-instructed patient can then maintain.

Radiotherapy, once popular, has largely been discarded since it caused an increased incidence of leukaemia in later years. However, radiotherapy may still be employed in cases genuinely unresponsive to other treatment.

Surgery

Posterior spinal osteotomy for spinal deformity is possible, but is both difficult and dangerous. Peripheral joint involvement may be treated by synovectomy and total hip replacement may dramatically alter a patient's life.

Prognosis

The prognosis is good and should encourage proper management. In general the mental attitude of the spondylitic is excellent and this should encourage the therapist. Almost all patients can remain at work and over half continue with their original employment. Problems mostly occur in those patients with insidious, long-standing disease who already have deformity and immobility when first seen. Early and continuing treatment is important.

REITER'S DISEASE

Reiter's disease is characterized by urethritis, sero-negative arthritis and conjunctivitis in young men.

Clinical features

Although the presence of urethritis and arthritis are essential for the diagnosis to be made, conjunctivitis is not, since it is found in only half the cases. Mouth and genital ulceration and a characteristic skin lesion – keratoderma blennorrhagica – each occur in 10 per cent of cases. In Great Britain and Western Europe the disease develops from non-specific urethritis which is transmitted sexually. In many tropical and developing countries and in time of war an identical disease follows various types of dysentery. The venereal type of the disease is rare in women and the

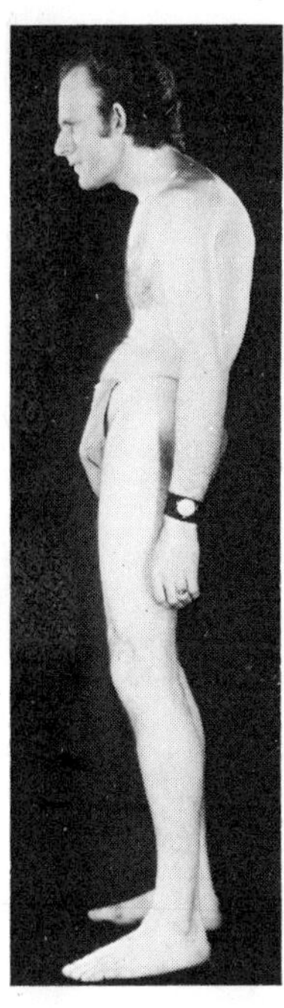

Plate 6/1 Spinal deformity, flat chest and ballooned abdomen in advanced case of ankylosing spondylitis (*see p. 52*)

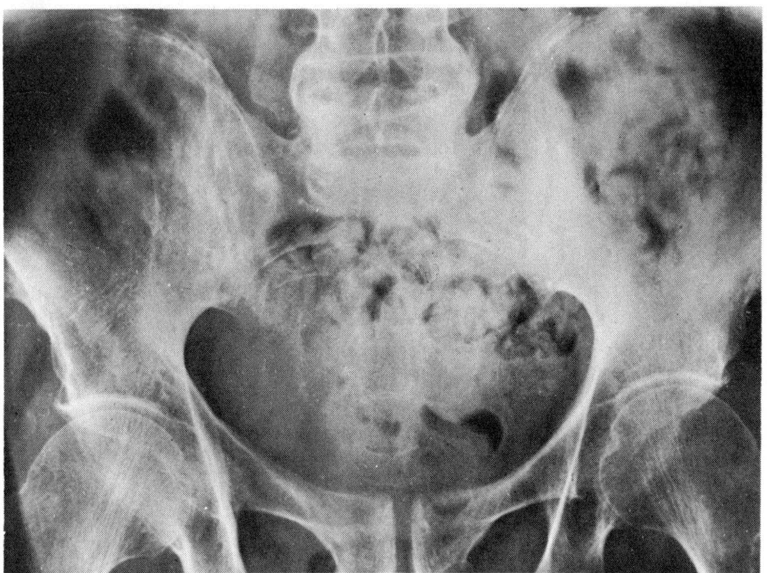

Plate 6/2 Radiograph showing bilateral ankylosis of sacro-iliac joints in ankylosing spondylitis (*see p. 52*)

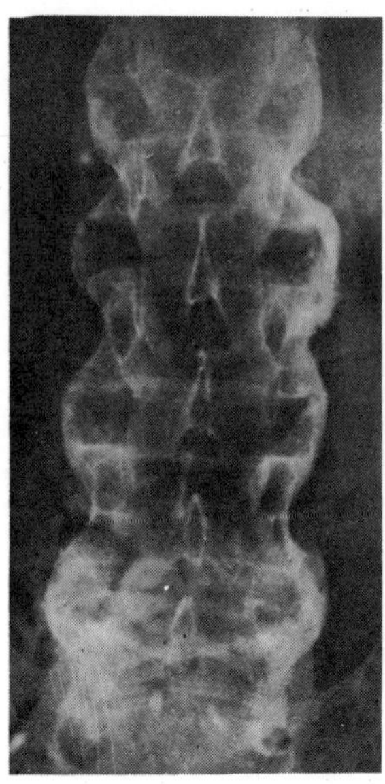

Plate 6/3 'Bamboo spine'. Bony bridges between vertebral bodies in ankylosing spondylitis (*see p. 53*)

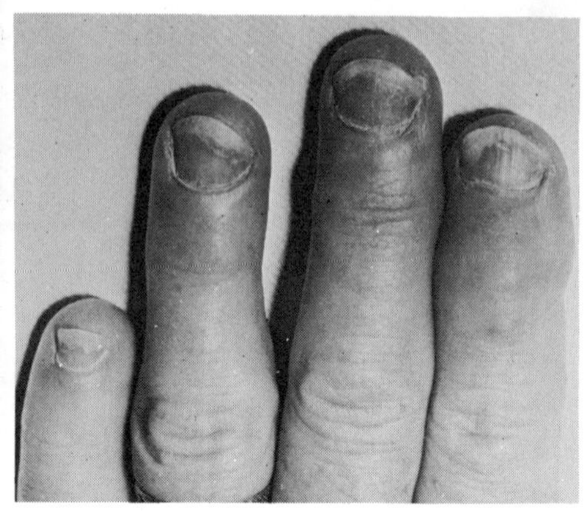

Plate 6/5 Psoriatic arthritis, with nail and distal interphalangeal joint involvement (*see p. 59*)

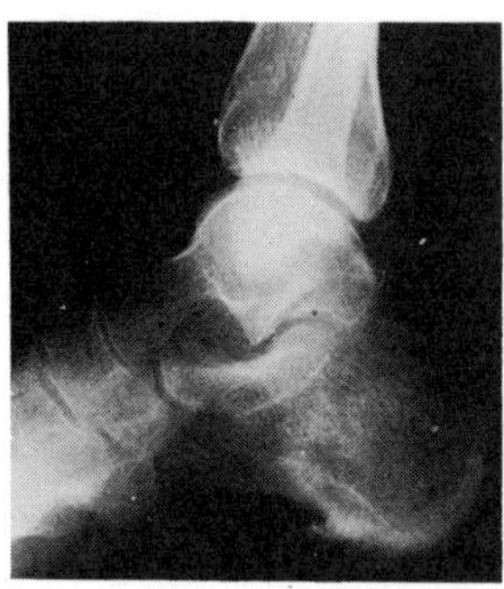

Plate 6/4 Plantar fasciitis in Reiter's disease with large plantar spurs, which appear fluffy due to the periosteal reaction (*see p. 57*)

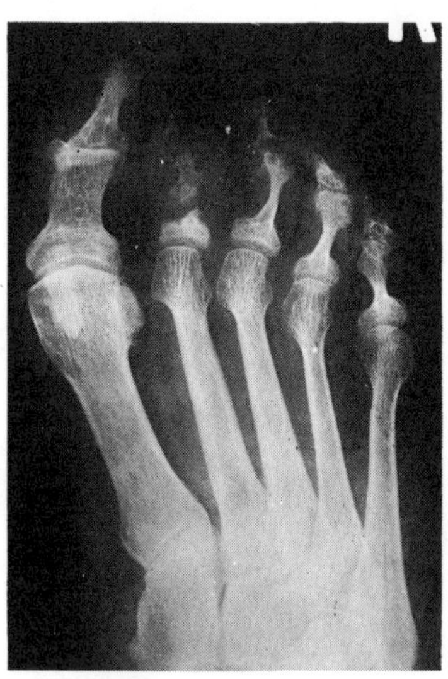

Plate 6/6 Radiograph of psoriatic arthritis showing erosions of distal interphalangeal joints of foot with marked bone loss in 2nd toe (*see p. 59*)

disease in children is always of the dysenteric type. Approximately one per cent of men with non-specific urethritis will develop other features of Reiter's disease after 10 to 21 days. The annual recurrence rate is about 15 per cent and can be precipitated by trauma and intercurrent infection as well as urethritis and dysentery.

URETHRITIS

A serous, sterile urethral discharge may be accompanied by dysuria and haematuria. Inflammation in other parts of the genito-urinary system with cystitis, prostatitis, salpingitis, etc. is not uncommon. Penile ulceration is common and the ulcers may coalesce to form the typical circinate balanitis in about 10 per cent of cases.

ARTHRITIS

This is an acute, asymmetrical sero-negative arthritis involving mostly knees, ankles and feet, although any peripheral joint may be affected. There is marked synovial proliferation and effusion and often serious disability. Tendinitis and fasciitis, particularly around the ankle and heel, is common (Plate 6/4). With persistent or recurrent disease sacro-iliac joint involvement occurs and may progress to a patchy spondylitis making the differentiation from ankylosing spondylitis difficult. An erosive arthritis similar to rheumatoid arthritis occurs in some cases and may lead to serious deformity, particularly of the feet.

EYES

Conjunctivitis with sterile eye discharge causing overnight 'gumming' of the eyelids is the usual ocular sign. Iritis, with the danger of permanent eye damage, occurs in persistent and recurrent cases, usually those with sacro-iliac joint involvement.

SKIN AND MOUTH LESIONS

Non-specific mouth ulceration is common but a more characteristic ulcerated area may be found on the roof of the mouth in 10 per cent of cases.

Keratoderma blennorrhagica develops on the palms and soles in 10 per cent of cases. The deep-seated sterile pustules resemble those of pustular psoriasis. The involved skin becomes much thickened and there are accompanying destructive lesions of the nails.

OTHER FEATURES

A systemic reaction with fever, weight loss and general malaise is usual. Heart, lung and neurological involvement have been recorded but death from Reiter's disease is extremely rare.

RADIOLOGY

Early radiographs may show evidence of periostitis due to joint and tendon involvement, but later the appearances are difficult to distinguish from rheumatoid arthritis and ankylosing spondylitis, depending upon whether peripheral or spinal joints are involved.

Diagnosis and aetiology

Blood tests show no characteristic features. The white cell count and ESR are raised and there is often a mild anaemia. Synovial fluid examination confirms the inflammatory nature of the disease but occasionally may show the presence of large macrophages, 'Reiter's cells'. All tests for infection are negative.

The important diseases to exclude are other venereal diseases, syphilis and gonorrhoea, which may produce urethritis and arthritis and which may co-exist with Reiter's disease. In later cases and especially in women, in whom the urethritis may be symptomless, the differentiation from ankylosing spondylitis and other causes of sacro-iliac joint inflammation is difficult. The skin lesions may be confused with those of psoriasis.

The cause is unknown although an infection seems likely. All attempts to reliably isolate an organism have failed. It is likely that genetic factors determine which patients with non-specific urethritis will proceed to Reiter's disease.

Management

Management will include: (1) rest and splintage; (2) anti-inflammatory drugs; (3) joint aspiration and injection; (4) antibiotics; (5) surgery.

The disease is self-limiting in almost every case, but the time to remission varies from three weeks to two years. The aims of management are to induce early remission and certainly prompt treatment shortens the course of the disease. Full bed rest, usually with splints, is the quickest and ultimately the kindest way to settle the arthritis in impatient young men. Aspiration of joint effusion and intra-articular corticosteroids will speed this process. It is vital that mobilization proceeds slowly as recurrence is common, especially if too much activity is allowed before muscle bulk has returned. The decision to mobilize must be taken clinically as the ESR is slow to settle and is a poor guide to management. Full dosage of an anti-inflammatory drug (page 159) should be given and in cases failing to improve corticosteroids or even immunosuppressive agents may be required. Antibiotics, ideally tetracycline, will control the non-specific urethritis but will have no effect upon the rest of the disease.

In persistent or recurrent cases *synovectomy* or even reconstructive surgery, particularly of the feet, may be undertaken.

PSORIATIC ARTHROPATHY

Psoriasis and rheumatoid arthritis are both common conditions each affecting 2 per cent of the population and may occur coincidentally in the same patient. However, a specific form of sero-negative polyarthritis is now recognized, and although the management is essentially the same as that of rheumatoid arthritis, the disease is associated with less systemic upset and has a better prognosis.

Clinical features

The presence of psoriasis is essential for the diagnosis. However, only small patches on the extensor surfaces of knees and elbows or in the scalp may be found. Nail involvement, with pitting, ridging and/or destructive lesions, is very common. Four patterns of joint involvement are recognized although two or more patterns may co-exist.

DISTAL INTERPHALANGEAL JOINT DISEASE

This severe erosive arthritis of the hands and feet is often associated with marked bone loss of the finger tufts (Plate 6/5). Involvement of these joints is rare in rheumatoid arthritis but the features may be confused with generalized osteoarthrosis with Heberden node formation if nails and skin are not carefully examined.

RHEUMATOID TYPE DISEASE

The pattern of joint involvement follows that of rheumatoid arthritis although tending to be less symmetrical and often accompanied by marked flexor tendon involvement producing a 'sausage' finger. The tests for rheumatoid factor remain negative.

SACRO-ILIAC JOINT DISEASE

Bilateral sacro-iliitis alone or in association with other patterns of disease is common, and may progress to spondylitis indistinguishable from ankylosing spondylitis.

ARTHRITIS MUTILANS

This is a rare, very destructive arthritis associated with marked bone loss which produces the appearance of telescoping of the soft tissues since their length is unaltered (Plate 6/6).

There are clear genetic influences in the disease since there is an increased incidence of psoriasis, psoriatic arthropathy and ankylosing spondylitis in the patients' relatives. There are probably links with Reiter's disease and the arthropathy of ulcerative bowel disease.

Management

Exacerbations in the skin and joint disease rarely coincide and each must be treated separately. Skin lesions should be treated initially with a descaling ointment and various tar-based preparations are suitable. Subsequently local corticosteroid therapy is employed. Treatment of the joints should follow the lines suggested for rheumatoid arthritis and ankylosing spondylitis. In most cases the benign nature of the disease means that an anti-inflammatory drug is all that is required, but more severe cases may require corticosteroids or even an anti-metabolite such as methotrexate. The therapist can help with exercise programmes, local therapy to finger joints and general advice. Surgical procedures of the type used in rheumatoid arthritis may occasionally be required and are associated with similar results. Active skin lesions are no bar to surgery but extra preparation of these infected areas is advisable.

ULCERATIVE COLITIS AND CROHN'S DISEASE

These distinguishable diseases which present with severe diarrhoea and general ill-health are associated with similar articular features. These include:

COLITIC ARTHRITIS

This is a self-limiting synovitis and effusion, usually of the knees and ankles. A simple programme of rest, splints, anti-inflammatory drugs and exercises will control symptoms and restore full function. The arthritis mirrors the activity of the bowel disease and remits completely after colectomy.

SACRO-ILIITIS

Twenty per cent of patients have sacro-iliitis, leading to an increased incidence of ankylosing spondylitis. Iritis is a common complication. The usual management of ankylosing spondylitis is applicable.

ERYTHEMA NODOSUM

Ulcerative bowel disease may be associated with erythema nodosum (see page 63).

For Bibliography see end of Chapter 9, p. 104.

Chapter 7

Inflammatory Arthritis

including arthritis due to infection, connective tissue diseases and crystal arthritis

by ALASTAIR G. MOWAT, MB, FRCP(ED)
and JOAN M. ABERY, MCSP

ARTHRITIS DUE TO INFECTIONS

Rheumatic fever

Rheumatic fever is a disease of declining incidence and severity which affects young people and which is caused by an abnormal immunological reaction to infection with β-haemolytic streptococcus. The streptococcal infection is usually in the throat and although this may have cleared by the time other features of the disease appear, a rising anti-streptolysin (ASO) titre in the blood can be taken as evidence of infection. The most serious effect of rheumatic fever follows inflammatory damage to heart structures, often leading to mitral and aortic valve disease and cardiac arrhythmias, which will produce increasing disability during the rest of the patient's life, especially during episodes of cardiac strain such as pregnancy.

The acute stage of the disease is characterized by fever, polyarthritis, subcutaneous nodules, skin rash, chorea and a raised ESR. The polyarthritis migrates through any peripheral joint, accompanied for two to three days by marked swelling and pain but causing no permanent damage.

MANAGEMENT

Rest is essential for both the heart and joints in the acute phase of the disease. Splintage of joints is rarely necessary. Aspirin and related drugs (see p. 159) dramatically relieve joint symptoms and control the fever. Corticosteroids are occasionally required for severe cases. Penicillin will eradicate any residual streptococcal infection and is generally given for five years to protect the patient against recurrent infection and subsequent rheumatic fever.

Septic arthritis

Septic arthritis may result from infection elsewhere in the body and from the introduction of bacteria directly into the joint by trauma, intra-articular injection or operation. Occasionally it may occur without obvious cause in a damaged joint. The presence of a metal prosthesis appears to increase the risk of such infection, and any debilitating disease, diabetes or treatment with corticosteroids and immunosuppressive agents, will further exaggerate the tendency to joint infection.

The patient is usually unwell, with fever, rigors and raised white cell count. The larger peripheral joints are usually affected but no joint is immune. Although the staphylococcus is the commonest infecting organism, infection with other organisms such as salmonella and meningococcus must be remembered.

MANAGEMENT

Prompt bacteriological culture of the synovial fluid, blood and any other potentially infected material is essential. Systemic treatment with the appropriate antibiotic and local support for the painful joint is given. Surgical drainage or irrigation of joints is seldom necessary. Repeated aspiration of a large effusion will make the patient more comfortable but local injection of antibiotic is unnecessary and may cause chemical irritation.

Gonococcal arthritis

Gonorrhoea, an increasingly common venereal disease, may cause articular disease. The arthritis is commoner in women, in whom the initial urethritis and other genito-urinary symptoms are often mild and untreated. The arthritis, most commonly in the knee, is a form of septic arthritis but is often preceded by a flitting arthralgia and accompanied by tenosynovitis and a rash. Diagnosis is more certain if it is suggested to the bacteriologist, as culture of the organism may be difficult. Antibiotic therapy should ensure a full remission.

Brucellosis

Despite testing of cattle, brucellosis may result from drinking unpasteurized milk. Direct contact with infected animals as a source of infection only applies to farmworkers, butchers and veterinary surgeons. There is intermittent fever, general malaise, myalgia and arthralgia of larger limb joints. A destructive, septic arthritis of hip, knee and spine may follow. Diagnosis is by serum agglutination test and treatment with streptomycin and tetracycline.

Tuberculosis

This is now a rare cause of arthritis, although the joint remains second to the lung as a site of infection. The disease is commoner and painful in children, but chronic, often relatively painless, monarticular disease should suggest tuberculosis in any age group, particularly in the elderly and in coloured immigrants. The hip, knee and lumbar spine are the commonest sites of infection and involvement of tendons and fingers and the tracking of a 'cold' psoas abscess to the groin are now all rare. Diagnosis may be delayed, often being made after biopsy of involved areas. Treatment is with standard anti-tuberculous drugs and immobilization. The patient should be referred to a chest physician, so that the patient and his contacts can be examined regularly for possible pulmonary tuberculosis, and given appropriate treatment. Without such referral, and the exclusion of tuberculous cows from milk production for public consumption, these two main forms of tuberculosis could again become widespread in the United Kingdom. Synovectomy of peripheral joints is indicated both for diagnostic and therapeutic reasons. Other surgical treatment is rarely needed in Britain.

Viral arthritis

It is important to remember that a transient, but often painful, synovitis may accompany many viral infections. Rubella (German measles) arthritis is the commonest, tending to affect the knees of young women, the group already at risk from this infection since it may cause fetal abnormalities. Diagnosis is often made after the symptoms have settled by finding a rise in the level of antibodies in the blood.

Erythema nodosum

Erythema nodosum is characterized by crops of large, red, tender, raised lesions over the shins, which gradually fade like bruises. The rash represents a hypersensitivity reaction to a variety of causes including sarcoid, tuberculosis, streptococcal infection, ulcerative colitis, Crohn's disease and drug allergy. However, in up to one half of cases no cause is found. A synovitis, usually of the knees and ankles, occurs in some 60 to 70 per cent of patients with erythema nodosum. Confusion may arise since the synovitis often precedes the skin rash by several weeks. The synovitis settles over weeks or months even, without treatment, but salicylates or even corticosteroids should usually be given.

CONNECTIVE TISSUE DISEASES

Disseminated lupus erythematosus

The disease, which is most common in young women, is associated with a characteristic facial rash, several types of serious and often fatal renal disease and serious damage to other systems. Myositis and synovitis of small, peripheral joints is common. The joints may resemble those of early rheumatoid arthritis but cartilage and bone damage is usual. A variety of abnormal antibodies have been found in this disease but the precise relationship of these to the inflammatory damage in blood vessels, which is responsible for most of the clinical features, is uncertain.

Anaemia and a raised ESR are common. Low white cell and platelet counts are common features of the disease and may result in intercurrent infections or purpuric or haemorrhagic episodes. The finding of anti-DNA (deoxyribonucleic acid) antibodies in the serum and altered white cells, so called LE cells, in the peripheral blood are the most helpful diagnostic tests.

The disease carries a serious prognosis and usually demands the use of large doses of corticosteroids or immunosuppressive agents.

Dermatomyositis

This is a rare disease characterized by chronic, inflammatory disease in muscles, especially the proximal limb muscles. The patient complains of muscle tenderness and progressive weakness, and the serum levels of muscle enzymes (aldolase, creatine phosphokinase) are raised. Heliotrope (bluish purple) discoloration of the face and extensor surfaces of the fingers is found in dermatomyositis but is absent from the otherwise identical polymyositis. Both diseases show evidence of widespread vascular abnormalities including synovitis of peripheral joints but motility disturbance and other gastro-intestinal symptoms are the commonest. The disease is commoner in women and there are peak incidences in childhood and again in the fourth and sixth decades. The incidence of underlying neoplastic disease increases with the age of onset of the disease, and a careful hunt for a tumour should always be made.

The prognosis is poor in children with only half surviving two years. Adults without tumour do better. High doses of corticosteroids are usually required.

Scleroderma (progressive systemic sclerosis)

This is a rare disease which affects skin, joints, gastro-intestinal tract, lungs and kidneys. The disease may be confined to the skin for many years producing a tight, shiny appearance in hands and face. Skin atrophy and calcification may lead to ulceration and gangrene. Joint deformities may be produced. Synovitis in joints is usually mild.

The disease is often preceded by Raynaud's phenomenon – a hypersensitivity to cold demonstrated by whiteness and 'deadness' of the fingers. Raynaud's phenomenon is common in children but late onset or increasing severity of the phenomenon should suggest scleroderma or other connective tissue disease.

The prognosis in scleroderma is related to the age of onset and the severity of anaemia, renal and lung symptoms. At present there is no effective treatment.

Sjögren's syndrome

This is a chronic inflammation of the lacrimal and salivary glands leading to dryness of the eye and mouth. In some two-thirds of cases rheumatoid arthritis or another connective tissue disease is present. Rarely there may be involvement of other glandular structures leading to reduced sweating, reduced bronchial and nasal secretions, reduced gastric and pancreatic secretions and vaginitis. The underlying connective tissue disease should be treated in the usual ways. There is no effective treatment for Sjögren's syndrome although corticosteroids may be tried. Eye damage can be prevented by using methyl cellulose drops ('artificial tears').

Polyarteritis nodosa

The features of polyarteritis nodosa are due to patchy, inflammatory damage in medium-sized arteries. These include haematuria, hypertension and renal failure, myocardial infarction and arteritis, gastrointestinal haemorrhage and perforation, skin nodules, hemiplegia and peripheral neuropathy and polyarthritis. Larger joints are usually involved, synovitis being migratory and rarely leading to erosive or permanent changes. The disease differs from the other connective tissue diseases in affecting more men than women and in involving rather larger arteries. A proportion of patients have asthma and lung infiltration on chest radiographs. Such patients usually have a raised eosinophil count in the blood. Otherwise investigations, apart from biopsy of the lesions, are not helpful. The disease causes early death and there is no definitive treatment.

Polymyalgia rheumatica

Polymyalgia rheumatica is a clinical syndrome of unknown cause in which severe pain, stiffness and tenderness of the muscles of the shoulder and pelvic girdles are accompanied by a variety of systemic symptoms and signs. These include general malaise, fever, loss of weight and appetite, headache and depression. The onset is frequently sudden, producing severe disability. Joint involvement is minimal. The ESR is markedly elevated but there are no other specific laboratory findings. There is no evidence of muscle disease.

An underlying vasculitis can be found by temporal or other artery biopsy in 25 per cent of cases and is probably the basis for the disease in all cases. Temporal (or giant cell) arteritis is a variant of the same disease. Corticosteroid therapy rapidly controls the muscular and generalized symptoms, and prevents the development of serious vascular symptoms (which include blindness). The disease, which occurs most often in patients over 60 years, is self-limiting and treatment can be reduced and ultimately stopped after two or three years.

CRYSTAL ARTHRITIS

Gout

Gout represents the inflammatory response of some patients, usually men, to a raised plasma uric acid level (hyperuricaemia) and to the deposition in tissues of monosodium urate crystals.

CLINICAL FEATURES

Gout occurs in males, usually after the age of 20, and is rare in women until the menopause. Recent studies of the beneficial effect of oestrogens on blood levels of uric acid and on the susceptibility of cells to damage by urate crystals explains this finding.

The disease presents as an acute attack of *crystal synovitis* which clears completely in a week or so, to be followed at intervals of weeks, months or even years by further attacks. After a time deposits of urate, *tophi*, appear on the ears, in tendons and in joints. The joint disease becomes more chronic and leads to secondary degenerative joint disease. The acute attack, which frequently involves the metatarsophalangeal joint of the great toe, causes severe pain, redness, and swelling. There is usually a *systemic reaction* with malaise, fever and a raised ESR and white cell count. Any joint, including the spine, may be involved but it is uncommon in the hip and shoulder. Two per cent of cases are chronic from the outset. The incidence of tophi increases with the length of the history of gout and in untreated cases may reach 90 per cent (Plate 7/1). Tophi are only occasionally visible on X-rays. They may involve many organs and although they are present in 10 per cent of kidneys, the major renal abnormalities of fibrosis and vascular damage leading to hypertension and renal failure are caused by ill-understood mechanisms. Renal disease is a major cause of death in patients with gout.

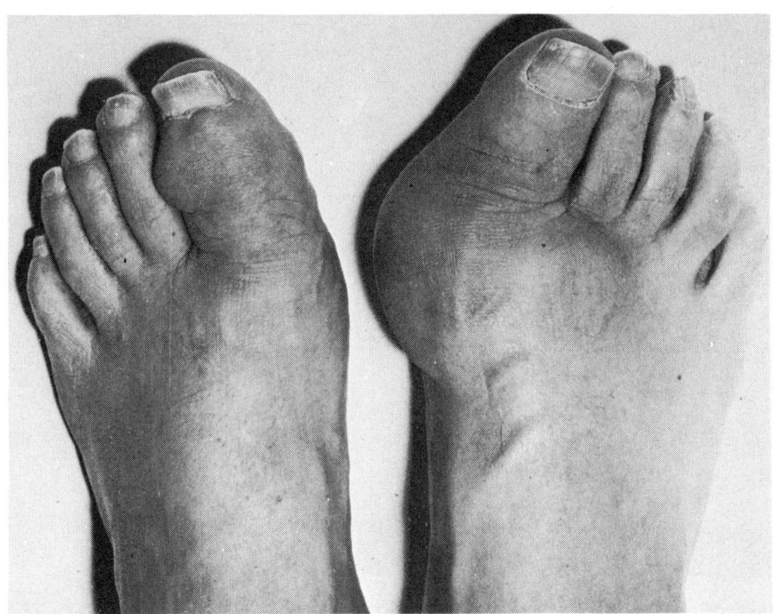

Plate 7/1 Gout. Typical swelling of right 1st metatarsophalangeal joint with tophaceous deposits in distal left great toe

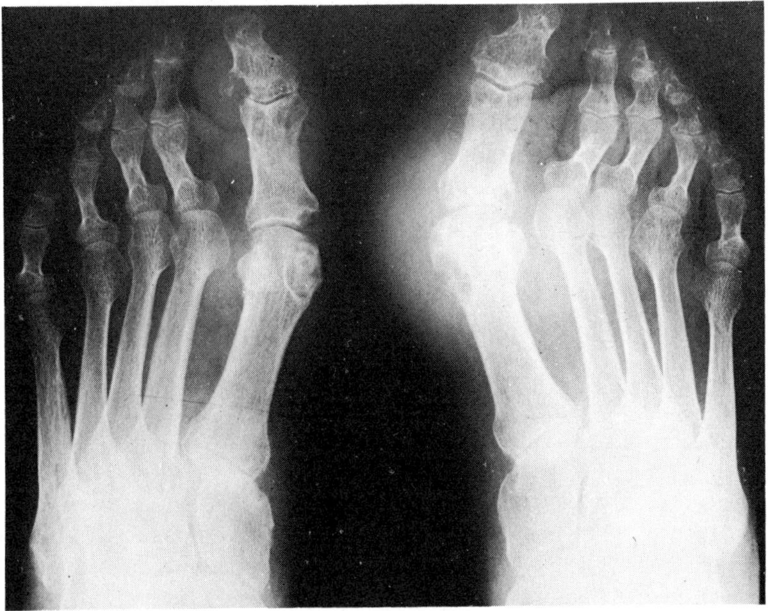

Plate 7/2 Radiograph of Plate 7/1 showing soft tissue swelling of acute gout and erosions associated with deposits of uric acid

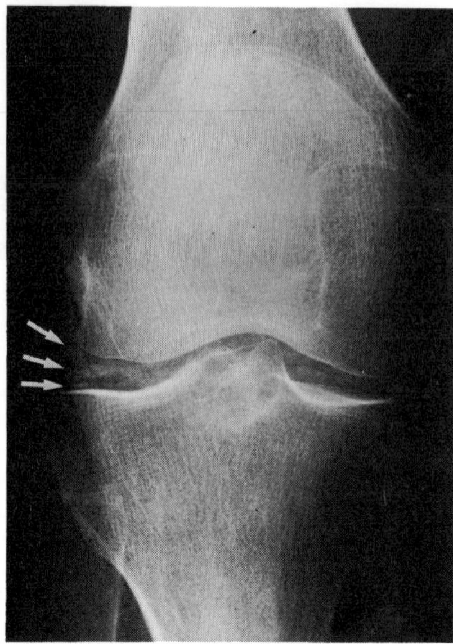

Plate 7/3 Pyrophosphate arthropathy. Calcium crystals are present in both hyaline cartilage of articular surface and fibrocartilage of meniscus (*see p. 71*)

METABOLIC AND PATHOLOGICAL MECHANISMS

Uric acid is the final breakdown product of purines and is excreted chiefly by the kidney. There are three major factors in purine metabolism: (1) the replacement and breakdown of body purines (endogenous); (2) the breakdown of ingested purines (dietary); (3) the renal excretion of uric acid.

The plasma uric acid level and the incidence of gout depends upon the interaction of these factors. The upper limits of normal are usually taken as 6 mg per cent for women and 7 mg per cent for men. Approximately 5 per cent of the population has higher values and is thus hyperuricaemic but only a small proportion will develop gout.

THE REPLACEMENT AND BREAKDOWN OF BODY PURINES

The major pathways in purine metabolism are shown in Fig. 7/1. The amount of uric acid resulting from the breakdown of body purines is at least partly controlled by the ability of enzymes to salvage various purine metabolites (dotted lines in figure). The absence or reduced activity of such enzymes will result in increased uric acid production. Such enzyme abnormalities are probably genetically determined. The last stages in purine breakdown from hypoxanthine to xanthine to uric acid are controlled by the enzyme xanthine oxidase. This fact is utilized in the management of gout with the xanthine oxidase inhibitor allopurinol. Hyperuricaemia with attacks of gout is due to the overloading of this delicately balanced system by an increase in endogenous purine

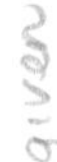

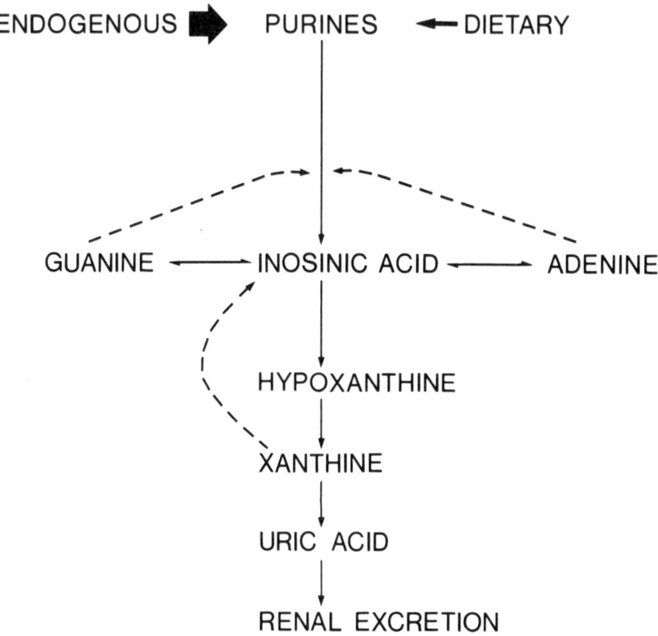

Fig. 7/1 Major pathways in purine metabolism

metabolism following a variety of stresses such as infection, surgery and trauma. Secondary gout is caused by excessive purine breakdown in the presence of a normal metabolic pathway and occurs in such diseases as the leukaemias, polycythaemia, myeloma and psoriasis.

BREAKDOWN OF INGESTED PURINES

This is not an important cause of gout as it is exceptional for patients to produce hyperuricaemia with even severe dietary excess unless there is some metabolic abnormality, of the type suggested above, already present. Dietary restriction is thus not necessary with current drug therapy.

RENAL EXCRETION OF URIC ACID

The rate of excretion of uric acid is genetically determined and is proportional to the plasma uric acid levels. The excretion rate increases as the plasma level rises but in some patients the excretion rate is set at a lower level and hyperuricaemia and gout result. Clearly, renal disease of many types can interfere with the excretion of uric acid and can consequently cause gout. Possibly more important, a variety of drugs and other factors can impair the ability of a normal kidney to excrete uric acid. These include diuretics, salicylates in low doses and ketosis due to starvation, diabetes or excessive alcohol intake. Moderation of alcohol intake is thus sensible in the management of gout. Other drugs, such as aspirin in high doses and uricosuric drugs such as probenecid, increase the excretion of uric acid and are used in treatment.

PATHOLOGY

The attack of gout is caused by the ingestion of micro-crystals of urate by white cells in the synovial fluid with a subsequent release of inflammatory enzymes. Such attacks occur either when the solubility of urate in body fluids has been exceeded and deposits are accumulating, particularly in articular and periarticular tissues, or when the plasma uric acid is lowered and such deposits are going into solution. The second mechanism explains why attacks of gout may occur during the first weeks of treatment.

DIAGNOSIS

The commonest diagnostic confusion is with septic arthritis since both diseases produce severe pain, marked local inflammation and a raised white cell count. The finding of an elevated plasma uric acid level indicates hyperuricaemia and hence the possibility of gout. The diagnosis is confirmed by the clinical features and the finding of uric acid crystals in a joint effusion. Large, 'punched-out', juxta-articular, bony lesions on X-rays are helpful but not diagnostic features (Plate 7/2).

Treatment of gout

The patient must understand the basic abnormalities in gout if he is to be persuaded to accept continuous treatment. Such treatment consists of: (1) relief of the acute attack; (2) prevention of further attacks.

RELIEF OF ACUTE ATTACK

Colchicine, although effective, produces diarrhoea in full dosage and is now rarely used. Phenylbutazone (800 mg per day) and indomethacin (200 mg per day) are very effective and the dose can be progressively reduced over one week. Systemic or intra-articular steroids are rarely required.

PREVENTION OF FURTHER ATTACKS

This follows the reduction in the plasma uric acid and can be achieved either with uricosuric drugs (probenecid 1–2 g per day), which increase the renal clearance of urate or by a xanthine oxidase inhibitor (allopurinol 300 mg per day). The use of the latter drug allows purine metabolites to be excreted as xanthines (Fig. 7/1) rather than uric acid, and since xanthines are excreted much better than uric acid, the drug has advantages in patients with severe gout or renal disease. Because of the risk of precipitating acute attacks it is usual to add a small dose of phenylbutazone or indomethacin for the first three months of treatment (see Pathology, p. 70).

Pyrophosphate arthropathy

This disease, sometimes called chondrocalcinosis or pseudo-gout, is due to synovitis caused by crystals of calcium pyrophosphate dihydrate. The pathological mechanisms and symptoms are similar to those of gout. The knee, shoulder and wrist are commonly involved and the characteristic radiological features may also be found in the pubic symphysis. These include calcification in both fibrocartilage and hyaline cartilage, but the presence of such calcification does not automatically make the diagnosis of pseudo-gout since many elderly people show such features (Plate 7/3). The term chondrocalcinosis is thus best used to describe the radiographic features and not the disease. The disease is occasionally associated with hyperparathyroidism and haemochromatosis. The most effective treatment is joint aspiration and instillation of local steroids. Indomethacin and phenylbutazone help to prevent and control acute attacks.

ARTHRITIS ASSOCIATED WITH MALIGNANT DISEASE

A variety of vague musculo-skeletal pains may be associated with any malignant disease, and bone pain from skeletal metastases is most common with lung, breast, thyroid and prostatic tumours. Leukaemia often presents with migratory polyarthritis and in children may be confused with rheumatic fever and juvenile rheumatoid arthritis. Myeloma may present with polyarthritis either by direct involvement or by causing the deposition of amyloid tissue in and around joints.

Hypertrophic pulmonary osteoarthropathy, characterized by chronic periostitis of the distal limb bones at the wrists and ankles, recurrent synovitis of large joints and clubbing of the fingers is usually associated with lung and gastric tumours. Other associated conditions include liver cirrhosis, lung sepsis, and bacterial endocarditis. The pathological mechanisms involved are not clearly understood.

Despite the capacity of synovial tissue to proliferate in response to many irritants, a synovial tumour is very rare.

ARTHRITIS ASSOCIATED WITH HAEMOPHILIA

The most crippling complication of haemophilia is arthritis. This disorder, due to a deficiency of a blood clotting factor (factor VIII or antihaemophilic globulin, AHG) is genetically determined, being transmitted by women but appearing as a clinical condition in men. The disease is characterized by repeated episodes of bleeding into joints and muscles and occasional bleeding from the kidney and gastro-intestinal tract, occurring from childhood onwards and often without an obvious cause. Joint and muscle haemorrhage causes severe pain, swelling and disability and if treated poorly or if the haemorrhages are frequent, permanent deformity results.

Management

The aims of management are to (1) control the bleeding; (2) relieve pain; (3) maintain and restore function.

CONTROL OF BLEEDING

Factor VIII must be replaced in sufficient quantity to allow normal blood clotting to proceed. With minor bleeding fresh plasma will suffice but with major bleeding some concentrate of plasma must be used. Factor VIII from animal sources can be used until antibodies develop and then a concentrate of human plasma prepared by various freezing techniques is employed. It is usual to employ factor VIII to control the initial haemorrhage and also to 'cover' the patient during early mobilization. In addition, considerable quantities of factor VIII are required for several days if reconstructive surgery is undertaken to improve the function in damaged joints. This is a developing field in orthopaedic surgery.

RELIEF OF PAIN

Routine analgesics are employed. Anti-inflammatory drugs such as aspirin and phenylbutazone should be avoided as they further alter blood clotting. Rest in plaster of Paris splints will relieve pain and assist in the control of bleeding and tissue swelling.

MAINTENANCE AND RESTORATION OF FUNCTION

A continuing programme of splints and slow, careful mobilization with suitable exercises, particularly for the quadriceps muscles, will maintain and restore function and for those with more severely damaged joints fixation splints may be needed (see Chapter 8).

ARTHRITIS ASSOCIATED WITH NEUROLOGICAL DISEASE

Paralysis of a limb may protect joints from both rheumatoid arthritis and osteoarthrosis. However, partial nerve damage may exaggerate osteoarthrosis, since unusual joint loading may occur. Damage to the neurological supply of a joint may lead to gross destruction and instability (Charcot joint). Although the joint usually becomes painless, contrary to popular belief, the recurrent episodes of swelling earlier in the disease are often painful. Syringomyelia is the usual cause of this type of arthritis in the upper limb, while syphilis (tabes dorsalis) and diabetes are common causes in the lower limb joints. Repeated intra-articular steroid injections may rarely be the cause.

For Bibliography see end of Chapter 9, p. 104.

Chapter 8

The Management of Inflammatory Joint Disease

by ALASTAIR G. MOWAT, MB, FRCP(ED)
and JOAN M. ABERY, MCSP

GENERAL PRINCIPLES OF MANAGEMENT

The same general principles of management apply to all forms of inflammatory joint disease in which the precise cause is unknown. However, the extent to which these principles are applied will depend upon the natural history, severity and chronicity of the disease. It is convenient to describe the general management of rheumatoid arthritis, and such treatment can be modified to suit each individual patient and disease. Indeed, the importance of planning the management of each patient cannot be over-emphasized. Better results are achieved in many forms of joint disease, particularly rheumatoid arthritis, if the patient is admitted to hospital early in the course of the disease. This reflects how important it is that the nature of the disease and the aims of treatment be fully understood by the patient, his family and his medical advisers from the onset.

There are considerable advantages in treating patients with inflammatory joint disease in a separate ward or unit as they can often help and advise each other and are not subjected to the pressures of bed turnover which inevitably prevail in general medical or surgical wards. These patients progress slowly and indeed may not improve if their treatment programmes are hurried. Further, since the diseases produce complex disabilities and are usually associated with domestic, economic, employment and social factors, team-work is essential in their management. The team is composed of general practitioner, physician, orthopaedic surgeon, physiotherapist, occupational therapist, nursing staff and medical social worker. A psychiatrist may often be added. A close liaison must be continued with the various domiciliary services.

The aim of management of chronic joint disease is simply to allow the patient to achieve and maintain the maximum functional capacity.

This will entail not only an accurate assessment of the initial status of the patient but a continuing assessment of the changing status of the disease and of the patient's reaction to the disease. It is important to appreciate that the patient's problem is not arthritis but rather the disability that the arthritis produces. Thus many patients, especially the elderly, are subjected to unnecessary hospital visits for examination and treatment when all they require is a simple, commonsense approach to their domestic difficulties. There are no general rules about management. Each patient must be treated as an individual.

Such management may include the use of:

(1) rest;
(2) exercise and other physical methods including walking aids;
(3) splintage;
(4) drugs (Chapter 14);
(5) nursing care and dietary advice;
(6) various appliances designed to overcome or reduce disability and dependence upon others;
(7) the introduction of changes in employment and in the pattern of daily living;
(8) orthopaedic surgery (Chapter 9).

These items will be described and discussed in subsequent pages.

Role of the physiotherapist (See also Chapter 11)

The physiotherapist is an important member of the management team and she has a varied role. The therapist's initial role must be (i) the assessment of the patient as a whole, temperamentally, socially and psychologically and, in particular, to try and determine which patients are likely to be able to co-operate fully with the therapist; (ii) the assessment and recording of muscle strength and quality according to standard scales, particularly around the joints with the major involvement; (iii) the measurement and recording of the ranges of active and passive joint movement, once again concentrating upon the joints chiefly affected.

Clearly, normal working time and the concentration of both patient and the therapist does not allow highly detailed measurements of all joints and muscles to be made. It is important that the therapist should have the ability to spot the problems and so limit her examination and measurements. Further, it is important that she be able to record her findings in a simple manner so that she contribute to the general discussion of a patient's needs during conferences of the management team. Some form of charting sequential information is valuable and can be included in the patient's records (e.g. Fig. 9/1, p. 102).

The physiotherapist can also do much to help the patient settle in hospital by explaining and amplifying basic disease information (p. 90).

Further, she must assist in the general assessment of the patient's attitude to his disease and disability. A general discussion of the patient's and family's roles, the degree of protection of the patient by the family and the extent of insight of the patient into his or her present and potential problems, can be undertaken at the same time as a detailed assessment of muscle quality and strength is made.

Rest

For the patient at home a period of rest each day may allow increased and more economical function during the remainder of the day. Such a rest may be combined with the use of a suitable splint for periods of prone and supine lying to prevent and/or correct deformity in the spine, hips and knees. For the patient with very active disease rest in hospital is required. The continued use of joints during a phase of active disease increases pain, muscle spasm and wasting and exaggerates any systemic symptoms, and tends to cause flexion deformities in weight-bearing joints. Bed rest relieves these symptoms and improves the general well-being of the patient. There are dangers, however, in uncontrolled bed rest in the form of general physical deterioration, muscle weakness and joint contractures.

Accordingly, splints for arms and legs are provided. The use of a firm mattress and a back rest to ensure adequate support, proper posture and comfort are necessary. A fixed bed cage with padded foot rest to keep the weight of the bedclothes off inflamed joints, to prevent foot drop during periods when leg splints are not worn, and to prevent the patient from slipping down the bed, is also necessary. Many patients prefer a continental quilt.

EXERCISE AND OTHER PHYSICAL METHODS INCLUDING WALKING AIDS

Exercise

There is little benefit in instituting physical exercises until joint activity has settled as it is very difficult to increase muscle bulk or strength around an actively inflamed joint. However, once the joint inflammation has settled, a planned programme of graduated exercises is essential as considerable muscle wasting occurs in association with joint disease. Elaborate exercise programmes are not necessary and will certainly not be undertaken by patients at home. Passive movements tend to produce protective muscle spasm and are discouraged. Active, isotonic exercises against increasing resistance are the most satisfactory; but where pain is still present on joint movement, and particularly for the knee joint, the exercises are performed isometrically.

Thus for the patient with painful knees associated with synovial proliferation and effusion, the period of rest in splints can be used by the therapist to discuss general aspects of his disease. The exercise programme is begun slowly, often allowing the patient to simply loosen up for the first two to three days. The use of a slippery board is helpful. The first exercises will be quadriceps contractions performed isometrically. The patient should be encouraged to achieve a modest target which can be repeated frequently during the day. When ten contractions can be achieved without fatigue, straight-leg raising and flexion exercises can be commenced. The patient slowly progresses to straight-leg raising with 2 to 4 lb weights (depending on body build) attached to the ankles before weight-bearing is allowed. The last few degrees of extension may be more readily achieved by supporting the knee over a small 'hump' (Plate 8/1). Weight-bearing initially involves standing by the bed and sitting down again, followed by marking time to allow the patient to regain balance and co-ordination. Early ambulation may require a walking aid.

Any increase in swelling, ache or pain, or any increase in morning stiffness, indicates that too much has been undertaken the previous day. Ice treatment will control these symptoms. The rate of increase in activity needs to be slower than many imagine.

Similar exercise programmes can be planned for any joint.

During any programme of rest and splintage for a joint or joints, general exercises designed to improve circulation and maintain muscular condition should be given to the remaining joints and trunk. The same considerations apply during the non-weight-bearing phase following orthopaedic surgical procedures (Chapter 9).

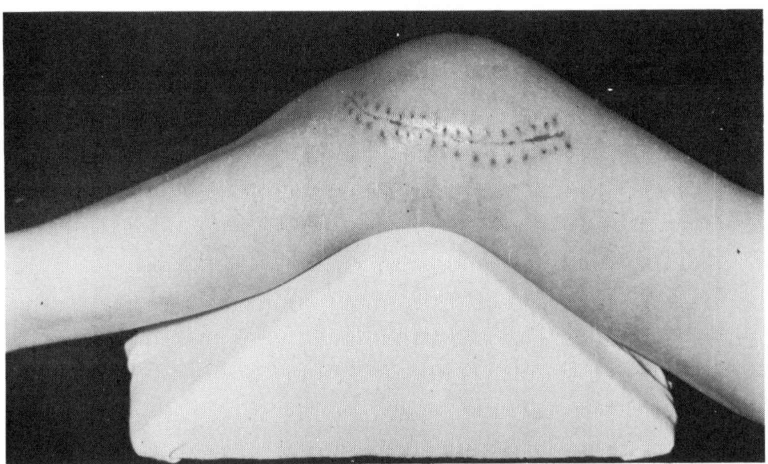

Plate 8/1 Use of a 'hump' to improve extension and quadriceps strength post-operatively (*see above*)

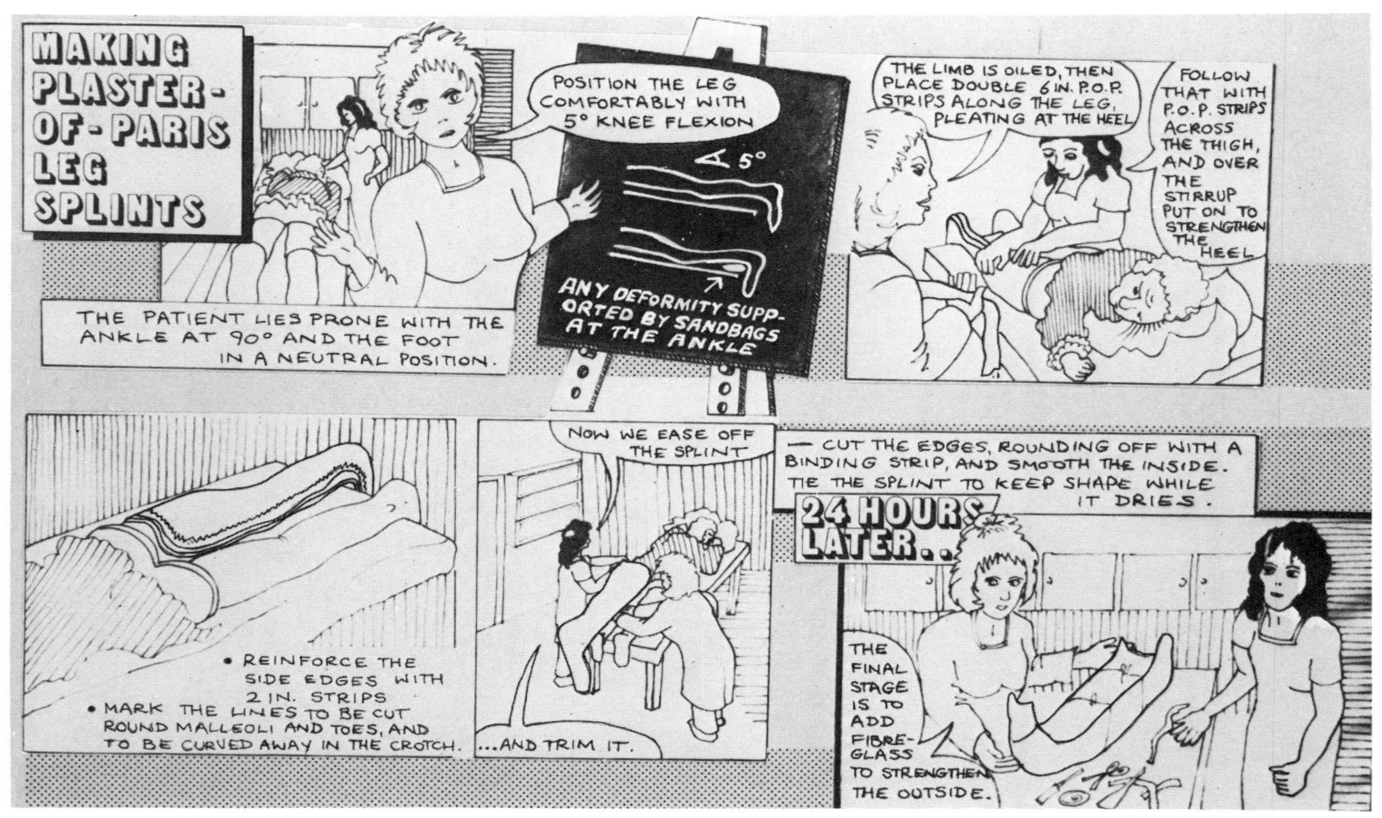
MAKING PLASTER-OF-PARIS LEG SPLINTS
THE PATIENT LIES PRONE WITH THE ANKLE AT 90° AND THE FOOT IN A NEUTRAL POSITION.
POSITION THE LEG COMFORTABLY WITH 5° KNEE FLEXION
5°
ANY DEFORMITY SUPPORTED BY SANDBAGS AT THE ANKLE
THE LIMB IS OILED, THEN PLACE DOUBLE 6 IN. P.O.P. STRIPS ALONG THE LEG, PLEATING AT THE HEEL
FOLLOW THAT WITH P.O.P. STRIPS ACROSS THE THIGH, AND OVER THE STIRRUP PUT ON TO STRENGTHEN THE HEEL
• REINFORCE THE SIDE EDGES WITH 2 IN. STRIPS
• MARK THE LINES TO BE CUT ROUND MALLEOLI AND TOES, AND TO BE CURVED AWAY IN THE CROTCH.
NOW WE EASE OFF THE SPLINT
...AND TRIM IT.
— CUT THE EDGES, ROUNDING OFF WITH A BINDING STRIP, AND SMOOTH THE INSIDE. TIE THE SPLINT TO KEEP SHAPE WHILE IT DRIES.
24 HOURS LATER..
THE FINAL STAGE IS TO ADD FIBRE-GLASS TO STRENGTHEN THE OUTSIDE.

Plate 8/2

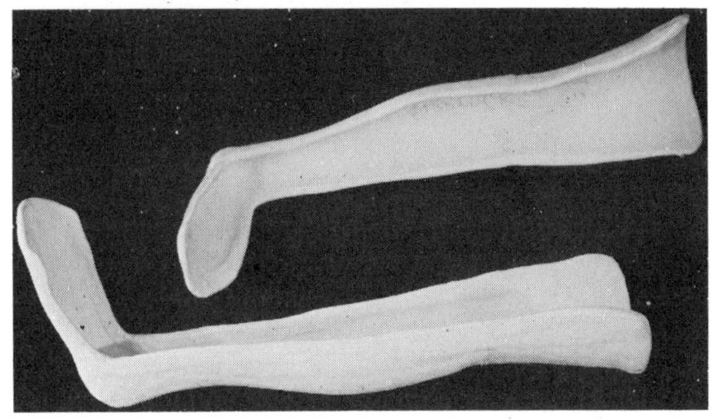

Plate 8/3 Plaster-of-Paris leg splints (*see p. 84*)

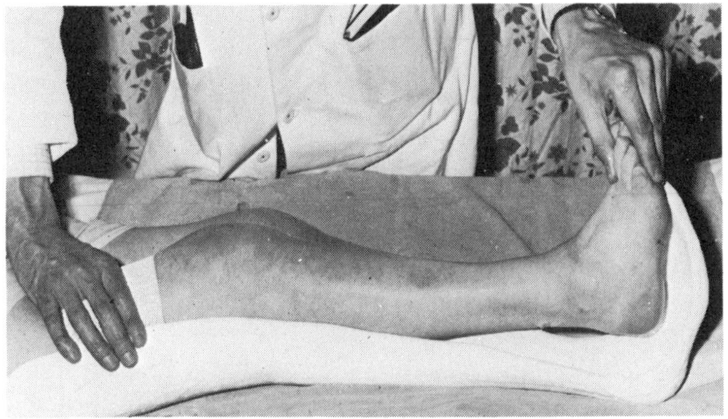

Plate 8/4 Plaster-of-Paris leg splints used to correct a flexion deformity at the knee-joint (*see p. 85*)

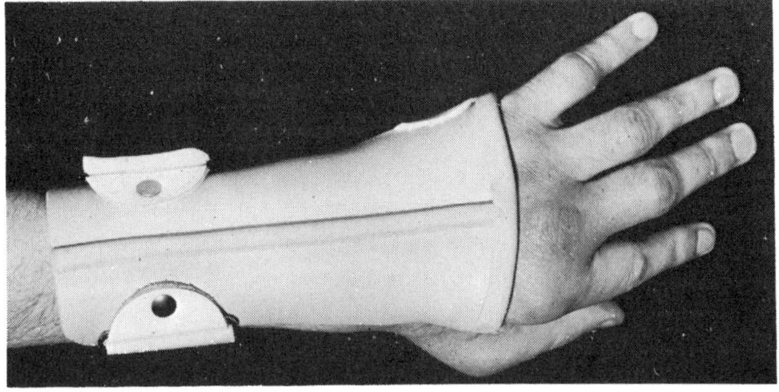

Plate 8/5 Lightweight Prenyl working wrist splint with Velcro fastenings. A thin palmar band does not impair hand grip

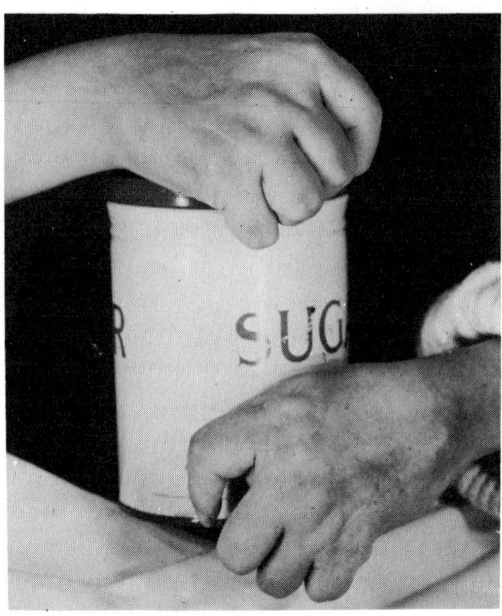

Plate 8/6 Holding a tin and removing the lid may be difficult with deformed fingers (*see p. 89*)

Heating and Cooling

Various forms of heating and cooling may be used to reduce joint swelling and muscle spasm before a period of active exercises. Short-wave diathermy or infra-red heat may be used for large joints, while paraffin wax (melting point 38 to 41°C) is the best heat treatment for hands.

However, many patients prefer ice therapy. Chipped ice in a towelling bag, which in turn is placed in a plastic bag, is put directly over the joint and left for 15 to 30 minutes. Ice treatment for the hands and wrists is best achieved by immersing them in melting ice for periods of up to 30 seconds until aching is produced. If this proves too painful, an ice-bag, as for larger joints, can be used. Ice treatment for the hands is best interspersed with exercises but for larger joints exercises are preceded by ice treatment.

Such ice treatment can be used at home, using a 2 lb bag of frozen peas in place of the chipped ice. The same application technique is used, and after use the peas may be returned to the deep-freeze to be re-used many times. At home heat is more readily applied by a hot-water bottle or small pad rather than with a lamp. For hands, wearing plastic gloves in hot water is a suitable substitute for wax therapy.

However, it is wisest for the therapist to assess the best treatment and instruct the patient. Certainly there are markedly different individual patient reactions and responses to heat and ice treatment, and it is vital to select the correct treatment for each patient.

Hydrotherapy is a form of treatment which produces widely differing results in different patients, and indeed there are marked differences among physiotherapists in their enthusiasm for and assessment of the value of such treatment. Such differences can be seen by comparing these comments with those on page 127. Unfortunately, there are no properly documented scientific studies of hydrotherapy and most comments are therefore personal in nature. These authors feel that hydrotherapy probably does not increase the final range of joint movement or reduce the time needed to achieve full weight-bearing, but it may improve a patient's morale.

Faradic foot pads combined with exercise shorten the period of foot stiffness after bed rest.

Crutches

Various forms of walking aids may be required and care must be taken in their selection. In many hospitals this is the responsibility of the physiotherapist. Many patients resist the idea of walking aids and a sympathetic explanation of the mechanics of weight-relief may be needed.

The traditional under-arm crutch is neither suitable nor necessary for most patients with joint disease. These crutches are designed largely or completely to relieve weight-bearing in one limb and impose considerable strain on upper limb joints and muscles, particularly the shoulder joint. A lightweight support which will provide some reduction in lower limb weight-bearing and increase confidence in walking is all that most patients require. Such supports may be used in one or both hands. The standard elbow crutch fills these needs (Fig. 8/1 A). However, the crutch cannot be used by patients with significant flexion deformity at the elbow, a painful wrist or very poor hand function. The alternative gutter crutch can be used by most of these patients since it demands even less of the upper arm joints; and, if fixed to the forearm by Velcro or other simple release fastening, can be managed even with severely affected hands (Fig. 8/1 B). The crutch height should always be adjustable and it is preferable to use crutches in which the length and position of the arm supports are also adjustable.

Other walking aids

Walking sticks or a sturdy umbrella help many patients once they have overcome their pride. A single stick or crutch can be used by patients with unilateral disease to relieve weight and should be used on the contralateral side. However, better weight relief and balance are provided by the use of two supports. The sticks should be of the correct height;

level with the greater trochanter with the patient erect in shoes or level with the lower end of the ulna with the arm held at the side. The handle of many sticks and crutches is too small for the arthritic hand to grip strongly, but soft padding, Sorbo-rubber or Plastazote can be used to provide the correct sized handle. Strong, lightweight, inexpensive metal

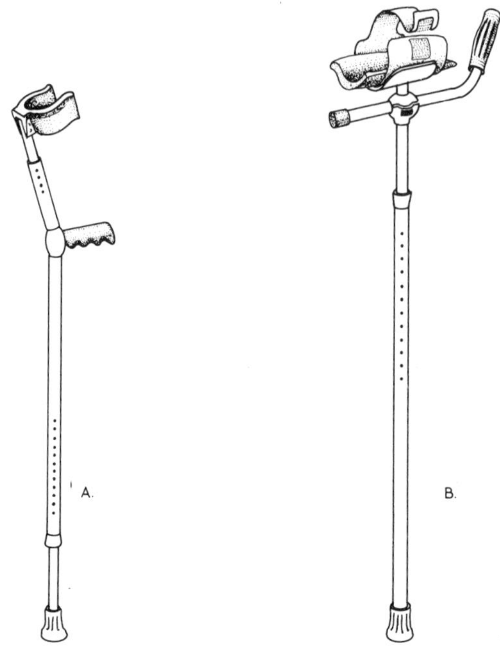

Fig. 8/1 A. Standard elbow crutch. B. Gutter crutch with Velcro fastening

sticks with suitable, moulded left or right handles are available and these can be cut to the correct length. A straight handle is often preferred to the traditional curved handle. A very hard grip or a stick which is too long, causing wrist extension, may lead to symptoms of local median nerve compression.

Sticks with four small legs (quadruped) provide more support and are particularly useful in those patients with poor balance whether due to neurological, eye or joint disease (Fig. 8/2 A). Most crutches and walking aids can be modified to provide a hook for a shopping basket or handbag. A lightweight, wide-based walking frame is favoured by many patients, particularly in the early stages of rehabilitation after surgery or severe disability. Occasionally patients with poor hand function cannot manage the walking frame, and a modified version with two small wheels on the leading legs and suitably adjusted arm supports should be provided (Fig. 8/2 B). However, such aids do not encourage a normal walking movement and are cumbersome in most small-roomed houses. Carefully positioned furniture will be found as useful in many homes, but in other cases, a small trolley may be preferred since it provides both a walking aid and a carrying surface. The patient may need to be shown how to walk with a normal gait, climb stairs and rise from a chair.

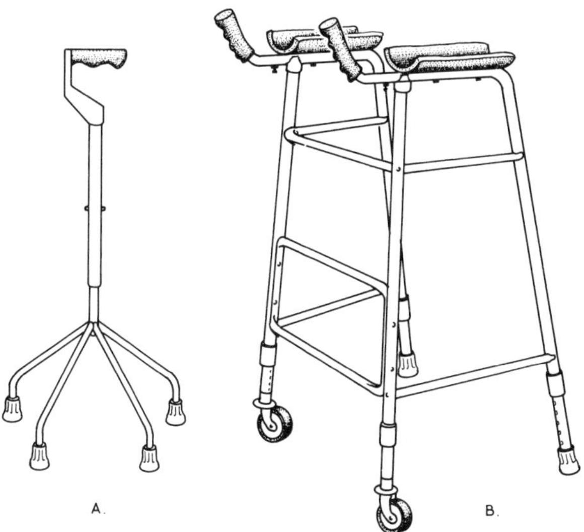

Fig. 8/2 A. Quadruped walking aid with hook for handbag. B. Quadruped walking frame with small wheels on leading legs, and arm supports

SPLINTAGE

Splints have three main functions: (1) rest and relief from pain; (2) prevention and correction of deformity; (3) fixation of a damaged joint in a good functional position.

Rest splints

Skin-tight, unpadded plaster of Paris splints which hold the limb in good position without muscle spasm are bandaged on at night and for periods of rest during the day as long as active disease persists. Contrary to what might be expected, morning stiffness is decreased by the use of night splints as inflammation is controlled. The fear of joint stiffness progressing to ankylosis leads many to combine splinting with exercises, even during the most active phases of disease. However, there is no substance in these fears and as long as cartilage remains, joints do not become ankylosed.

Continuous immobilization by fixing the splints to the limb with plaster cuffs, perhaps for three weeks, has a place in the early stages of rheumatoid arthritis (Fig. 8/3). It is probably best avoided in those with severe joint damage and in elderly patients who more readily develop complications such as venous thrombosis, fluid retention, hypostatic pneumonia, constipation and osteoporosis. After removal of the rest splint from the limb, no formal exercises are performed for two to three

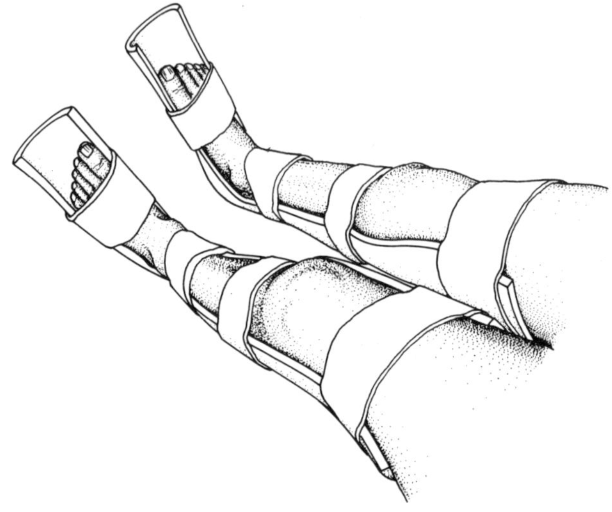

Fig. 8/3 Rest splints fixed to limbs with plaster cuffs

days. However, gentle flexion is allowed and the use of a slippery board facilitates this in lower limb joints.

These splints are comfortable and allow no significant movement. They are made by direct application of plaster of Paris to a limb previously oiled with olive oil. Posterior shells extend from the gluteal creases to the heels with right-angled foot-plates and with knees in 3 to 5° of flexion. The patient lies prone with the leg supported on a sandbag. Some knee flexion must be allowed so that muscles relax and so that the foot can be held in mid-flexion without inversion (Plate 8/2). Posterior arm splints extend from the elbow to the finger tips with the wrist held in mid-pronation and a few degrees of extension. It is usual to leave one elbow free or the patient cannot reach her mouth. If the wrist and fingers are very deformed, anterior splints are easier to make and use. The minimum amount of plaster, consistent with the patient's weight and strength, is used. Care is taken in the finishing stages to remove all rough areas and the application of a fibreglass backing increases their strength and useful life (Plate 8/3).

Corrective splints

Correction of deformity before contractures have occurred can be achieved at any joint, especially the knee, with the use of serial splints. The posterior shell, made as described above, is applied in the position of deformity, and no force, traction or manipulation is used. The shell is fixed to the limb with plaster cuffs. Symptoms settle rapidly and new splints which accommodate the gain in extension can be made at weekly intervals (Plate 8/4). When no further extension can be achieved, routine muscle strengthening exercises are used as a prelude to either walking or surgical treatment.

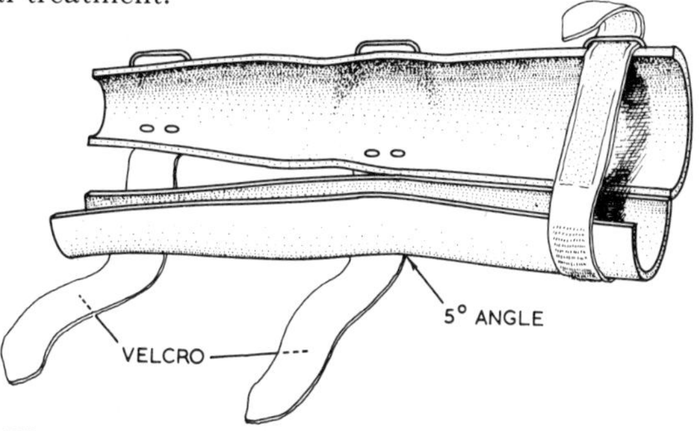

Fig. 8/4. Fibreglass bivalved cylinder for support of knee-joint. The splint has Velcro fastenings

A similar correction may be achieved with dynamic slinging, but it is important to ensure that excessive force is avoided lest joints be damaged or encouraged to sublux.

Fixation splints and other appliances

Static support for a persistently painful, unstable or permanently deformed joint can be provided by a removable splint. The splint is used to hold the joint in a position of function. Thus, to improve walking it may be necessary to use such splints on the knee or ankle and in addition splints can be used at the wrist and elbow joints, to improve the handling and value of suitable walking aids. Splints of this type allow the activity in a single joint or limb to settle without the need for complete rest. In addition, they can be used to reassure patients that any planned surgical fixation of a joint will not produce the disability that they fear. They are particularly useful long-term aids to function in patients who for various reasons may not be considered suitable for surgical treatment.

A variety of suitable materials exists such as Polythene, Orthoplast, leather and fibreglass, all of which combine lightness, strength and durability with ease of construction and use. Plastazote, although possessing some of these qualities, generally lacks the strength necessary for limb fixation; plaster of Paris is too heavy and many newer plastics are unnecessarily rigid and tend to cause local sweating. Velcro or similar simple fastenings should be used and care taken to ensure they are placed so that the patient can use them.

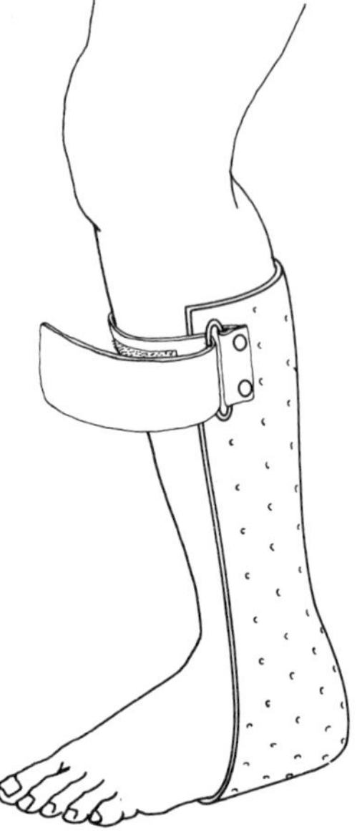

Fig. 8/5 Moulded posterior plastic splint for fixation of the ankle and sub-talar joints

It is important that the splints should be fitted in the optimal position. Ideally an elbow should be held in 90° of flexion with the forearm in mid-pronation, and a wrist should be held in 10° of extension with the thumb left free and finger flexion allowed, by using a dorsal splint with a thin palmar band (Plate 8/5). A knee is best supported by a full cylinder with the joint held in 5° of flexion and this can be removed for sitting (Fig. 8/4). Although, theoretically, the knee can be supported by a hinged caliper which allows the patient to sit easily, in practice it is often difficult to produce a cosmetically acceptable lightweight caliper and the multiple straps and hinge mechanism often cannot be managed by arthritic hands. Flexion deformities should be corrected as far as possible before supporting splints are provided for lower limb joints. Thus uncorrected knee deformities will tend to produce similar compensatory deformities at the hip and ankle joints in the same limb, and unless the inequality in leg length is corrected, similar deformities will develop in the opposite limb. Unfortunately many knee joints have a valgus deformity, and this makes the provision of a splint difficult since it will inevitably rub on the opposite knee.

Adequate fixation splints with simple fastenings are difficult to produce for the ankle joints. It is often simplest to provide a pair of boots or bootees. An alternative is to use a moulded posterior plastic splint stretching from mid-calf to mid-tarsus. This splint, which is fixed with a Velcro strap round the calf, also fixes the sub-talar joint (Fig. 8/5). Fixation of the sub-talar joint or correction of the common valgus deformity may also be achieved by the use of small plastic heel cups (Fig. 8/6), suitable insoles or firmly heeled shoes. An outside leg iron with or

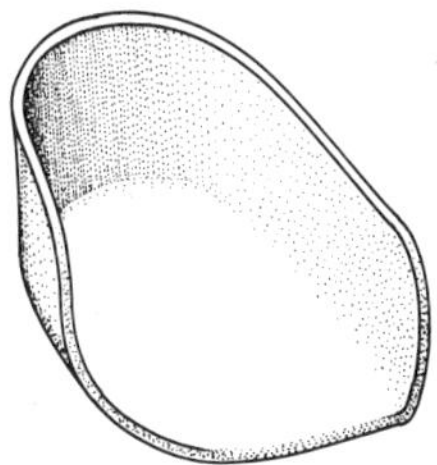
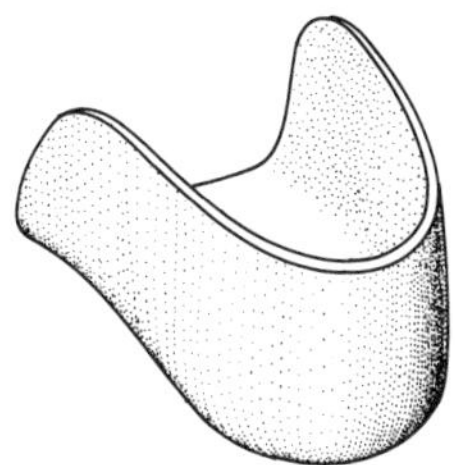

Fig. 8/6 Moulded heel cups for fixation of sub-talar joint or correction of common valgus deformity

without a 'T' strap is very satisfactory but is not always cosmetically acceptable.

Broadening and rigidity of the forefoot with clawing of the toes and the developing of plantar callosities is particularly common in inflammatory joint disease, and can be helped by the use of metatarsal domed insoles. Great care must be taken to place the dome just proximal to the metatarsal heads, otherwise the insole will be ineffective or even increase foot pain. Since these insoles take up space in shoes, new, larger shoes may be required if the insoles are to be used properly.

The greatest improvement in walking may be achieved by the provision of satisfactory shoes. In the early stages wider and deeper shoes with rigid soles and good supporting heel cups can be obtained from normal retail sources. With progressive disease it may be necessary to provide custom-made shoes. There has been some controversy over the advantages and disadvantages of seamless or 'space' shoes versus traditional surgical shoes. Seamless shoes are cheaper and tend to become available to the patient sooner but are unsightly to many wearers and tend to increase sweating of the feet. Local arrangements often determine decisions; the speed of delivery, the accuracy of fitting and the ease of alteration are the key factors and these will vary from supplier to supplier. Patients with poor peripheral circulation, whether due to arteriosclerosis or vasculitis, should be provided with soft, fur-lined boots.

Finally every patient with lower limb joint or lower spinal involvement should have their legs measured. Real and/or apparent shortening of one leg is a common cause of symptoms in the contralateral, 'long' leg and in the lower back. The shoe should be raised approximately one-half the leg length difference in young patients and three-quarters of the difference in elderly patients. Such raises should not significantly increase the weight of the shoe. Raises of over $1\frac{1}{2}$ to 2 in. (4 to 5 cm) will need to be combined with sub-talar joint support, usually as a boot. With higher shoe raises some tapering of the sole allows the patient to walk more easily.

NURSING CARE AND DIETARY ADVICE

Nursing care

The pain, stiffness, deformity and disability of joint disease make heavy demands on the nursing staff. The first few hours of each day can be difficult as this is the period of greatest disability for the patient. There is little value in demanding much of the patient in terms of washing, dressing, physical therapy, visits to X-ray, etc. until this period has passed. It is desirable that the beds should be of an adjustable height to facilitate the movement of patients and it is useful to have available hoists and other lifting devices. Toilets and bathrooms must be provided with adequate grab-rails, adjustable seats and non-slip mats. Many patients find showers simpler to use.

Patients who are immobilized in bed require regular turning; and if their limbs are fixed in splints, they may require assistance with feeding, washing, etc. Particular care must be paid to the condition of the skin or pressure sores will develop, particularly in those patients receiving steroid drugs and in those with systemic disease. The presence in the bed of small fragments of plaster of Paris is an added hazard. However, with proper nursing care, pressure sores should not develop and they certainly should not be accepted as an inevitable sequel to sustained bed rest in these patients.

Diet

Many patients suggest that an abnormal diet may have contributed to their development of rheumatoid arthritis or other joint disease. There is no evidence to support these suggestions. Patients require only a good balanced diet. It should be remembered that a number of patients are overweight and that this is an added burden to inflamed or damaged joints. A programme of weight reduction can usefully be instituted in hospital.

DOMESTIC AND OCCUPATIONAL FACTORS

Consideration of domestic and occupational factors produced by joint disease involves chiefly the occupational therapist and medical social worker, but satisfactory adaptation to disease depends upon the efforts of the whole medical team. In addition, these efforts are wasted unless the full co-operation of the patient and his family is obtained.

The traditional role of the occupational therapist has been to provide diversional activities during the patient's hospital stay. There remains a place for this in patients who may be in hospital for several weeks, but the activity should be chosen to ensure that it develops and improves functions in which the patient has become inefficient. The therapist should assess the patient's functional capacity in considerable detail as it is only in that way that sensible programmes of management can be arranged. It is helpful if there are facilities for the practice of routine activities such as dressing, bathing, cooking, ironing and the use of electrical equipment. Consideration can also be given to the provision of a wide range of gadgets to assist the patient with washing, dressing, eating, cooking, turning taps, etc. Ideally the patient should also be studied in his or her own home (Plate 8/6). Most of these gadgets and appliances are very simple and physiotherapists should familiarize themselves with the general range. They will then be better able to spot the patient who can be helped and if there is no occupational therapist in their hospital they can then contact a therapist attached to the local authority.

Alterations in the home

Unless the furniture is required for support, it should be moved to provide a clear floor area for walking. The use of crutches and other aids in confined spaces is difficult. Easily held, strong rails should be placed beside all stairs and steps, and banisters should be fitted to both sides of the main house stairs. Rails may also be required outside the house to provide extra support during wet or snowy weather, and this is particularly important if the patient needs to use an outside toilet. For the severely disabled the ideal answer inside the home is to provide a ground-floor bedroom and bathroom, and outside to replace all steps by suitably inclined ramps. For flat dwellers a change of accommodation may be necessary.

Patients with knee or hip joint involvement have difficulty in sitting down and rising from chairs, beds and toilets of the normal height, and this is particularly so if a supporting knee joint splint is used. Appropriate alterations in height can easily be undertaken, but many patients prefer a special chair which is not only of the correct height but which has firm arms, a high moulded back and a seat of reduced depth.

Alterations to a patient's home and the selection of furniture is clearly a personal matter and for the patient to gain the greatest benefit from such changes there must be a close collaboration between the hospital and local authority. Much of the assessment for the detailed work must necessarily be done in a patient's own home, with the combined advice of staff based in the hospital and of domiciliary workers based on the local authority.

Transport and travel may become an increasing problem for the arthritic, and those with a very limited walking ability may be eligible for a powered three-wheeled vehicle or a mobility allowance. Those persons with walking ability restricted enough to bring them within this group, but who are not employed, may also be eligible for a vehicle if it is necessary to enable them to carry out household duties, including shopping. The lists of those eligible for assistance with outdoor transport is under continuing review and thus if an arthritic patient appears to be eligible for assistance they should be referred to the nearest Department of Health and Social Security appliance centre.

Many patients will require advice in planning a pattern of daily living which is more economical of work output, so that heavier and more difficult tasks are spread over the week. Patients are reluctant to accept that routine tasks such as washing need not be done on fixed days, and that there are different ways of ironing, cooking, etc. They must learn to constantly adjust to their disease, increasing activity slowly, resting as required and enrolling help from the family without feeling that their independence is endangered. The physiotherapist and occupational therapist will find it useful to work together with more disabled patients to practise transfers from bed to chair to toilet, and to plan simple ways of coping with functional problems.

The medical social worker should assess the patient's reaction to the disease, simplify the general explanation, advice and encouragement given by other members of the team, identify any special domestic, social or psychiatric problems, and assist in finding suitable employment. The medical social worker can often discuss, particularly with women, sexual problems created by the disease. However, in many cases this advice is best given by the hospital consultant or the general practitioner. Advice about a change of employment should not be given hurriedly as lighter jobs are usually less well paid. The prognosis in many forms of joint disease is often better than is imagined and the patient should be encouraged to return to his original employment. When the patient is determined on a change of job every help should be given him. A personal approach to an employer is always worthwhile. Assistance from the Disablement Resettlement Officer may be required, especially for men, so that arrangements for re-employment, assessment of employment potential and retraining can be arranged.

Wheelchairs

At the present time there are more than 100,000 wheelchair users in the United Kingdom. These chairs are supplied through the Department of Health and Social Security's Artificial Limb and Appliance Centres (DHSS ALAC), although many patients may be assessed in hospital clinics with a technical officer from the nearest centre in attendance. Increasingly, remedial therapists attend such clinics with their patients, realizing that a wheelchair is not a sign of disability but merely an aid to mobility and that they are often the best people to advise on the type of chair to be provided.

Clearly an extensive description of wheelchairs is beyond the scope of this book and those interested should read the Supplement on wheelchairs in *Equipment for the Disabled* (see Bibliography, p. 104).

In choosing a wheelchair the aims and needs of the patient must be carefully reviewed and a visit to the patient's home is invaluable. The chair should increase a patient's mobility and independence, but unfortunately many chairs are so badly selected that they do neither. In the same context it is important that a patient should not use all her energy propelling a chair if an electrically-propelled chair would really allow greater independence. Genuine effort by a patient must be encouraged but it must not be allowed to become wasteful effort. (There is a danger that the increased use of the upper limb joints and the shoulder girdle required to propel a chair leads to an increased rate of damage in these joints.) The correct assessment of this moment of transition should dictate the change from walking to using a chair, and again from using a self-propelled to an electrically-propelled chair.

TYPES OF WHEELCHAIRS

Indoor chairs are designed for manoeuvrability and can be rigid or folding. They are usually self-propelled by large, 22 inch diameter, front or rear wheels. The front-wheeled type are the more easily handled indoors, especially on carpets, but the wheels impede side transfers. Rigid outdoor chairs, designed to be pushed by an attendant, are very comfortable, while the more commonly used folding chair is ideal for most cars but is tiring to push for long distances.

Modifications can be made to standard chairs and a range of backrests, footrests, arms, cushions and brakes is available. Patients should not only be comfortable but able to produce their maximum function.

Electrically-powered chairs are available for both indoor and outdoor use and the position and type of control can be modified to suit any patient.

Patients must be instructed in the proper and most efficient manner of using their chair. Too many chairs are unused either due to poor choice on the part of the medical team or due to lack of confidence and ability on the part of the patient.

For Bibliography see end of Chapter 9, p. 104.

AGENCIES WHICH HELP PATIENTS SUFFERING FROM ARTHRITIS

Arthritis & Rheumatism Council for Research,
Faraday House,
8–10 Charing Cross Road,
London W.C.2.

British Red Cross Society,
9 Grosvenor Gardens,
London S.W.1.

British Rheumatism & Arthritis Association,
1 Devonshire Place,
London W1N 2BD.

Central Council for the Care of the Disabled,
34 Eccleston Square,
London S.W.1.

Disabled Living Foundation,
346 Kensington High Street,
London W.14.

Chapter 9

Orthopaedic Surgical Treatment of Inflammatory Joint Disease

by ALASTAIR G. MOWAT, MB, FRCP(ED)
and JOAN M. ABERY, MCSP

Surgical procedures are being increasingly used at all stages of joint disease, particularly rheumatoid arthritis, but it is essential that such procedures should form part of the continuing management of the patient by the whole medical team. If surgical procedures are undertaken after a full assessment of the patient's needs and a detailed assessment of the likely improvement in function in the light of other joint involvement, inappropriate operations and postoperative rehabilitation problems will be avoided (see also Chapter 11).

Corticosteroid therapy is not a contra-indication to surgery, although an increase in dosage for 48 hours over the period of operation may be required. Special problems posed by surgery in this group of patients are few. There is no change in the incidence of wound infection or the rate of wound healing even in patients on steroids. The possible danger of atlanto-axial subluxation has been mentioned (p. 44). The use of prostheses should be preceded by a careful hunt for and eradication of any infection, as such foreign bodies are especially liable to become infected. Postoperative mobilization should begin early because of the risk of losing movement in the operated and other joints by sustained immobilization. Finally, the involvement of multiple joints may impose difficulties in the selection of suitable crutches and other walking aids. This involvement of many joints means that patients with rheumatoid arthritis make lesser demands on their joints than patients with other forms of chronic arthritis, and the life of various procedures and prostheses may be longer than expected. The indications for surgery are simply relief of pain and swelling and restoration of function. It is convenient to consider surgical procedures under the general headings of synovectomy and reconstructive surgery.

This chapter will not include a description of the detailed physiotherapeutic regimes used for each surgical operation. It is assumed that the therapist is familiar with the basic principles of, and the methods employed in, the development of muscle strength and control. This chapter only includes details of patient management where these have been found to be valuable or important. Further, such management must be considered against a background of total management as described in Chapters 8 and 12. It must also be appreciated that many orthopaedic surgeons advocate highly individualized programmes of management and that the programmes described in this chapter are not necessarily the only or the 'correct' forms of management. They have, however, been shown to be effective.

SYNOVECTOMY

Removal of the synovial membrane is employed in those joints in which this tissue is readily accessible and this includes the knee, elbow and the small joints of the fingers. In addition synovectomy of tendon sheaths, particularly those of the flexors and extensors of the fingers, may be undertaken.

Tendon synovectomy relieves pain and improves tendon function and in some cases may be required urgently to protect the extensor tendons of the fingers from stretching or rupture.

Joint synovectomy is carried out in patients in whom radiological evidence of disease is minimal or absent, in the presence of pain and swelling unresponsive to all other methods of treatment (properly and conscientiously employed) for about six months. It is rarely possible to remove all synovial tissue from a joint. In the knee it is unusual to attempt to remove more than two-thirds of the tissue since this amount is all that can be achieved by the usual anterior, parapatellar incision. The mechanism by which pain and swelling is relieved in over 90 per cent of cases is not clear, since regeneration of the synovial tissue occurs within a few months. Whether the operation prevents further damage is debatable. Certainly joint synovectomy should not be undertaken only on the basis of a prophylactic effect since some loss of movement occurs in most patients. This is especially the case in the small finger joints, particularly the proximal interphalangeal joints, and any improvement in function produced by pain relief may be offset by loss of movement. Synovectomy is performed using a tourniquet, and a firm supporting bandage of the Robert Jones type is applied. Movement inside the bandage is encouraged and full mobilization follows after suture removal at about the fourteenth postoperative day. In the knee early movement is encouraged by using a slippery board, and in the hand an exercise splint is useful. Such splints assist full extension, and active flexion is encouraged against the splint.

RECONSTRUCTIVE SURGERY

The surgical procedures considered under this heading are of four types and one or more of these may be applied to each joint. They are:

(i) *Arthroplasty without a prosthesis* – usually involving synovectomy and removal of some bone to achieve pain relief, improved function and joint realignment;

(ii) *Arthroplasty with a prosthesis* – such operations are being increasingly employed, with the prosthesis replacing part of, or the whole of, the joint;

(iii) *Osteotomy* – division of the bone near a damaged joint with re-alignment of the cut ends in order to alter or correct the line of transmission of load through the joint;

(iv) *Arthrodesis* – obliteration of a severely damaged joint.

Operations in this group are undertaken to relieve pain, restore function, correct deformity and provide stability. A series of operations may be necessary. Thus the full benefit of knee surgery may not be achieved without the addition of an operation on the hip. The patient may not be the best judge of her surgical requirement. The considerations and the increasing availability of satisfactory arthroplasties have reduced the number of joints that are arthrodesed.

The importance of the physiotherapist in the success of any surgical procedure cannot be over-emphasized. The role of the therapist in patient selection and assessment has been discussed (p. 75). Furthermore, the pre-operative bulk and strength of the muscles around the operated joint may significantly affect the rate of postoperative recovery and the quality of the final result. Thus it is often valuable to spend some time before an operation on educating the patient about muscle control, improving muscle bulk and strength and, if necessary, correcting joint deformities, especially flexion deformities, by the use of serial splints (p. 85). Finally, many orthopaedic surgical procedures impose heavy demands upon patients because of the continued need for graduated exercises which often must be performed in the face of considerable discomfort. The patient who has confidence in a sympathetic but firm therapist will do well.

Individual joints will now be discussed in more detail.

Hand and wrist

In the fingers, periarticular, tendon and muscle involvement as well as joint disease contribute to the symptoms and the characteristic ulnar deviation, swan neck and boutonnière deformities (p. 42). In addition to synovectomy of the metacarpophalangeal and proximal interphalangeal joints, soft tissue release, repair of the extensor apparatus and realignment of the tendons may be required. Although such procedures produce cosmetically satisfactory results, there is usually some loss of movement, and finger function is not always improved. Many surgeons prefer to delay operating until more extensive changes have taken place, often with subluxation of the metacarpophalangeal joints, since an improvement in function is then achieved. The various types of excision arthroplasty available and the recently introduced 'plastic' prostheses of several types (Swanson, Calnan-Nicolle, Niebauer) offer equally satisfactory results. Flexion of the fingers is usually limited but adequate grip and pinch movements result. Arthrodesis of an unstable interphalangeal or metacarpophalangeal joint of the thumb may substantially improve pinch movements.

Arthrodesis of a joint is followed by six weeks in plaster of Paris. The postoperative management of prosthetic finger surgery varies considerably, some surgeons keeping the joints in extension with plaster support for 10 to 14 days, while others encourage early flexion. However, most agree that a lively splint which keeps the resting joints in extension and encourages active flexion against the splint is useful, once movement is allowed (Plate 9/1).

Synovial proliferation and capsule stretching results in anterior subluxation of the wrist with disruption of the inferior radio-ulnar joint, and prominence, tenderness and springing of the lower end of the ulna. Excision of the distal three-quarters of an inch (2 cm) of the ulna with synovectomy of the distal radio-ulnar joint and extensor tendons relieves pain and increases strength without reducing wrist or forearm movement (Plates 9/2, 9/3). Indeed rotation is often increased. Postoperative movement especially of the fingers and forearm is encouraged to reduce swelling. Such swelling is often a problem after finger and wrist surgery and is due to lymphatic damage, but can be rapidly relieved by elevation while allowing free arm movement by using a balanced sling. The old-fashioned roller towel sling should not be used.

In those with very severe wrist damage arthrodesis remains a useful procedure. The loss of movement is more than offset by the gain in hand power. Carpal tunnel decompression may be required in those with evidence of median nerve compression.

Elbow

Synovectomy may be useful. Excision of the radial head increases the range of pain-free movement, especially pronation and supination. Although joint stability may be reduced, this is rarely important, as these patients have reduced requirements. Various types of arthroplasty have been used in the elbow joint with excision of the ends of the humerus and/or ulna and radius. In some instances the insertion of a strip of tensor fascia lata will achieve a reasonable range of pain-free movement. Experience with metal or plastic hinge arthroplasties (McKee, Dee, Swanson), is still at an early stage but suggests that a stable, pain-free joint with no loss and often gain in movement will result (Plate 9/4). Arthrodesis may occasionally be required; the optimum position is 90° of elbow flexion with the forearm in the neutral position. Such a procedure demands good shoulder function.

Shoulder

Excision of the acromion and the underlying bursa relieves pain and improves movement. However, joint stability may be impaired and abduction is often severely restricted. Arthrodesis of the shoulder is technically difficult to achieve but may improve upper limb function if care is taken in selecting the optimum position for fusion. The replacement of the humeral head (Neer's prosthesis) is rarely used, and probably relieves pain rather than increases movement. Total shoulder prostheses are currently being evaluated.

Toes

Synovitis of the metatarsophalangeal joints and the associated structures results progressively in broadening and rigidity of the forefoot; loss of the transverse arch; hallux valgus and lateral deviation of the other toes; clawing of the toes; subluxation of the joint and development of callosities over prominent areas particularly the metatarsal heads in the soles (Plate 9/5). Synovitis of the other toe joints, unlike the hand, is minimal.

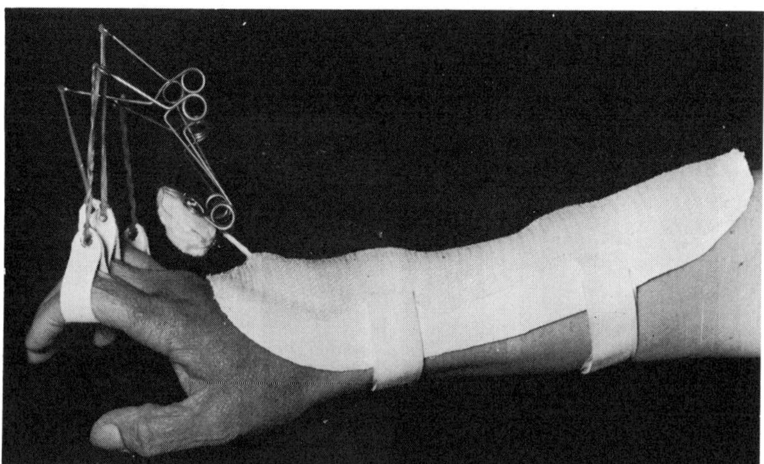

Plate 9/1 A lively splint allows finger flexion against the resistance of springs and the supporting elastic bands

Plate 9/2 Pre-operative radiograph of rheumatoid wrist showing widening and erosions of distal radio-ulnar joint due to synovitis (*see p. 96*)

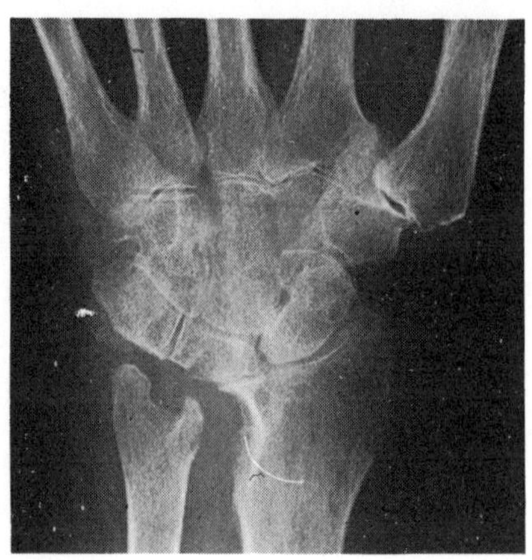

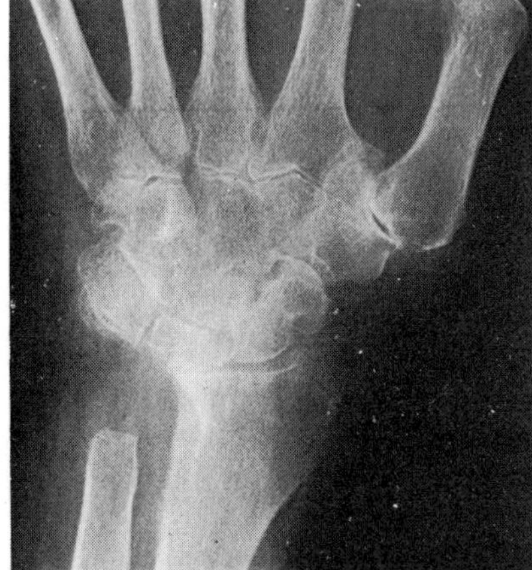

Plate 9/3 The same wrist as in Plate 9/2, after excision of the lower end of the ulna (*see p. 96*)

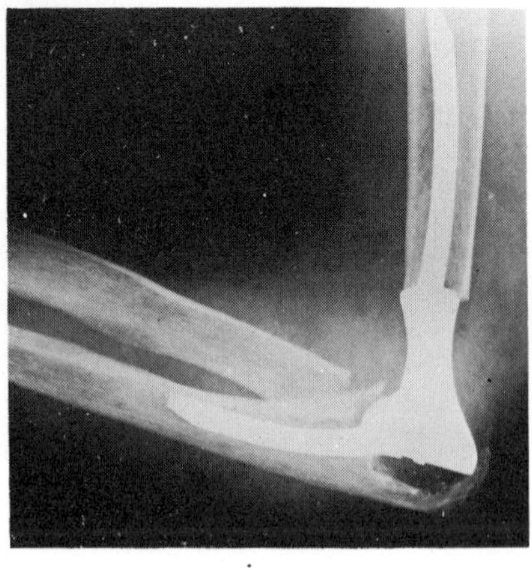

Plate 9/4 Radiograph of rheumatoid elbow joint replaced with a Dee metallic hinge (*see p. 97*)

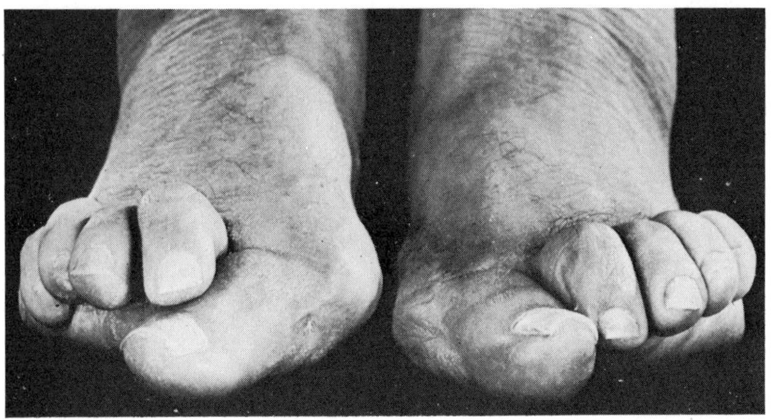

Plate 9/5 Typical deformities in a rheumatoid foot (*see p. 97*)

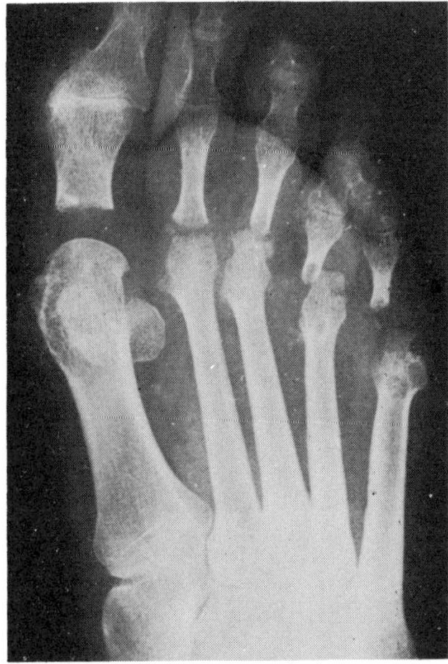

Plate 9/6 Postoperative radiograph of excision arthroplasty in a rheumatoid foot. Bases of proximal phalanges have been excised and toes manipulated into better alignment (*see p. 101*)

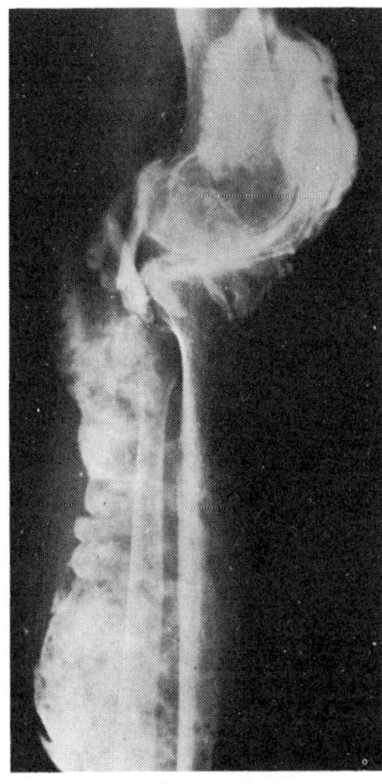

Plate 9/7 Knee arthrogram (lateral aspect right knee) showing a proliferated synovial lining in joint and a large posterior cyst extending down the calf (*see p. 101*)

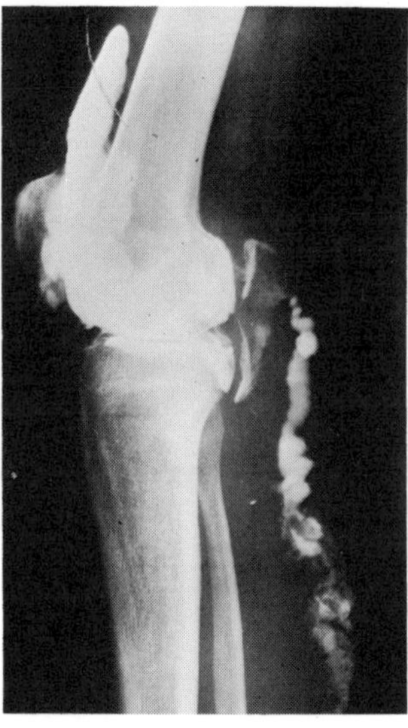

Plate 9/8 Knee arthrogram (medial aspect right knee) showing rupture of joint with leakage of dye into calf. Note appearance is not cystic and margins are not distinct (*see p. 101*)

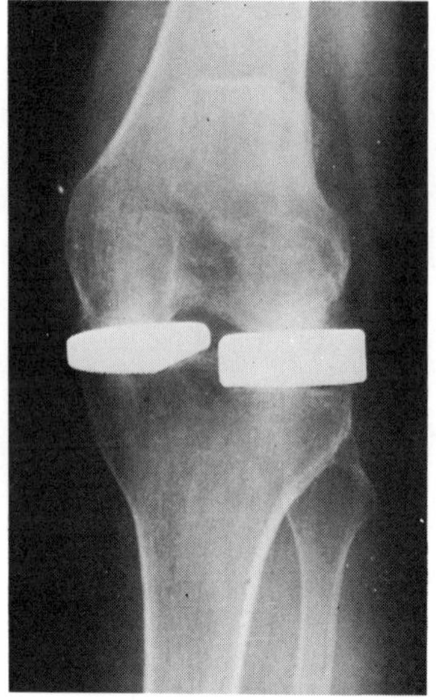

Plate 9/9 Bicompartmental MacIntosh arthroplasties in rheumatoid knee. Prostheses of different depth allow replacement of damaged tibial surfaces, correction of deformity and restoration of joint stability (*see p. 101*)

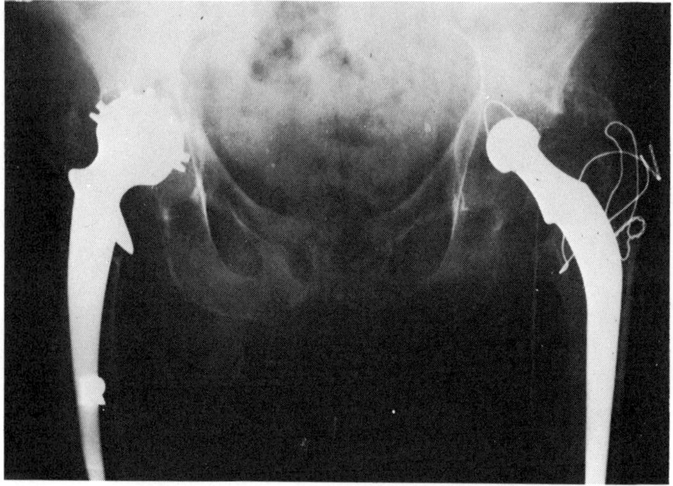

Plate 9/10 Bilateral total hip replacement in rheumatoid arthritis. A McKee-Farrar prosthesis has replaced the right hip and a Charnley prosthesis the left. Wire is used to reattach the greater trochanter, removed to facilitate insertion of prosthesis (*see p. 103*)

In the early stages the provision of suitable shoes to accommodate the feet and prevent the development of pressure areas and of suitable domed insoles to redistribute the weight is all that is required (p. 87). Synovectomy of the metatarsophalangeal joints is rarely performed. Excision arthroplasty with removal of the metatarsal heads and/or the bases of the proximal phalanges and manipulation of the toes into normal alignment produces satisfactory results in 90 per cent of cases (Plate 9/6). Poor results are due to insufficient or irregular excision of bone. Grossly deformed toes may be amputated. Swelling may occur following foot surgery, with some impairment in wound healing and consequently a delay in walking. The swelling can be reduced by performing Buerger's exercises several times daily.

Mid-tarsal, sub-talar and ankle joints

Involvement of these joints is best treated by the provision of suitable shoes or boots with valgus insoles. Various forms of anklet, plastic heel cups and even a leg iron and 'T' strap may adequately support these joints (p. 87). Occasionally, simple manipulation under anaesthesia reduces pain and restores movement. Arthrodesis is the most satisfactory operation. The ankle should be fused in 5° of plantar flexion in men and 10° in women. The foot and heel should be fixed in neutral position.

Knee

Synovectomy is an excellent, well-tried operation for early disease in the knee. Anterior synovectomy is usually performed and may also be valuable in those with an enlarged posterior cyst. Such cysts, which are usually extensions of the normal semi-membranosus-gastrocnemius bursa, may become grossly enlarged, prevent full knee extension and cause venous obstruction (Plate 9/7). In addition, since they are connected to the knee joint by a one-way valvular mechanism, they are subjected to markedly increased fluid pressures. This may result in the enlargement of the cyst into the calf or the sudden rupture of the cyst with the release of irritant synovial fluid. Symptoms and signs of joint rupture, which have also been recorded at the wrist and elbow, mimic those of a deep venous thrombosis. Arthrography should be used to establish the diagnosis (Plate 9/8). Rupture of the cyst should be treated by rest. A large calf cyst may be excised but synovectomy of the joint will treat the cause of both a small cyst and rupture.

Partial replacement arthroplasties are available for the treatment of the moderately damaged joint. Full extension, flexion to 90°, realignment and return of joint stability can be achieved in most cases. Metal replacements for one or both tibial condyles (MacIntosh, McKeever) are available (Plate 9/9). Total replacement operations employing metal hinges with or without cement (Walldius, Shiers and Young operations) produce similar results. However, because of various technical difficulties and the occasional need for removal of the prosthesis they should probably be regarded as the operation of choice only in those with very severe joint damage. More recently a second generation of total knee prostheses (Freeman-Swanson, Geomedic, Gunston) have attempted to mimic the rocking and gliding motions of the normal joint and initial results suggest that they will largely replace the hinges. Arthroplasties of the knee are undertaken using a tourniquet and a firm bulky supporting bandage applied after wound closure. Movement within the bandage is encouraged from the start of the recovery period and full mobilization follows removal of the sutures at about the fourteenth day (Fig. 9/1).

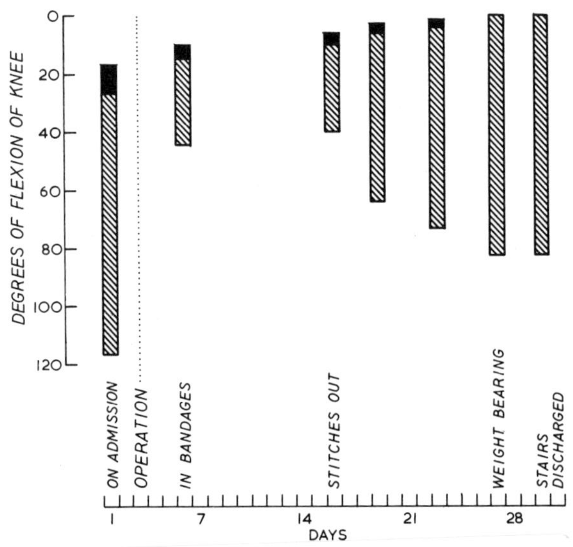

Fig. 9/1 A simple method of recording the flexion deformity, the extension lag (represented by the black parts of the bars), and the range of flexion in the knee joint. Similar charts can be used for any joint

Manipulation under anaesthesia

It is occasionally necessary to manipulate an operated joint under anaesthesia because of a delay in the return of movement. No rules about the timing of such a procedure can be given as knowledge about the normal rate of return of movement after an operation is acquired by experience. The knee is the joint most commonly manipulated and it is important that the manipulation is not performed too late or the benefit will be minimal. In general, some 60 to 80° of flexion should be achieved within three to four weeks following a knee operation; significantly less movement indicates the need for prompt manipulation.

These authors believe that pain can best be controlled and better final results achieved by leaving the joint supported in the fully flexed position for the first day while a series of ice-bags is applied. Movement to full extension is allowed on the second post-manipulation day.

OSTEOTOMY AND ARTHRODESIS

Osteotomy of the femur and/or tibia near the joint margins seems to relieve pain in some patients but it is best avoided in those with active disease since the delay in mobilization necessary to ensure bony union usually results in serious loss of joint movement. Arthrodesis of the knee, which provides a stable pain-free joint, albeit with 1 to $1\frac{1}{2}$ in. (3 to 4 cm) of leg shortening, remains a suitable procedure in those patients with limited involvement of other joints. It may prove very disabling for those with significant limitation of hip movement.

Hip

Synovectomy is rarely employed. Arthrodesis should never be employed in this joint in rheumatoid arthritis. Displacement osteotomy has not proved of value. Some form of arthroplasty should be employed. In younger patients some surgeons continue to use cup arthroplasty until the long-term results of hip replacement are known. However, since these patients demand less of their joints than those with osteoarthrosis, total hip replacement can be considered in any patient. The prostheses of McKee-Farrar and Charnley, together with their modifications are very satisfactory, producing painless movement in over 90 per cent of cases (Plate 9/10). The range of final movement may be less than in patients with osteoarthrosis due to permanent soft tissue changes. In these hip operations some limp may persist due to weakness of the abductor muscles, and even the distal displacement of the greater trochanter and its muscle insertions does not always remove the limp. Postoperative, non-weight-bearing movements are encouraged from the first or second day. Some surgeons use balanced slings while others leave the patient free with an abduction pillow. A good range of strong abduction is essential for the success of hip operations, and therapists must use a progressively more demanding routine to achieve this. Flexion is encouraged with a slippery board. Immediate weight-bearing is possible with the total hip replacement but many surgeons believe that better functional results are achieved if this is delayed a few days. These patients can return home after three weeks. There is a risk of subluxation of the total hip prostheses in the early postoperative weeks until fibrous tissue has developed. Patients should avoid flexion-rotation movements and thus they must be warned not to sit on low chairs, toilets, beds, etc. With the cup arthroplasty a more gradual increase in weight-bearing is allowed and the patient progresses through a series of walking aids until normal walking is allowed at about six months.

Many patients require both hip and knee surgery. In general, more satisfactory results are achieved since the patient can more readily mobilize the operated joints, if the hip is treated first.

Thromboembolic phenomena, always a problem with hip surgery, can be reduced by the routine use of anticoagulants. Deep sepsis, which may be delayed many years, is a problem with these arthroplasties. Antibiotic cover is often given over the operative period to eliminate staphylococci, the usual infecting organism, and further reductions in the incidence of sepsis may be achieved using special theatre techniques.

The excision arthroplasty of Girdlestone is used rarely because although movement is good, the resulting joint is rather unstable, particularly in heavier patients and up to 2½ in. (6 cm) of leg shortening may result. The operation is particularly useful as a simple, quick procedure for the relief of pain in a patient confined to a wheelchair. Many such patients exist in whom more complicated surgery is wasteful since the involvement of multiple joints will prevent any increase in function.

BIBLIOGRAPHY

Boyle, J. A. and Buchanan, W. W. *Clinical Rheumatology*. Blackwell, 1971.

Copeman, W. S. C. (ed.) *Textbook of the Rheumatic Diseases*. Churchill Livingstone, 4th ed. 1969.

Day, B. H. *Orthopaedic Appliances*. Faber & Faber, 1972.

Goble, R. E. A. and Nichols, P. J. R. *Rehabilitation of the Severely Disabled, Vol. 1 Evaluation of a Disabled Living Unit, Vol. 2 Management*. Butterworth, 1971.

Hollander, J. L. and McCarthy, D. J. (eds.) *Arthritis and Allied Conditions: A Textbook of Rheumatology*. Lea & Febiger, Philadelphia, 8th ed. 1972.

Mason, M. and Currey, H. L. F. (eds.) *An Introduction to Clinical Rheumatology*. Pitman, 1970.

'Wheelchairs and Outdoor Transport', a special supplement to *Equipment for the Disabled*. Published by the National Fund for Research into Crippling Diseases, Vincent House, Vincent Square, London, S.W.1.

Chapter 10

Osteoarthrosis

aetiology, pathology and clinical features

by B. M. GRAVELING, MCSP, DIP.TP

Osteoarthrosis is a disease of synovial joints. The condition has been known as osteoarthritis, which erroneously implies an active inflammatory disease. It is more accurately called osteoarthrosis or degenerative joint disease.

Degenerative changes occur with ageing but there are often other predisposing factors responsible for the changes seen in osteoarthrosis. The disease is best divided into three types: primary, secondary and idiopathic.

Primary osteoarthrosis

(nodal multiple osteoarthrosis or generalized osteoarthrosis)

This type of degenerative change may have a familial incidence, occurs in middle-aged and elderly women, and affects more than one joint. A characteristic feature is the presence of Heberden's nodes at the terminal interphalangeal joints of the fingers. There may be associated flexion and lateral deformity at these joints. Involvement of the carpometacarpal joint of the thumb causes an adduction deformity (Plate 10/1) and the appearance of a 'square' hand.

Secondary osteoarthrosis

Degeneration may occur secondary to mechanical, metabolic, vascular or inflammatory disorders of the synovial joint.

MECHANICAL FACTORS

Alteration in the mechanics of a joint will cause abnormal loading of its surfaces. Changes in the nutrition and structure of the hyaline cartilage result, and degeneration is precipitated. Alteration in the mechanics can be due to the following:

(a) Fractures or dislocations of the joint which damage the articular surfaces;

(b) Repeated minor trauma as seen in the shoulders of coalminers, elbows of pneumatic drill workers or ankles of footballers;

(c) Structural deformities such as kyphosis and scoliosis of the spine, valgus or varus deformities of the knee, and coxa vara lead to malalignment of joint surfaces;

(d) Repeated minor trauma to a joint which has lost its protective sensory mechanism may result in rapid degeneration of that joint. These so-called neuropathic joints occur in tabes dorsalis, syringomyelia and diabetes mellitus. Prolonged treatment with anti-inflammatory agents such as corticosteroids may have a similar effect;

(e) Congenital abnormalities of joints. Congenital dislocation of the hip and club foot are examples;

(f) Perthes' disease and osteochondritis dissecans, joint disorders of childhood and adolescence produce incongruity of articular surfaces which predispose these joints to premature degeneration;

(g) Patients with rare dystrophies and dysplasias such as chondro-osteodystrophy (Morquio-Brailsford disease) and multiple epiphyseal dysplasia, develop early osteoarthrosis.

METABOLIC FACTORS

Gout, alkaptonuria and chondrocalcinosis may predispose a joint to degenerative changes. Obesity, another metabolic disease, can aggravate osteoarthrosis in weight-bearing joints.

VASCULAR FACTORS

Avascular necrosis may affect the surfaces of a joint and result in osteoarthrosis. The blood supply to the joint may be affected by fractures, irradiation and, rarely, Caisson disease.

INFLAMMATORY FACTORS

Inflammatory diseases of joints such as rheumatoid arthritis will damage articular cartilage and result in osteoarthrosis.

Idiopathic

Osteoarthrosis may be present in the absence of any of the above predisposing causes. It is possible that some of these so-called idiopathic cases may represent formes-frustes of such conditions as rheumatoid disease, slipped upper femoral epiphysis or Perthes' disease.

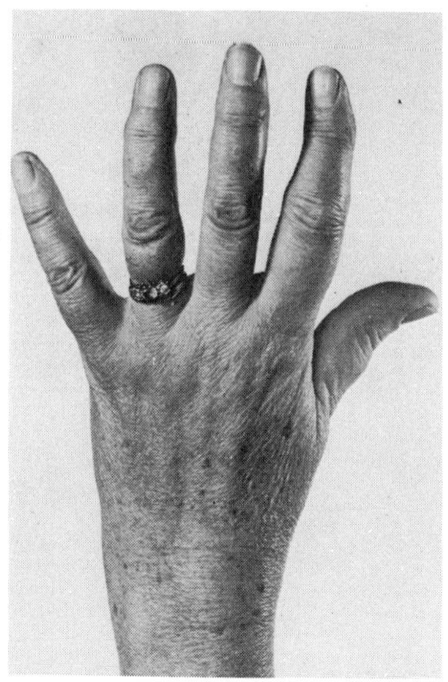

Plate 10/1 Generalized osteoarthrosis, showing Heberden's nodes and adducted thumb (*see p. 105*)

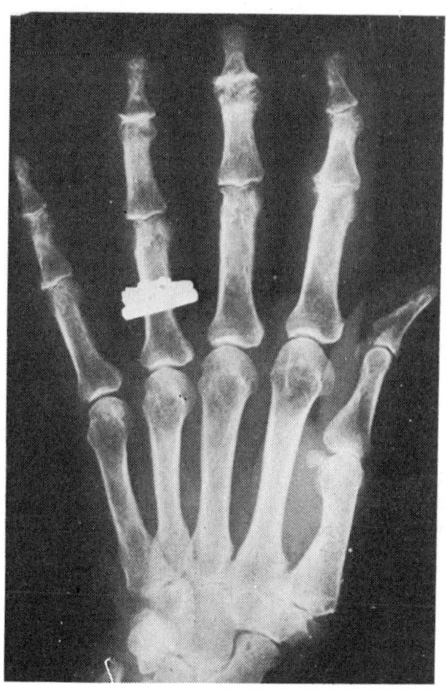

Plate 10/2 Radiograph of hand shown in Plate 10/1

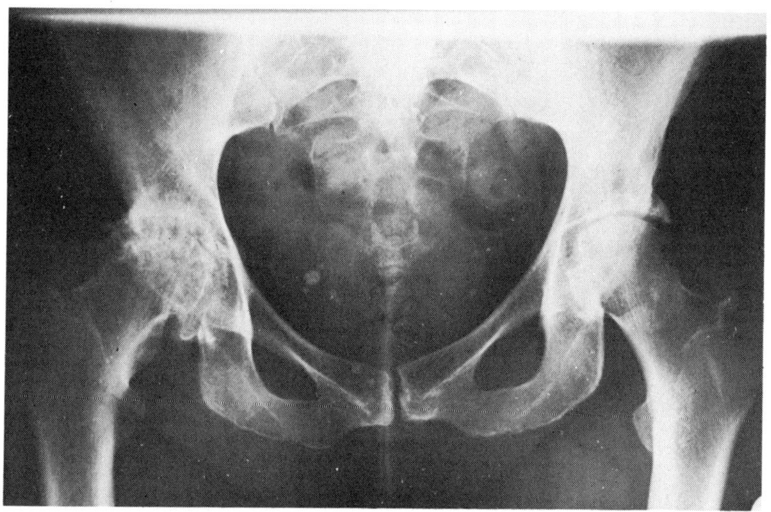

Plate 10/3 Radiograph of bilateral osteoarthrosis of hips, showing diminished joint space, cystic change, sclerosis and osteophyte formation (*see p. 111*)

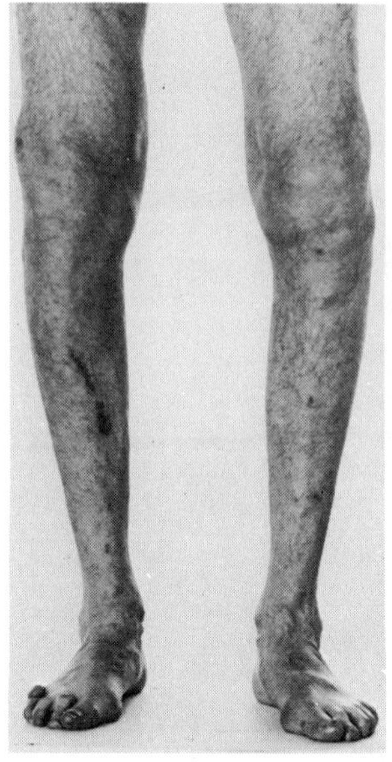

Plate 10/4 Bilaterial osteoarthrosis showing varus deformity (*see p. 111*)

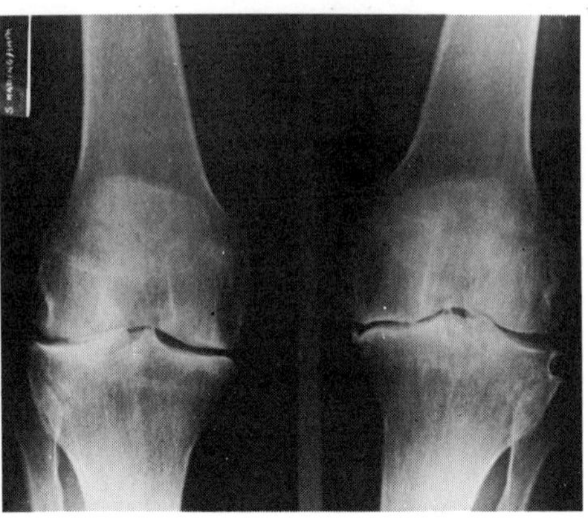

Plate 10/5 Anterior radiograph of patient in Plate 10/4

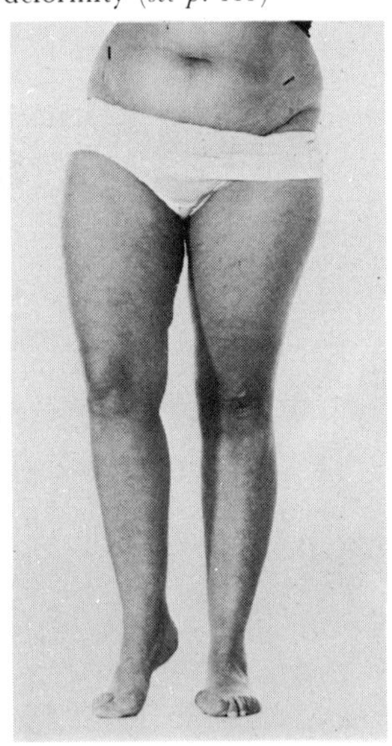

Plate 10/6 Osteoarthrosis of right hip. The pelvis is tilted on the right to compensate for adduction deformity

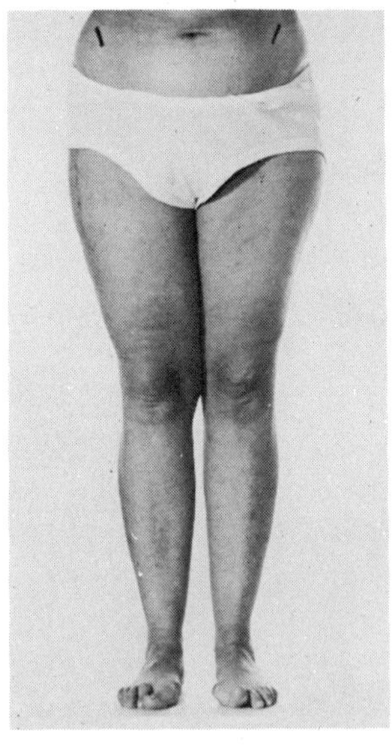

Plate 10/7 The same patient with corrected deformity after hip arthroplasty (*see p. 113*)

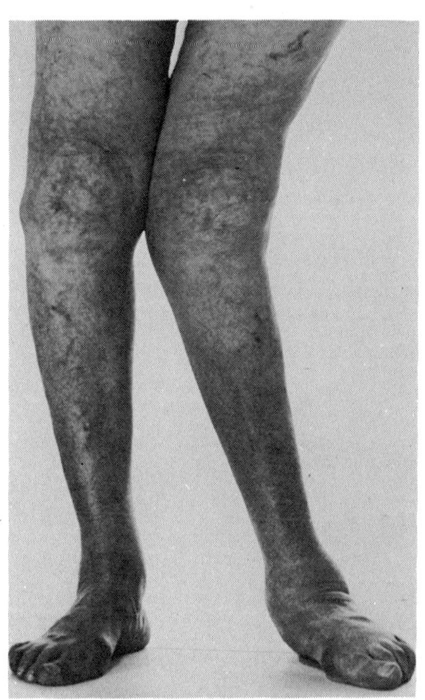

Plate 10/8 Bilateral osteoarthrosis showing gross valgus deformity of left knee and subluxation of right (*see p. 115*)

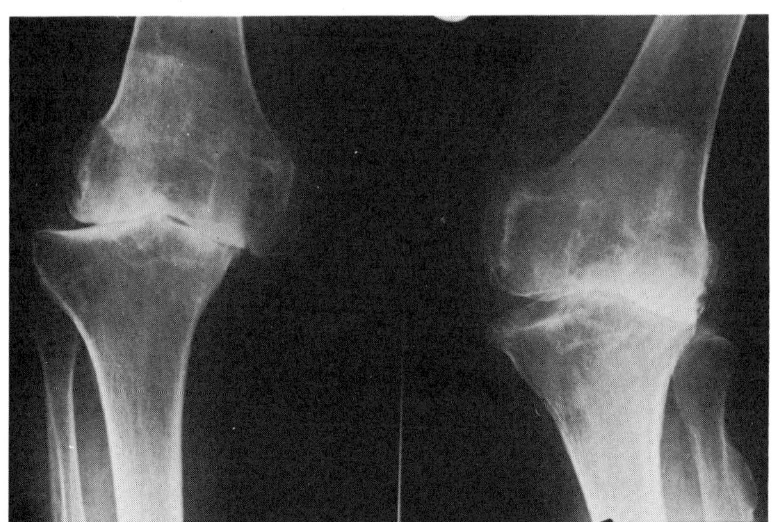

Plate 10/9 Anterior radiograph of patient in Plate 10/8

PATHOLOGY

Osteoarthrosis involves all the structures in and around a joint including the capsule, cartilage, synovial membrane and bone. There are no systemic effects or changes in other tissues and organs as seen in rheumatoid disease.

The pathological changes begin in the hyaline articular cartilage which acts as a compressible cushion between the bone ends and allows free and frictionless movement. The depth of the articular cartilage varies from joint to joint and in the normal adult may range from 2 to 6 mm in thickness. Further, cartilage depth is not uniform, being often thickest in the weight-bearing areas of a joint. Cartilage receives its nutrition from the synovial fluid and the subchondral vessels. Intermittent compression and movement of the joint enables synovial fluid to be absorbed into the cartilage. Trueta (1953) has shown that degeneration occurs more readily in the areas of cartilage which are subjected to least pressure. The earliest pathological changes in the cartilage are softening, flaking and eventual separation of fibres or fibrils from the superficial layer into the joint cavity, a process termed fibrillation. The subchondral vessels hypertrophy and invade the cartilage which calcifies and later ossifies. Gradually the cartilage becomes thinner until there is exposure of the subchondral bone. With continued friction the subchondral bone becomes hardened and polished, or eburnated. The subchondral bone thickens and bony outgrowths or osteophytes develop at the joint margins. Occasionally, bone infarction may cause partial collapse of the articular surface. This often occurs in the femoral head. Cyst formation and microfracture of the trabeculae are common. Hypertrophy of the synovial membrane and fibrosis of the joint capsule produce thickening of the joint and limitation of movement. Complete loss of movement can sometimes occur and this is called ankylosis.

Radiographic changes

There is often no correlation between the radiographic appearance and the symptoms of the patient with osteoarthrosis. Patients with radiographs showing minor changes may have severe symptoms whilst patients with advanced joint changes may have surprisingly few symptoms. The six radiographic features are described below:

DIMINISHED JOINT SPACE

As the cartilage becomes thinner there is approximation of bone ends which eventually may be in apposition.

OSTEOPHYTE FORMATION

Sharpening and pointing of the articular margins can be seen in early cases, and later, larger bony growths or osteophytes develop.

SCLEROSIS OF SUBCHONDRAL BONE

The hardened or eburnated subchondral bone, together with abnormal trabeculation, may give a sclerotic appearance on radiographs adjacent to the joint surfaces (Plate 10/3).

CYSTS

Cysts located in the subchondral bone vary in size and shape, and may reach 2 cm in diameter. They are round or oval in shape.

LOOSE BODIES

Loose bodies within the synovial cavity are formed by very small fragments of cartilage becoming detached and growing in the synovial fluid. They may become ossified and apparent on the radiograph. Loose bodies are commonly seen in the knee and elbow.

DEFORMITY

Subluxation of a joint may be apparent on a radiograph. This is seen in the carpometacarpal joint of the thumb, where the metacarpal head is displaced laterally. Subluxation may occur in the severely degenerative knee (Plates 10/4, 10/5).

SIGNS AND SYMPTOMS

The progress of the disease may be insidious with minimal symptoms or advance rapidly. Minor trauma frequently provokes an acute exacerbation of symptoms in a disease which is progressive and chronic in nature.

Symptoms

PAIN

In the early stages of the disease, pain is present only during activity, but in advanced disease the patient may experience constant pain. Venous congestion may contribute to rest and night pain. The fibrous capsule is richly supplied with pain nerve endings and stretching of this tightened fibrous capsule produces a dull ache. This may occur at night when muscle tone is reduced or, inadvertently, when active movement goes beyond the range permitted by the capsule. Hyperaemia and the exposure of the subchondral bone may contribute to pain. Although muscle spasm around the joints is a protective measure to prevent movement and pain, it in itself may produce pain.

REFERRED PAIN

There may be evidence of referred pain and a very common example of this is pain referred to the knee from osteoarthrosis of the hip.

STIFFNESS

Stiffness is present initially after rest but with progression of the disease, may be more persistent. Significant morning stiffness is unusual, being a feature of inflammatory joint disease.

Signs

LOSS OF MOVEMENT

Movement is always restricted. In the early stages there may be a minimal loss of range, but gradually as the disease progresses the joint may become completely immobile.

Adjacent joints may lose range particularly where one joint is dependent upon the function of another, e.g. patients with osteoarthrosis of the hip often lose movement of the lumbar spine.

The loss of movement in joints is due to: (1) bone changes; (2) contracted capsules and ligaments; (3) muscle spasm and pain.

LOSS OF FUNCTION

Due to loss of movement the patient is unable to manage the normal activities of daily living and can lose independence.

CREPITUS

This is grating and grinding felt on movement of the joint and is indicative of roughening of the opposing articular surfaces. In more advanced cases this roughening may involve only bone.

DEFORMITY

The pathological changes described result in deformity. There is a pattern of deformity for some joints, e.g. the hip is usually flexed, adducted and laterally rotated, the first carpometacarpal joint is usually adducted. The knee may show valgus or varus deformity.

MUSCLE CHANGES

Due to loss of movement and function the muscles working over the involved joint become weak and wasted, and in addition, muscle function of the whole limb may be diminished.

In an attempt to prevent movement and pain, muscles go into protective spasm. This is more apparent in the long tendinous muscles such as the adductors of the hip. Persistent shortening of muscle will lead to contracture of the fibrous tissue of muscle and atrophy of muscle fibres.

APPEARANCE OF JOINT

Moderate effusions may be visible in superficial joints. Synovial and capsule thickening may be seen, and the presence of new bone and osteophytes may give the bone an enlarged appearance.

CLINICAL FEATURES OF INDIVIDUAL JOINTS

Hip

In up to 50 per cent of patients with degenerative joint disease of the hip, no obvious cause or predisposing factor is evident. Secondary osteoarthrosis may develop in a hip previously affected by any of the following conditions. These include:

Perthes' disease.
Slipped upper femoral epiphysis.
Congenital dislocation or subluxation.
Rheumatoid arthritis.
Protrusio acetabuli (Otto pelvis).
Fracture or fracture dislocation of the neck of the femur with avascular necrosis of the femoral head.
Fractures of the acetabulum.

SYMPTOMS

PAIN

This is felt in the groin, in the region of the great trochanter, in the anterior aspect of the thigh and in the knee.

LOSS OF FUNCTION

The disabilities are mainly those resulting from the lack of flexion. These are: (i) Putting on the shoes and socks; (ii) Cutting the toenails; (iii) Sitting and standing from a chair or lavatory; (iv) Getting into bed and sitting up in bed; (v) Going up stairs; (vi) Getting into a bath.

Walking any distance is also difficult.

SIGNS

LOSS OF RANGE AND DEFORMITY

Internal rotation is usually the first movement to be lost but gradually *all* movements are diminished and the leg is held in flexion, adduction and lateral rotation (Plate 10/6).

True shortening of the limb will follow collapse or deformity of the femoral head and neck. Apparent shortening is due to the pelvis being raised on the affected side. The pelvis adopts this position in an attempt to bring the adducted leg vertical and parallel with the other. To keep the trunk vertical and to compensate for the fixed flexion deformity of the hip, the lumbar spine adopts a position of lordosis and the pelvis tilts forwards. Scoliosis of the lumbar spine may be secondary to the lateral tilt of the pelvis.

PROTECTIVE MUSCLE SPASM

This occurs mostly in the adductors and psoas and contributes to the position of deformity.

STANCE AND GAIT

A positive Trendelenburg sign is common and this occurs as a result of weakness of gluteus medius or mechanical instability of the hip. This instability plus the shortening of the leg produces a limp which is less obvious when a stick is used. The patient walks on the toes with shortened steps and with the leg held in the position of deformity. The foot may be everted in an attempt to clear the floor when flexion of the hip is particularly limited.

Knee

The knee is a common joint to be affected by osteoarthrosis of both the primary and secondary types and any one of the three compartments can be affected: the medial, lateral and patello-femoral.

The causes of secondary osteoarthrosis are as follows:

(1) Injury of bones, ligaments or articular cartilage;

(2) Undiagnosed semilunar cartilage injury;

(3) Long-standing deformity of the knee as in genu varum or valgum;

(4) Loose bodies which may have damaged the articular cartilage and could occur in osteochondritis dissecans.

Osteoarthrosis of the patello-femoral compartment is common in young people and may be a sequel to chondromalacia patellae or result from repeated injury as in recurrent subluxation or dislocation of the patella.

SYMPTOMS

PAIN

Pain is felt around the knee, but may be more marked on one side. It is felt on movement and particularly when the patient goes up or down a step or stairs. Sudden pain is caused by nipping of loose bodies in the joint.

STIFFNESS

The joint feels stiff after rest, and the patient complains of difficulty in moving, particularly after sitting for any length of time.

INSTABILITY

Many patients have instability of the knee and a common complaint is of the knee 'letting them down'.

SIGNS

LOSS OF RANGE AND DEFORMITY

The knee is often in a varus deformity which is more marked on weight-bearing. Valgus and flexion deformities can occur (Plates 10/8, 10/9).

Full range of extension and flexion is often lost and movements of the patella are diminished.

APPEARANCE

The joint is often enlarged and effusion may be seen. All muscle groups of the leg may be weak and wasted and in particular the quadriceps and hamstrings.

PALPATION

Crepitus may be felt on movement and tenderness may be elicited around the joint and patella.

RADIOGRAPHS

These show loss of joint space which is frequently unequal in the medial and lateral compartments. Erosion and irregularities in the deep surface of the patella may be seen.

Metatarsophalangeal joint of the great toe

HALLUX RIGIDUS

This is a condition occurring in young adults affecting the metatarso-phalangeal joints of the great toe. The aetiology is uncertain, but there is often a history of trauma. It may be an example of premature primary osteoarthrosis. Rotational deformity of the forefoot is often evident. The disease is usually bilateral and seen more in men.

Pain is often severe and worse on walking. The patient is unable to hyperextend the metatarsophalangeal joint. To compensate for this immobility the patient develops hyperextension of the interphalangeal joint.

Ankle and other foot joints

Primary osteoarthrosis in these joints is rare but secondary osteoarthrosis can follow long-standing deformity, trauma or inflammatory disease.

Shoulder joint

Primary osteoarthrosis is seldom seen in this joint. Secondary osteoarthrosis may occur in manual workers such as miners.

Pain is usually felt around the joint and after strenuous movement. There is gradual loss of all movements, and tasks which involve rotation such as brushing the hair, washing the back of the neck and putting on a jacket become very difficult.

Acromioclavicular joint

This joint is involved in primary osteoarthrosis; secondary osteoarthrosis may occur as a result of previous injury. Pain is felt around the shoulder and may radiate into the cervical regions, particularly on elevation of the arm. The joint may be tender and enlarged. Radiographs show sclerosis and lipping.

Sternoclavicular joint

Primary osteoarthrosis affects this joint but does not produce severe symptoms. Pain is felt over the joint and sometimes over the base of the neck. There may be localized tenderness and enlargement of the joint.

Elbow

Osteoarthrosis of this joint may be asymptomatic and is often discovered by chance. Employment in heavy work is a predisposing factor. Miners, carpenters and men who work pneumatic drills seem to be prone to develop degenerative changes in this joint. Movement of the radio-ulnar joints may be diminished. Occasionally entrapment of the ulnar nerve may occur, producing ulnar neuritis (see also Chapter 15).

Wrists

Primary osteoarthrosis rarely involves the wrist joint. An ununited fracture of the scaphoid, or fracture of the lower end of the radius involving the articular surface, may produce a secondary osteoarthrosis pattern. Pain occurs in the region of the joint and there is limitation of all movements.

The first carpometacarpal joint

This joint is often affected in primary osteoarthrosis. It is a very painful and disabling condition in that it limits many gripping activities. Women complain amongst other things of their inability to hold the kettle or teapot.

Weakness and wasting occurs in the muscles of the thenar eminence. In the same condition of primary osteoarthrosis, Heberden's nodes on the distal joints of the fingers may cause pain, diminished sensation and hence a 'clumsy' hand and concern over the hand's appearance.

For Bibliography see end of Chapter 12, p. 139.

Chapter 11

Physiotherapy in Osteoarthrosis

by B. M. GRAVELING, MCSP, DIP.TP

The physiotherapist may be asked to treat patients with varying degrees of osteoarthrosis, from those with minimal joint changes to those with advanced changes awaiting surgery. Whatever type of case is treated, it is essential to make an assessment before treatment is commenced.

Assessment

There must be a planned system of examination and recording.

As much information as possible should be obtained from the patient's notes and radiographs. Such information as age, distance of residence from the hospital, occupation, drugs prescribed and any other medical or social information which is relevant to the understanding of the patient's problems, must be recorded.

Subjective examination

The physiotherapist should question the patient regarding pain, stiffness and functional loss.

PAIN

In order to understand the degree of irritability of the joint the physiotherapist should know the severity, position and nature of the pain. A very irritable hip joint will be painful on walking a few yards and the pain will continue into the night, preventing sleep. A less irritable joint will be fairly symptom-free until jarred or strained and the pain will subside after a few hours.

STIFFNESS AND LOSS OF FUNCTION

The patient should be asked about stiffness and how much this prevents normal activities being carried out. He or she should be asked to relate the activities which are difficult or impossible to perform. These may be putting on a sock, and getting into a bath, if the hip is involved; holding a kettle if the carpometacarpal joint of the thumb is involved, or brushing the hair if the shoulder joint is affected. There may be problems in getting into a car or onto a bus or difficulties at work.

Many of these functional activities should later be observed by both the physiotherapist and occupational therapist. The occupational therapist will advise and supply appropriate aids and adaptations in the home and place of work and will also assess the suitability of the type of work for the individual.

Objective examination

This part of the examination includes observation, palpation and testing of movement.

OBSERVATION

Observation begins as the patient enters the department and continues as the patient removes any clothing, sits down or gets onto the couch.

The gait, stance, performance of movement and use of aids is noted. The size and shape of the joint, the presence of deformity and muscle wasting are all noted and compared with the other limb.

PALPATION

Where possible the joint should be palpated. The physiotherapist feels for soft tissue thickening, effusion, temperature, bony enlargement and any tender areas. Crepitus particularly in the knee may be felt on passive movement.

ACTIVE MOVEMENT

All ranges of the joint should be tested by active movement and recorded as described in the book *Joint Motion, Method of Recording* (American Academy of Orthopaedic Surgeons, 1966).

The physiotherapist should decide whether movements are being limited by pain, muscle spasm and joint stiffness. Adjacent joints must be immobilized so that the range of movement of the joint being examined is not augmented (Plate 11/8). When testing hip flexion the patient can increase the range of apparent flexion by flexing the lumbar spine. The maintenance of firm extension of the contralateral leg will avoid this pitfall.

PASSIVE MOVEMENT

When examining passive movements, care should be taken to avoid exacerbating pain. The range of passive movement may exceed active movement when the muscles are weak, or if active movement produces pain.

ACCESSORY MOVEMENT

These are passive movements which the patient cannot perform voluntarily. Accessory movements include gliding at the intercarpal, intertarsal and acromioclavicular joints. Investigation of these movements will often help to localize the origin of the patient's pain.

MEASUREMENT OF LEG LENGTH

Apparent and true shortening of the leg should be measured, where the hip is involved. True shortening is measured from the anterior superior iliac spine to the medial malleolus. Apparent shortening is measured from the umbilicus to the medial malleolus.

TREATMENT

Instruction in self-care and management

Instruction in self-care is very important and should be given to the patient at the first attendance following assessment. A careful examination of what the individual should aim to achieve will enhance co-operation between the patient and physiotherapist. Many patients can learn to avoid unnecessary trauma to the joint and prevent pain by adjusting their activities and giving the joint appropriate rest. Function can be maintained by daily performance of carefully graded exercises and positioning.

Instruction will vary according to age, occupation and the severity of the disease. A patient with a degenerative hip should avoid jarring the joint such as landing heavily when going downstairs, walking over rough ground or prolonged walking. Many patients with involvement of the knees or hips derive benefit from a stick or elbow crutches.

It is important that patients with osteoarthrosis of weight-bearing joints should lie flat for definite periods each day and position their limbs whilst resting, to maintain maximum stretch of the joint capsule, ligaments and muscles. For example, a patient with osteoarthrosis of the hip should lie prone to stretch the anterior part of the capsule. Many patients find that they can increase the range of movement after maintaining these positions for a while.

Home exercises must be carefully planned and taught. They should be few in number and use the maximum pain-free range of all movements. Patients should exercise all muscle groups without causing pain and the performance of these exercises should be checked at subsequent attendance.

It is advisable to include exercises for the whole limb as other joints are often limited in range. Patients with osteoarthrosis of the knee should have exercises to include the hip and ankle. If the hip is affected, exercise should be given for the lumbar spine and knee. Other exercises can be included in the patient's daily programme and if patients understand what they are trying to achieve they can be encouraged to think these out for themselves. Such exercises include isometric contractions of gluteal muscles; standing with pelvis forward to maintain full extension of the hip, and maintaining a good stride when walking. Patients with osteoarthrosis of the knee should practise quadriceps contraction with the knee in maximum extension whenever they are standing and flexion and extension when sitting. Many patients complain of stiffness after rest and patients should understand the importance of exercise before getting out of bed, out of a car and standing up from a chair.

Hot baths, electric pads or blanket, wax or ice are symptomatic methods of treatment that can be used at home. The physiotherapist will need to give guidance in their use.

Overweight patients require advice from the dietician.

The occupational therapist will assess and equip patients with all necessary aids to enable them to maintain independence. For example: a raised chair and long handled tongs and shoe horn for a patient with an osteoarthrotic hip (see p. 89). The physiotherapist must assess, equip and teach the use of all walking aids, and instruct the patient in the use of splints. For example: a caliper for an osteoarthrotic knee or plastic splint for the carpometacarpal joint of the thumb (see Chapter 8).

Physiotherapy techniques

The careful assessment of the patient guides the physiotherapist in the selection of treatment. Specific techniques of treatment are adjusted at subsequent attendances following appropriate re-assessment.

THE AIMS OF TREATMENT

The aims of treatment are to: (a) reduce pain; (b) improve movement; (c) achieve functional independence.

It must be understood that in osteoarthrosis there is a defect of movement and this manifests itself in faulty patterns of movement, pain and functional loss. Treatment must therefore be aimed to regain as much movement as possible.

To reduce pain

Pain is the reason for most patients seeking the doctor's advice and although improvement in movement will help to reduce pain other methods may be necessary.

DRUGS AND HYDROCORTISONE INJECTION

See Chapter 14.

ICE

See also page 80.

Ice packs or towels placed over the painful joints are found to ease pain. Benefit can be increased by appropriate exercise whilst these are in place. Ice baths are often helpful for the small joints of the hands and feet.

HEAT

Heat from infra-red irradiation, short-wave diathermy, hot packs, electric pads and wax can all be given to reduce pain and protective muscle spasm but it must always be remembered that these treatments are only used as adjuncts to movement and are not in themselves of much therapeutic value.

The benefit from short-wave diathermy is debatable and some patients complain that their symptoms are worse when receiving this treatment. It is possible that it aggravates the already hyperaemic bone and congested joint.

HYDROTHERAPY

See pages 81, 127.

ULTRASOUND

This can be used to reduce pain and is indicated where there are localized tender areas of the soft tissue around the joint.

To improve movement

Tucker has said that 'a joint with limited movement especially if painful is bound to deteriorate unless the range of movement and muscle power have been restored to as nearly normal as possible'.

The factors to be considered in improving movement can be discussed under the following headings: (1) reduction of muscle spasm; (2) mobilization of tight structures; (3) facilitation of muscle action; (4) improvement in proprioception; (5) facilitation of postural and equilibrium reactions.

REDUCTION OF PROTECTIVE MUSCLE SPASM

Muscle spasm should be reduced as soon as possible, otherwise it can become established and persist long after pain has ceased.

Hydrotherapy, an extremely valuable technique for reducing muscle spasm, is discussed on pages 81 and 127.

A second method is to use ice towels placed along the length of the muscle from origin to insertion and appropriate exercises are given whilst these are in place.

Various methods of relaxation exercise can be used. Techniques such as 'hold, relax', and 'slow reversal hold, relax' are described by Margaret Knott in *Proprioceptive Neuromuscular Facilitation* techniques. Simple suspension exercises can also be helpful.

MOBILIZATION OF TIGHT STRUCTURES

Restriction of movement due to tight ligaments and capsule can be helped by careful positioning and stretching as already described. Perseverance in the correction of both dynamic and static posture will help to prevent further tightness occurring.

Passive mobilizing techniques should form an important part of the treatment to relieve pain, to free restricted movement and to improve function. Grieve (1972), Mennell (1949) and Maitland (1970) have described the techniques (Plates 11/1–11/7).

The choice of technique is governed by the examination and assessment. Passive mobilization can be given in either functional or accessory ranges and the grades of movement selected will depend upon the joint irritability. Where pain is present at rest or is initiated by slight movement, mobilization techniques are kept to the low grades. As pain and movement restriction diminishes, higher grades are indicated.

Traction is a form of passive mobilization and can be given either manually or using apparatus. It has been found to reduce pain and improve range. When given to an osteoarthrotic hip which is painful the traction can be given in flexion (40 to 50°) and as pain eases the limb is brought down into extension. A suggested form of apparatus used for sustained traction is that described by Flewitt (1969). Weights of between 20 and 38 lb are used. Flewitt described this method using short-wave diathermy; others have found traction alone beneficial.

Hydrotherapy (pages 81, 127).

FACILITATION OF MUSCLE ACTION

Muscle action can be facilitated by techniques based on sensory-motor stimulus. These include the proprioceptive neuromuscular facilitation (PNF) techniques, and techniques based on the concept of Rood.

The patterns of movement used in PNF are valuable in that they are functional and have a rotary component. The extensor abduction medial rotation pattern is particularly beneficial in the treatment of an osteo-arthrotic hip.

As the range and patterns of movement are improved the muscles must be strengthened throughout the range by selection of appropriate

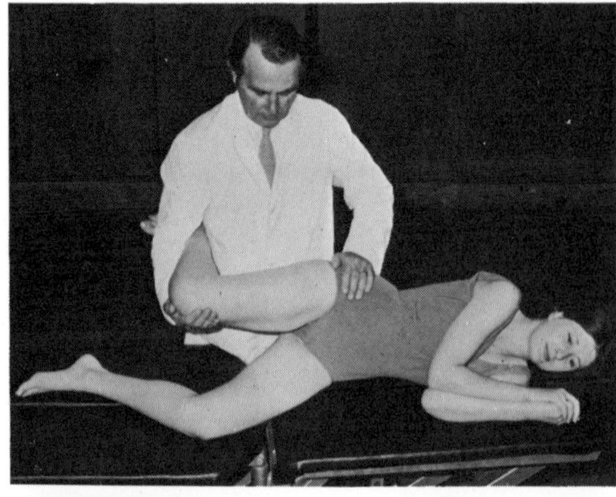

Plates 11/1–11/7. Passive mobilizing techniques (see p. 123)

Plate 11/1 Mobilizing abduction (grades I–II)

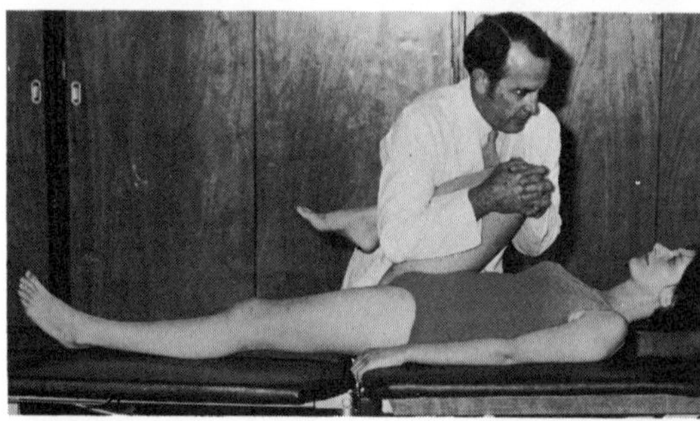

Plate 11/2 Examination and mobilization in flexion-abduction quadrant of right hip

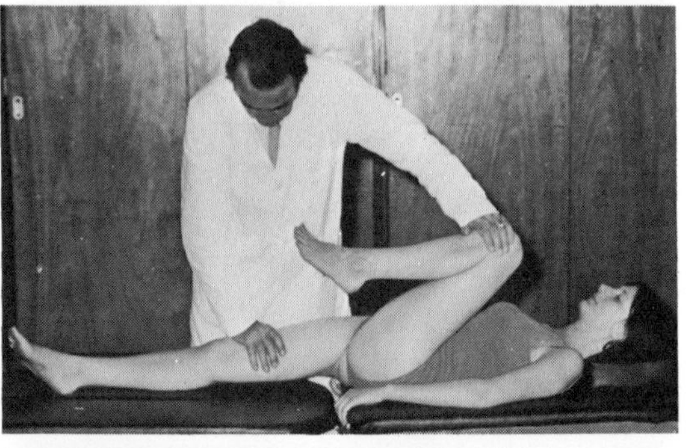

Plate 11/3 Extension of right hip

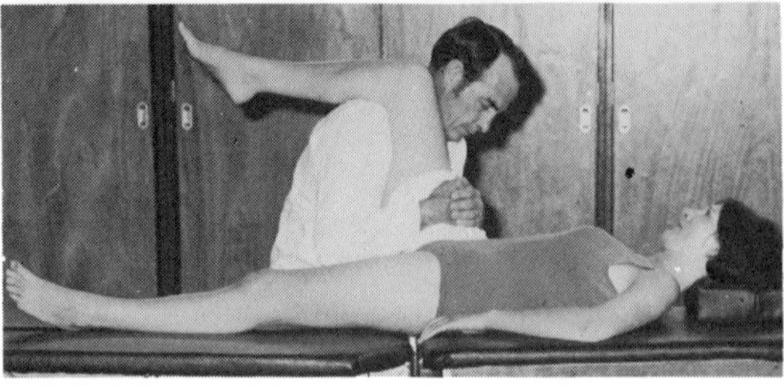

Plate 11/4 Distraction of right hip

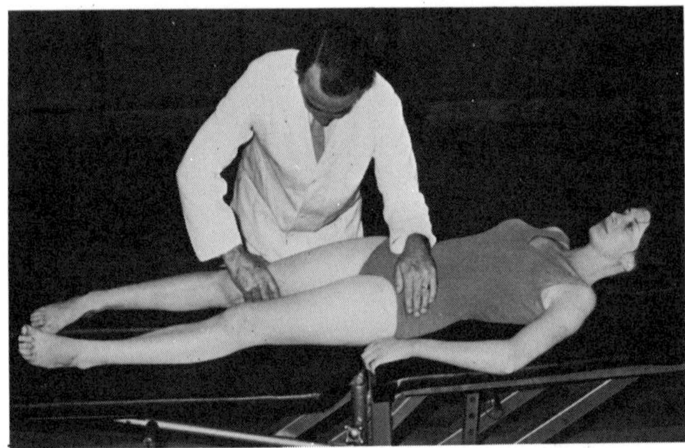

Plate 11/5 Mobilizing internal rotation (grade III)

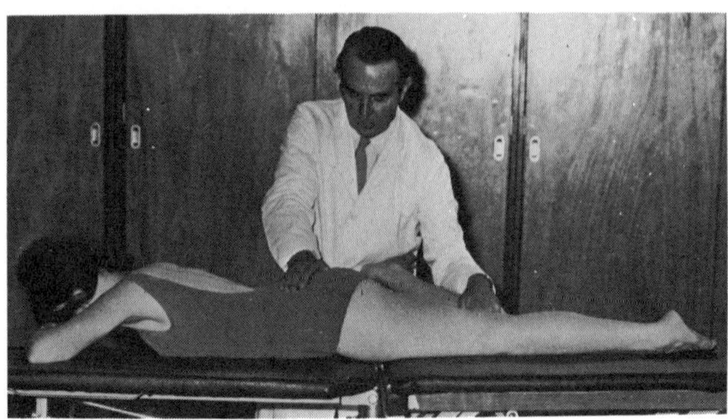

Plate 11/6 Mobilizing internal rotation (grade IV)

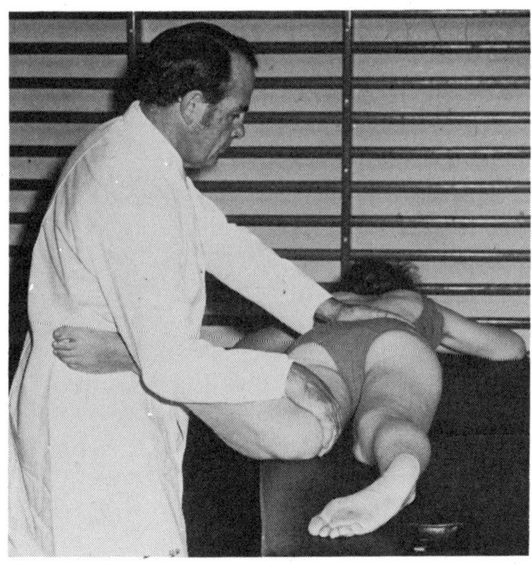

Plate 11/7 Mobilizing internal rotation (grade IV)

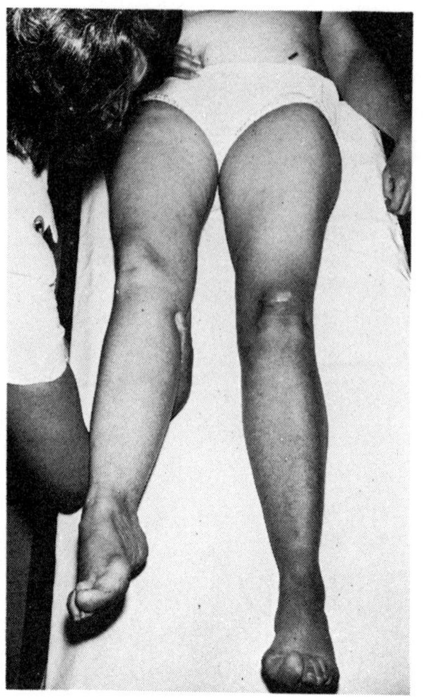

Plate 11/8 Testing abduction. Other hand must always be on the pelvis to detect any pelvic movement (*see p. 119*)

methods. These may include slow reversals, repeated contractions and rhythmic stabilizations.

Pulley exercises using a weight as resistance can be used to strengthen muscle groups and are best performed in proprioceptive neuromuscular facilitation patterns. Mat work exercises involving the trunk help to regain movement in joints which have become stiff through lack of use.

All movements should be performed in pain-free ranges but if pain is such that little or no movement is allowed then isometric contractions should be given. The principles of irradiation can be used when isotonic or isometric contraction of another part of the limb or of the other limb is given in order to achieve contraction of muscles around the painful joint.

IMPROVEMENT IN PROPRIOCEPTION

The patient can be made more aware of movement patterns and position by repetition, training 'to feel' and the use of mirrors.

FACILITATION OF POSTURAL AND EQUILIBRIUM REACTIONS

Many patients suffering from osteoarthrosis have difficulty in adjusting their posture to changes of position and this lack of postural reaction can limit their activities. By improving their mobility they can become much more able to adapt to changes in position.

Maintenance of the mobility of joints other than the affected one will enable the patient to move confidently whilst sparing the affected one.

Appropriate exercises selected to promote functional activities will also help to train postural reactions.

To achieve functional independence

Throughout the treatment programme techniques should be selected to assist functional independence (see p. 89 *et seq.*).

Consideration must be given to all joints involved in a functional activity and techniques selected to include these.

A patient with osteoarthrosis of the hip may require training in sitting up from lying, turning over and getting out of bed, standing from sitting, sitting from standing and guidance in getting into and out of a car.

Gait training should be included and this can be done first in the pool and in the parallel bars. Progression can be made to the use of crutches (see p. 81), or sticks, aiming to achieve a heel strike, correct weight transference and push off.

The use of sticks or elbow crutches is encouraged in order to save the joint and prevent aggravation of symptoms and where there is shortening of the leg the shoe can be raised (see p. 88).

Most patients need help and training in the use of steps and stairs. Many patients with osteoarthrosis of the hip or knee find it easier to walk up stairs with the non-affected leg going up first and down last.

When patients cannot achieve independence by their own movement then much help can be gained by the use of aids and adaptations (see also Chapter 8).

HYDROTHERAPY

The advantages of hydrotherapy for patients suffering from osteoarthrosis are manifold. The warmth and support of the water will reduce muscle spasm and pain and therefore increase the range of movement. Exercises can be given using the water to assist or resist movement and functional activities such as sitting to standing, walking and step training are often easier to train first in the water.

More than one joint can be exercised in the water and this is of considerable value for patients with osteoarthrosis of the hip who also require mobilization of the lumbar spine.

Most patients enjoy exercises in the pool and are greatly encouraged by the movement they achieve in the water.

Over recent years methods based on proprioceptive neuromuscular facilitation techniques have been in practice. These were developed by Dr Zin at Bad Ragaz and have now become known as Bad Ragaz techniques (Davies, 1967). By using appropriate floats the patient is completely buoyant. The physiotherapist positions her hands to facilitate the required movement and provides a fixed point around which the patient moves through the water.

These techniques are found to be very valuable in the treatment of osteoarthrosis of the hip.

Physiotherapy must be adjusted to every individual according to age, debility and joint involvement. It would be unwise to treat an 80-year-old in the same way as a 45-year-old with the same condition.

Many patients can learn to cope with their problems, if the symptoms are acceptable, for a considerable period, provided they are given adequate training and appropriate treatment.

For some patients symptoms deteriorate as the disease advances and surgery is then indicated.

Drugs in the treatment of osteoarthrosis

The types of analgesics and other drugs suitable for use in osteoarthrosis are described in Chapter 14. Although oral corticosteroids have no place in the treatment, local steroid injections are occasionally helpful (p. 162).

For Bibliography see end of Chapter 12, p. 139.

Chapter 12

Surgical Management of Osteoarthrosis

by B. M. GRAVELING, MCSP, DIP.TP

PHYSIOTHERAPY IN RELATION TO THE SURGERY OF OSTEOARTHROSIS

The physiotherapist should see the patient before surgery to assess movement and functional loss and to give the patient some understanding of postoperative treatment. Respiratory function should be assessed, especially in any cases where there is a history of respiratory disease. Postural drainage and breathing exercises should be given where necessary. The importance of moving all joints and muscles to prevent venous stasis after operation is stressed.

The therapist must have an understanding of the operation and be familiar with the regime of after-care recommended by the surgeon. She must observe all muscle and joint action, oedema and any undue pain or discomfort and report to the surgeon. Progression of treatment must be discussed regularly with the surgeon and in particular permission should be obtained before standing and walking a patient. Knowledge of whether the patient should be full weight-bearing or non-weight-bearing is obligatory.

Before discharge from in-patient care, functional activities such as getting in and out of bed and going to the lavatory should be practised and, where necessary, advice from the occupational therapist given. Arrangements with the appropriate authority for alterations in the home should be made for those patients who are not independent and instruction and guidance should be given to other members of the family on ways in which the patient can be helped at home (see also Chapter 8).

The need for physiotherapy as an out-patient should be discussed with the surgeon and instruction in exercises to be continued at home given.

The failure of conservative treatment may warrant surgical intervention in osteoarthrosis. The specific indications for surgery are disabling pain, instability and deformity.

SUMMARY OF OPERATIONS FOR OSTEOARTHROSIS

Soft tissue surgery

Soft tissue operations are seldom used in the treatment of osteoarthrosis. These operations do not influence the natural history of the disease and symptomatic improvement is rarely sustained. A closed adductor tenotomy alone or in conjunction with manipulation and intra-articular hydrocortisone may be used in the treatment of osteoarthrosis of the hip joint.

Debridement

The removal of intra-articular loose bodies, osteophytes and degenerate semilunar cartilages is sometimes indicated in the arthritic knee joint. At the same time, cartilage and subchondral bone may be drilled in order to stimulate repair. Removal of loose bodies is often necessary in the elbow joint. Debridement will relieve symptoms of mechanical origin such as locking of the joint, but the results are unpredictable.

Osteotomy

In this operation bone is divided close to a degenerate joint. Deformity may be corrected by excising an appropriate wedge of bone. Internal fixation is often used to stabilize the bony fragments and thereby allows early mobilization of the joint. Relief of pain is variable and the range of movement seldom increased. The mechanics by which osteotomy relieves pain are by altering the interosseous blood flow and by redistributing forces passing through the articular surfaces of the joint.

Arthrodesis

Arthrodesis or surgical fusion of a joint guarantees pain relief and stability at the expense of mobility. The remnants of the articular cartilage and underlying bone are excised and the bone ends are placed in the position of function. Bone grafts and internal fixation are used to promote union and maintain position. External splintage is retained until the fusion is solid. When a joint is considered for arthrodesis the function of surrounding joints must be assessed. Fusion is only carried out when these joints have good function.

Excision arthroplasty

Excision of a joint relieves pain, allows movement, but results in instability. This operation can be used in the hip joint as a primary procedure (Girdlestone's operation) but more commonly as a salvage operation following removal of a failed total replacement. Keller's and Mayo's operation on the metatarsophalangeal joint of the hallux and trapezectomy for osteoarthrosis of the carpometacarpal joint are other examples of this type of operation.

Interposition arthroplasty

The principle of this operation is to allow the prepared bearing surfaces of the joint to articulate with foreign material. Cup arthroplasty is the best example of this procedure. After reaming both the femoral head and the acetabulum, a highly polished vitallium cup is inserted between the two prepared bone surfaces. A smooth surface layer of fibrocartilage forms on the articulating bone surface. Pain relief is unpredictable and the functional results are inferior to those of total joint replacement. This operation is occasionally preferred in patients considered to be too young for total hip replacement.

Partial joint replacement

The articular surface of part of a joint may be replaced. Although partial replacement is not an ideal concept, good functional results may be obtained. The MacIntosh tibial plateau replacement is an operation of this type.

Total replacement arthroplasty

The introduction of cold-curing cement to securely anchor the components of prostheses to bone has enabled great advances to be made in the technique of joint replacement. Total hip replacement is now a well-established procedure in osteoarthrosis.

Total joint replacements for the knee, elbow and shoulder are being developed but at the present time are used primarily in rheumatoid arthritis.

A total replacement arthroplasty gives pain relief, mobility and stability and the postoperative treatment is demanding neither of patient nor physiotherapist.

SURGERY FOR PARTICULAR JOINTS

Almost all orthopaedic surgeons employ the same general principles with regard to surgical technique and to programmes of postoperative management. Clearly there will be many individual variations. Commonly employed methods are described in this chapter but differences must be expected when working in different hospitals. Such differences exist in postoperative treatment of joints, especially the knee joint and in periods of immobilization of the joint. Comparison can be made of the procedure described in this chapter with a similar or the same operation described in Chapter 9.

HIP

Total replacement arthroplasty is now the salvage operation of choice in the osteoarthrotic hip. There are indications for other operations which will be described briefly. The postoperative programme varies with each operation, but in all cases the physiotherapist must give exercises for all other joints and in particular for the lumbar spine, which is nearly always stiff.

Total joint replacement

A number of different prostheses are currently available for use in the hip joint since the original designs were introduced by McKee, Watson-Farrar and Charnley in the early 1960s. Most orthopaedic surgeons nowadays use metal to plastic implants.

The approach to the hip joint may be anterolateral (McKee-Farrar), lateral (Charnley) or posterolateral. There is potential instability with each of these approaches. In the anterolateral and lateral, the joint may be unstable in extension, adduction and external rotation and in the posterior approach in flexion, adduction and medial rotation.

ANTEROLATERAL APPROACH

There is no division of muscle. External splintage is not used and early mobilization is encouraged. Static contractions of the gluteal and quadriceps muscles and assisted flexion and abduction of the hip can be given on the first day after operation. Gradually the range of hip movement is increased and other exercises included to strengthen all hip muscles.

Lumbar spine exercises can be given from the first few days and the patient can sit with the legs over the edge of the bed three to four days after the operation. All patients should be encouraged to lie flat for a definite period each day and where possible prone. Standing is allowed after three to four days when attempts to correct posture are made. Leg length discrepancy is corrected where necessary by adjustment of the shoe height. Most patients need to be instructed to move the joint when they walk because they tend to retain their previous gait pattern of holding the hip stiff. The selection of walking aids will depend upon the general mobility of the patient. Although the joint can take full weight, many older patients with multiple joint involvement will require elbow crutches or sticks.

Gradually, instruction and training in steps, stairs, slopes, sitting, standing and managing the lavatory can be given.

The patient is usually discharged about three weeks after the operation when instruction should be given as to what he or she can or cannot do. Normal activities should be encouraged but jarring the joint should be avoided.

LATERAL APPROACH

The greater trochanter is osteotomized. After insertion of the components, the trochanter is reattached more distally to enhance the action of the hip abductors. There is a disadvantage in removing the trochanter in that it may fail to join or may give pain. The Charnley operation can be performed without removing the trochanter in some hips.

POSTOPERATIVE TREATMENT

An abduction pillow is kept between the legs for one week. Assisted knee and hip flexion is begun on the second day. The patient stands out of bed with the legs abducted twice daily on or after the fourth day in preparation for walking. The patient returns to the abduction pillow on getting back to bed. At about the fourth day, active knee and hip flexion is commenced and on the seventh day walking is allowed using an appropriate walking aid.

Abduction exercises on a polished board or with roller skates are started in the second week and 'hip updrawing or hitching' exercises in the third week if the opposite hip has a good range of abduction.

Sitting is permitted during the third week. Postoperative rehabilitation is dominated by encouragement to walk rather than to strive for range of movement or muscle building, and patients do not require physiotherapy on discharge from hospital. They are, however, given instructions not to sleep on the operated side for two months and to avoid forced flexion of the hip and crossing their legs.

Upper femoral osteotomy

This operation is restricted to young patients with pain-free hips that retain relatively good movement, i.e. 90°, and whose radiographs show congruent articular surfaces.

The femoral osteotomy is made at the level of the lesser trochanter. The osteotomy is fixed with a splint or nail and plate and compression may be used. Medial displacement of the distal shaft is avoided so that total replacement can be offered in the event of failure of the osteotomy.

POSTOPERATIVE TREATMENT

External splintage is not required and the patient carries out graduated hip movements in bed until the wound healing has occurred. The patient is then allowed to walk, taking partial weight until the osteotomy is united. This may take three to four months.

Arthrodesis of the hip joint

The position of fixation varies with the age and occupation of the patient. In young active people the hip is fixed in about 15° external rotation. Nowadays the operation is seldom done over the age of 60, but in the elderly the hip is fixed in a more flexed position so that sitting is easier. The lumbar spine and knee have to compensate to some extent for the fixation of the hip joint.

There are two main methods of arthrodesis:

(1) intra-articular, where the articular cartilage is removed from the head of the femur and the acetabulum and the joint fixed with either a Trifin nail or a Lag screw;

(2) extra-articular, where the joint is fixed with a nail and plate and a bone graft inserted below the joint joining the upper end of the femur to the ischium. This method is called an ischio-femoral 'V' arthrodesis. (Its advantage is that the hip joint is not opened or disturbed in any way.)

In both types of arthrodesis the joint is fixed securely and no plaster fixation is necessary. The patient can start knee movements a day or two after the operation. This is important because full movements of the knee are essential to compensate for the fixation of the hip joint.

The patient is allowed up on crutches when the wound has healed, usually about three weeks after the operation, and full weight can be put on the affected leg.

Radiological fusion takes about three months to occur, and during this time patients will need guidance and instruction in dressing and undressing and sitting. Most patients after an arthrodesis can sit in anything but very low chairs and can put on and take off shoes and socks.

Arthrodesis relieves all pain in the hip joint and is permanent. It can be carried out on only one side and is indicated only in unilateral hip joint disease.

Cup arthroplasty

See page 131.

POSTOPERATIVE TREATMENT

Traction is usually with or without a splint and care must be taken to prevent any outward rolling of the leg. (A plaster shoe with a piece of wood fixed to the heel in a transverse direction helps to prevent this.)

Movement is encouraged in a few days and the patient can be mobilized out of bed in four weeks.

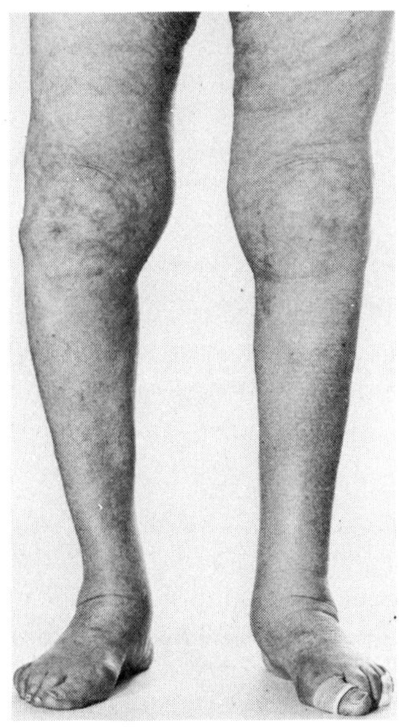

Plate 12/1 Corrected deformity after high tibial osteotomy held with two staples (*see below*)

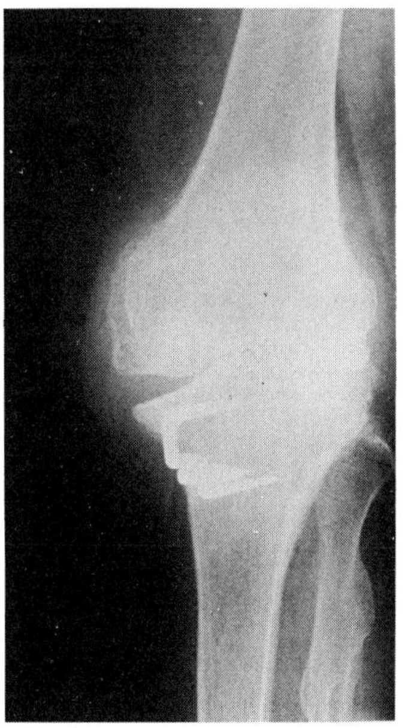

Plate 12/2 Anterior radiograph of left knee of patient shown in Plate 12/1

The procedure can be used in the younger patient in order to postpone the need to insert a total hip replacement.

KNEE

High tibial osteotomy

Degenerative joint disease often affects the tibio-femoral compartments of the knee unequally and deformity results. An osteotomy, with removal of a suitable wedge of cancellous bone from the tibia, above the level of the tubercle, allows correction of lateral deformity and usually ameliorates pain. The best results are obtained when the range of flexion is at least 90° before operation. Internal fixation of the osteotomy with staples enables the knee to be mobilized early (Plates 12/1, 12/2). Fibular osteotomy may be necessary in order to achieve firm correction of deformity.

POSTOPERATIVE TREATMENT

No external splintage is applied and static quadriceps and gluteal exercises can be commenced immediately. Gradual mobilization of the knee is commenced in two or three days and continued for six weeks when the patient is allowed to walk taking weight through the limb. Once up, the patient will require walking, step, standing and sitting training. Some surgeons use external splintage until there is union of the osteotomy. Others employ delayed splintage, plaster immobilization being used after a good range of movement has been accomplished.

Double osteotomy

This operation is sometimes advised in osteoarthrosis, where there is lateral deformity and particularly if the synovium is hypertrophic.

The tibia is divided through cancellous bone above the tibial tubercle and the femur within the joint at the upper margin of the articular cartilage.

POSTOPERATIVE TREATMENT

A plaster cylinder is applied and the patient allowed up in a few days using crutches and taking as much weight through the limb as is comfortable. Whilst in plaster, static quadriceps should be practised.

The plaster is removed after five weeks and the knee is manipulated to 90° under a general anaesthetic. After the manipulation, mobilizing and strengthening exercises are given to maintain the range and strengthen all muscles and the patient progresses to full weight-bearing.

Debridement

This operation will often relieve symptoms. It should only be performed when the knee is stable and in the absence of deformity. A parapatellar approach is made to the joint, osteophytes are removed, the irregular articular cartilage is smoothed and the eburnated bone is drilled in an attempt to revascularize the subchondral bone. Torn degenerate semilunar cartilages are removed.

POSTOPERATIVE TREATMENT

The knee is immobilized in plaster for five to seven days and static quadriceps and hip exercises should be practised. Mobilizing exercises are commenced after removal of the plaster and hydrotherapy when the wound is healed. The patient is allowed to walk non-weight-bearing at four to six weeks, progressing to full weight between six to eight weeks. Some patients may need a manipulation after six weeks.

Arthrodesis of knee

This operation guarantees pain relief and stability at the expense of loss of movement. It is best performed where there is monarticular disease, as considerable strain is placed on other joints to compensate for the immobility. The operation is indicated in a young patient who requires years of use of the knee.

A transverse incision is used and Steinmann's pins passed through the tibia and femur from side to side and compression is applied.

POSTOPERATIVE TREATMENT

A plaster cylinder is applied until union of the arthrodesis. The patient will need some instruction in managing with the stiff knee. For example, in ascending stairs the non-affected leg leads and follows when descending.

Patellectomy

This operation is performed where osteoarthrosis is confined to the patello-femoral joint. A transverse incision is made and the patella is excised; the quadriceps expansion is preserved.

POSTOPERATIVE TREATMENT

The leg is immobilized in plaster for six weeks and quadriceps contractions, foot and hip movements are practised. The knee is then mobilized. It is important to train good extension control of the knee as a lag can easily occur due to the surgery involving the extensor mechanism. Mobilization exercises can be performed in the pool.

Arthroplasty of the knee

Prosthetic replacement of the knee is now being accepted as a salvage procedure in advanced rheumatoid disease and occasionally is offered to patients with severe osteoarthrosis. Partial joint replacement, interposition arthroplasty and hinge arthroplasty are being superseded by the non-linked metal to plastic type of prosthesis (Gunston, 1971 and Swanson, 1972). The early results of these newer prostheses are promising.

POSTOPERATIVE CARE

Irrespective of the type of arthroplasty, wound healing is of paramount importance, and the limb is usually immobilized in a plaster of Paris cylinder for a fortnight or so until this has been achieved. The plaster cylinder is removed at two weeks and the wound inspected. The knee is then mobilized and the patient rapidly progresses to full weight-bearing.

METATARSOPHALANGEAL JOINT OF THE GREAT TOE

The following operations can be performed:

KELLER OPERATION

The base of the proximal phalanx is excised and the exostosis bevelled off. The patient is allowed to walk on the heel within a few days. After the stitches and dressings are removed all movements of the toes and foot can be encouraged and correction in standing and walking given. It is important to retain the mobility of the joint and to strengthen all intrinsic and extrinsic muscles, in particular abductor hallucis. Many patients need advice regarding correct shoes and stockings.

MAYO OPERATION

The head of the first metatarsal is excised and the exostosis removed. The postoperative treatment and physiotherapy are the same as for the Keller operation.

FUSION OF THE METATARSOPHALANGEAL JOINT

The joint surfaces are excised and screw fixation aids fusion. Plaster is applied for six to eight weeks until the fusion is solid and during this time the patient can walk but with non-weight-bearing on the joint. After removal of the plaster, exercises can be given particularly to mobilize all other joints to compensate for the lack of extension at the metatarsophalangeal joint. Instruction in posture and walking should be given.

SURGERY FOR OSTEOARTHROSIS OF THE UPPER LIMB

Acromioclavicular joint

Osteoarthrosis of this joint usually responds to conservative treatment, but in severe cases an excision of the lateral end of the clavicle can be performed. Mobilization of the shoulder can be commenced in a day or two after the operation.

Shoulder joint

Surgery for osteoarthrosis of this joint is rarely indicated.

ARTHRODESIS

The joint is fused in a position of 70 to 90° abduction, 15 to 25° forward flexion and 25 to 30° external rotation above the horizontal; various techniques are used to achieve fusion.

POSTOPERATIVE TREATMENT

A plaster spica is applied for four to eight weeks. On removal of this, exercises must be given to mobilize the elbow and scapula and particular attention given to exercise the trapezius and serratus anterior muscles.

Elbow

Very rarely is surgery indicated for osteoarthrosis of this joint. Removal of loose bodies may be necessary. An arthrodesis may be used in a painful joint when fairly heavy work is required.

Carpometacarpal joint of the thumb

Two operations can be performed to relieve symptoms arising from degenerative changes in this joint.

EXCISION ARTHROPLASTY

The trapezium is excised and the resulting gap allowed to fill with fibrous tissue. The hand is in plaster for three weeks and during this time finger, elbow and shoulder movements should be practised. Mobilizing and strengthening exercises are commenced on removal of the plaster. Particular attention should be given to the re-education of opposition of the thumb, because the patient will have avoided this movement before operation.

ARTHRODESIS

The trapezio-metacarpal joint is fused. The hand is put into a scaphoid type plaster for four months with the thumb in mid-position. Mobilization of *other* joints is given on removal of the plaster.

BIBLIOGRAPHY

Apley, A. G. *A System of Orthopaedics and Fractures.* Butterworth (London), 1968.

Benjamin, A. 'Double osteotomy for the painful knee in rheumatoid arthritis and osteoarthritis.' *Journal of Bone and Joint Surgery*, **51B**, 694, 1969.

Boyle, J. A. and Buchanan, W. W. *Clinical Rheumatology.* Blackwell, 1971.

Brittain, H. A. and Howard, R. C. 'Arthrodesis.' *Journal of Bone and Joint Surgery*, **32B**, 282, 1950.

Charnley, J. 'Total prosthetic replacement of the hip.' *Physiotherapy*, **53** (12), 40, 1967.

Charnley, J. 'Arthrodesis of knee.' *Clinical Orthopaedics*, **18**, 37, 1960.

Copeman, W. S. C. *Textbook of the Rheumatic Diseases.* Churchill Livingstone, 1969.

Davies, B. C. 'A technique of re-education in the treatment pool.' *Physiotherapy*, **53** (2), 57, 1967.

Duffield, M. H. *Exercises in Water.* Baillière Tindall, 1969.

Flewitt, B. 'Traction and s.w.d. for early osteoarthrosis of the hip.' *Physiotherapy*, **55** (12), 507, 1969.

Freeman, M. A. R. and Swanson, S. A. V. 'Total prosthetic replacement of the knee.' *Journal of Bone and Joint Surgery*, **54B**, 170, 1972.

Goff, B. 'The application of recent advances in neurophysiology to Miss M. Rood's concept of neuromuscular facilitation.' *Physiotherapy*, **58** (12), 41, 1972.

Golding, D. 'General management of osteoarthrosis.' *British Medical Journal*, **3**, 575, 1969.

Grieve, G. P. 'The hip.' *Physiotherapy*, **57** (5), 212, 1971.

Gunston, F. H. 'Polycentric knee arthroplasty.' *Journal of Bone and Joint Surgery*, **53B**, 272, 1971.

Haines, J. 'A survey of recent developments in cold therapy.' *Physiotherapy*, **53** (7), 222, 1967.

Helal, B. 'Pain in primary osteoarthritic knee, its cause and treatment by osteotomy.' *Postgraduate Medical Journal*, **41**, 172, 1965.

Jackson, J. P. and Waugh, W. G. 'High tibial osteotomy for osteoarthritic knee.' *Journal of Bone and Joint Surgery*, **51B**, 88, 1969.

Knott, M. and Voss, D. *Proprioceptive Neuromuscular Facilitation*. Harper and Row, 1969.

Maitland, G. D. *Peripheral Manipulation*. Butterworth, 1971.

Mason, M. and Currey, H. F. L. *An Introduction to Clinical Rheumatology*. Pitman Medical, 1970.

McKee, G. K. and Watson-Farrar, J. 'Replacement of arthritic hips by McKee-Farrar prosthesis.' *Journal of Bone and Joint Surgery*, **48B**, 254, 1966.

McMurray, T. P. 'Osteoarthritis of the hip joint.' *British Journal of Surgery*, **22**, 716, 1935.

Mennell, J. B. *The Science and Art of Joint Manipulation*. Churchill Livingstone, 1939.

Muller, G. M. 'Arthrodesis of the trapezio-metacarpal joint for osteoarthritis.' *Journal of Bone and Joint Surgery*, **31B**, 540, 1949.

Murley, A. H. G. 'Excision of the trapezium in osteoarthritis of the first carpo-metacarpal joint.' *Journal of Bone and Joint Surgery*, **42B**, 502, 1960.

Murray, R. O. 'The aetiology of primary osteoarthritis of the hip.' *British Journal of Radiology*, **38**, 810, 1965.

Patrick, M. *Ultrasonic Therapy*. Elsevier, 1964.

Saywell, S. *Physiotherapy in Major Knee Surgery*. Heinemann Medical, 1964.

Trueta, J., Harrison, M. H. M. and Schajowicz. 'Osteoarthritis of the hip. A study of the nature and evolution of the disease.' *Journal of Bone and Joint Surgery*, **35B**, 598, 1953.

Tucker, W. E. 'Manipulative techniques employed in the treatment of injury and osteoarthritis of the fingers and hands.' *Physiotherapy*, **57** (6), 255, 1971.

Tucker, W. E. *Home Treatment and Posture in Injury, Rheumatism and Osteoarthritis*. Churchill Livingstone, 1969.

Tucker, W. E. 'Treatment of osteoarthritis by manual therapy.' *British Journal of Clinical Practice*, **23** (1), 1969.

Wright, V. 'Treatment of osteoarthritis of knees.' *Annals of Rheumatic Diseases*, **23**, 289, 1964.

Chapter 13

Degenerative Arthritis of the Spine and Intervertebral Disc Disease

by ALASTAIR G. MOWAT, MB, FRCP(ED)
and JOAN M. ABERY, MCSP

ANATOMY, PATHOLOGY, INCIDENCE AND CAUSE

The spinal apophyseal joints

The spinal apophyseal joints are diarthrodial, synovial joints and are thus susceptible to be involved in the same inflammatory and degenerative processes which affect larger, peripheral joints. The apophyseal joints lie posteriorly on each side of the vertebral pedicles providing articulation with the adjacent vertebrae, and so each vertebra carries four articular surfaces (Plate 13/1). In addition each thoracic vertebra has four small articular surfaces for the articulation of the ribs with the sides of the vertebral body and the transverse processes. The atlas and axis (the first and second cervical vertebrae) carry similar posterior apophyseal joints, but in addition there are synovial joints between the anterior arch of the atlas and the odontoid process of the axis. The third to the seventh cervical vertebral bodies differ from those elsewhere in the spine in having small synovial joints on the posterior edge of the upper and lower surfaces of the bodies – neuro-central joints.

The spinal movements which take place at each vertebra are flexion, extension, lateral flexion and rotation, the latter two being associated movements. The extent of these movements at each part of the spine depends upon the thickness of the intervertebral discs, the tension in the interspinal ligaments and the angle of contact of the intervertebral joints. In consequence, greater movements occur in the cervical and lumbar spine than in the thoracic spine and for practical purposes none occurs in the sacral region. The joints between the atlas and the skull allow flexion, extension and lateral flexion of the skull while rotation of the skull upon the cervical spine is almost entirely carried out by the axis.

Degenerative arthritis in these joints, with loss of cartilage, eburnation of underlying bone and the development of marginal osteophytes, accompanied by a very variable amount of pain and decreased function, is a very common feature of advancing age (Plate 13/2). Surveys based upon radiographic findings show that some 70 per cent of the population has such changes by the age of 60 years and that the incidence steadily increases with age. Occupational factors tend to affect the incidence, since degenerative changes are commoner in men, particularly those engaged in manual work. Further, the incidence especially of cervical spinal lesions, is exaggerated in those patients, mostly women, with primary generalized osteoarthrosis with Heberden nodes around the distal interphalangeal joints of the hands. However, it must be emphasized that there is no correlation between the radiographic findings and the presence or severity of clinical symptoms and signs.

The intervertebral discs

The intervertebral discs, lying between successive vertebral bodies from the second cervical vertebra downwards, are composed of fibrocartilage, the outer portion of which consists chiefly of concentric rings of fibrous tissue, the annulus fibrosus, while the centre of the disc, the nucleus pulposus, is softer and gelatinous. The normal disc is capable of withstanding heavy loads with relatively little deformation and serves as an efficient 'shock absorber'. It can adapt to spinal movements and should distribute rapidly changing stresses evenly up and down the spine. Recent work suggests that many spines fail to achieve even distribution of stresses.

The discs account for one-quarter of the spinal length, and are not of uniform thickness, being of gradually increasing thickness from above downwards. The frequency of symptoms, which arise most commonly from the C5–6, C6–7, L4–5 and L5–S1 discs, is due to greater stresses being present at the junctions of very mobile and relatively immobile spinal segments. By early adult life the discs are avascular and degenerative changes set in accompanied by a progressive reduction in water content. Such degenerative changes are accompanied by a tendency for the contents of the nucleus pulposus to be extruded through weakened portions of the annulus fibrosus. Such extrusion may occur through the vertebral plate into adjacent vertebrae. These Schmorl's nodes are usually symptomless, but if multiple may be associated with degenerative arthritis and a loss of height.

Extrusion of the disc in other directions is influenced by the attachment of the disc to the vertebral ligaments. The disc is loosely attached to the anterior longitudinal ligament which in turn is firmly attached to the vertebral bodies, but the disc is more firmly attached to the posterior longitudinal ligament which in its turn is only loosely

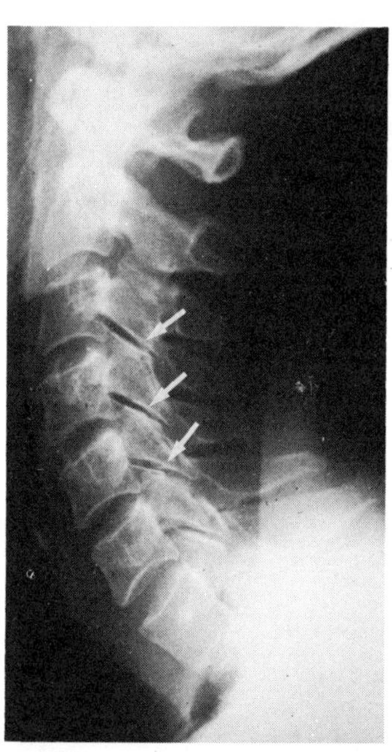

Plate 13/1 Normal lateral radiograph of cervical spine. The discs are well-preserved, there is little evidence of osteophyte formation on the anterior or posterior margins of the vertebral bodies, and apophyseal joints (arrowed) are normal (*see p. 141*)

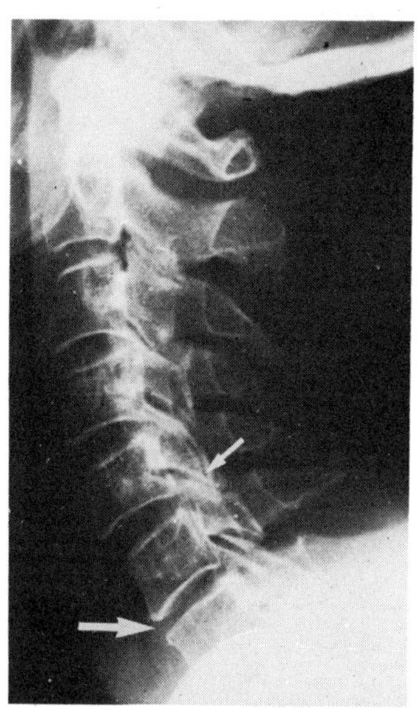

Plate 13/2 Narrowing of C6–7 disc and apophyseal joint arthritis (*see p. 142*)

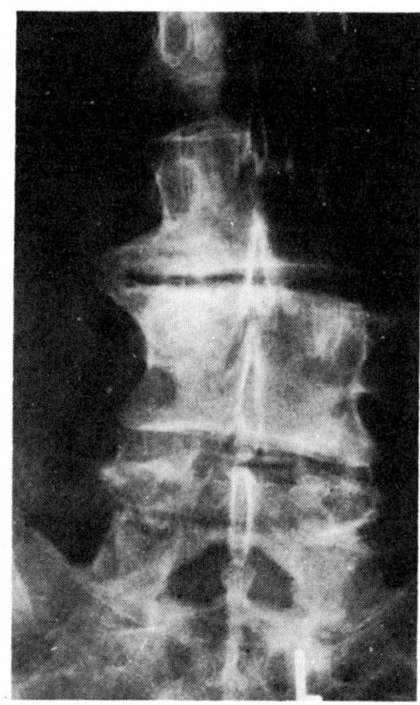

Plate 13/3 Antero-lateral osteophytes from adjacent vertebrae have united. Note associated disc degeneration and narrowing

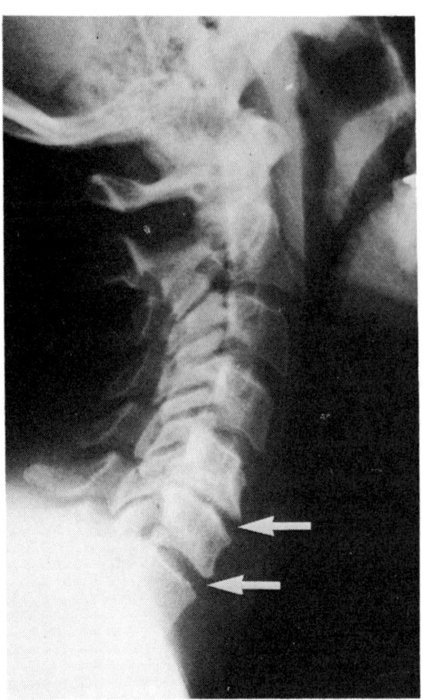

Plate 13/4 Narrowing of C5–6 and C6–7 discs with anterior and posterior osteophyte formation. The apophyseal joints are well-preserved (*see p. 146*)

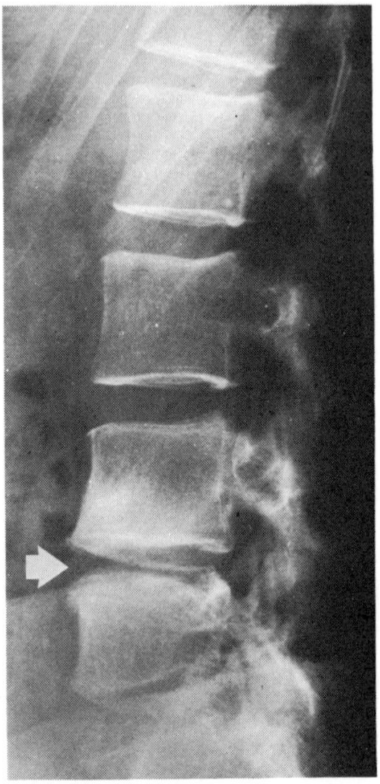

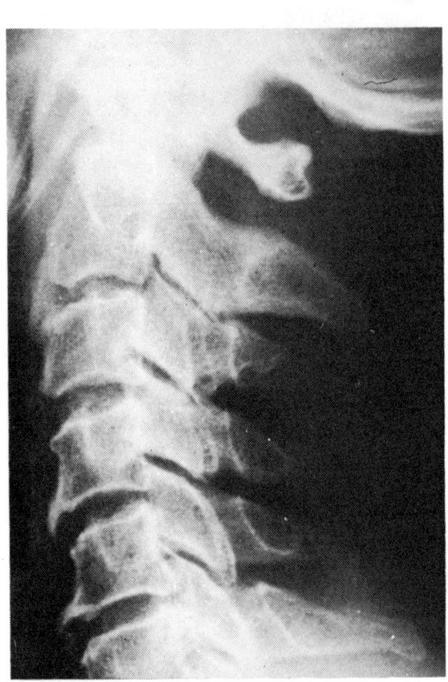

Plate 13/5 Marked anterior osteophyte formation in cervical spine (*see p. 146*)

Plate 13/6 Degenerative changes with narrowing of L4–5 disc, with loss of lumbar curve due to protective muscle spasm (*see p. 151*)

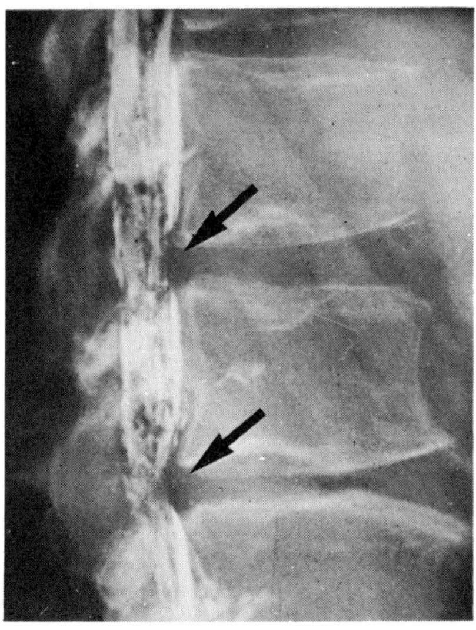

Plate 13/7 Lateral myelogram showing disc protrusion at L4–5 with less marked protrusion at L3–4 level (*see p. 154*)

attached to the posterior aspect of the vertebral bodies. Extrusion of the disc anteriorly or laterally causes anterior or lateral osteophyte growth which may be so marked as occasionally to unite and so fuse two vertebrae with consequent loss of movement of the apophyseal joints (Plate 13/3). Extrusion of the disc contents posteriorly causes greater problems. Fixation to the posterior ligament usually means that disc extrusion occurs postero-laterally, at which site symptoms will depend upon whether the extrusion is acute or whether it occurs slowly and is accompanied by osteophyte formation. In either event the disc contents and/or the osteophytes may press upon the spinal cord, the nerve roots either as they travel downwards or through the intervertebral foramina, or upon the vertebral artery in the cervical spine.

The phenomenon of disc degeneration, with or without osteophyte formation and extrusion of disc contents is very common, with 60 per cent of the population having significant radiological changes in all spinal segments by the age of 60 years. The incidence in all spinal segments is higher in men. Degeneration of discs is often associated with degeneration in the apophyseal joints and once again the radiographic and clinical presentations cannot be correlated (Plate 13/2).

The incidence of acute disc prolapse, commonest in the lumbar spine and which tends to occur in patients aged between 30 and 50 years, is difficult to determine, since the diagnosis of 'slipped disc' is a fashionable one, particularly by patients. Although acute disc prolapse produces a characteristic clinical picture, the diagnosis is medically proven relatively rarely.

Ligaments and muscles

As with joint disease elsewhere, there may be related or independent symptoms arising from associated muscles and ligaments. In addition to the anterior and posterior longitudinal ligaments, there are a variety of other spinal ligaments, the most important of which are the ligamentum flava connecting the laminae of adjacent vertebrae, and the interspinous ligaments joining the vertebral spines. A large number of muscles are attached to the spinal column, and these attachments may be the site of chronic inflammation secondary to trauma and abnormal or unbalanced loading.

THE CAUSES OF DEGENERATION IN THE SPINE

The causes of degenerative changes in the spine, sometimes called spondylosis, as with degenerative arthritis in other joints, are not clearly determined. In some patients the association with trauma, either as a single severe episode or related to repeated minor episodes over many years, usually determined by the nature of or the posture adopted at work, will be clear. In others obesity may be a major factor. However, in many patients the cause is unclear although developmental abnormalities and endocrine and metabolic factors may be involved. In the group of patients with widespread generalized osteoarthrosis genetic factors are dominant, the inheritance among female members of the family often being clearly seen. It is obvious, therefore, that only some of the potential causes can be influenced during management of the patient.

CERVICAL SPINE

Clinical features (Plates 13/4, 13/5)

Three main groups of symptoms are produced by degenerative arthritis and intervertebral disc disease in the cervical spine. (a) Symptoms due to pressure of osteophytes or postero-lateral disc protrusion on the spinal nerves. These are by far the commonest symptoms. (b) Symptoms due to pressure of osteophytes or central disc protrusion on the spinal cord. (c) Symptoms due to pressure of osteophytes or lateral disc protrusion on the vertebral artery.

Degeneration in the neuro-central joints of the third to seventh vertebrae may contribute to both spinal cord and nerve compression.

Symptoms may be produced by acute or chronic disc changes. Acute disc prolapse usually follows trauma in younger patients and produces sudden severe pain with a further increase in intensity over a few days. Changes associated with chronic disc disease are more gradual and frequently episodic in their production of symptoms.

SPINAL NERVE ROOT COMPRESSION

Spinal nerve root compression produces pain in the distribution area of the root, but it is important to remember that the pain may be wider spread than imagined, with C4 root pain being felt in the scapular region and C7 root pain in the anterior chest. Typically, acute spasms of pain are added to a background of dull aching. The pain may produce muscle

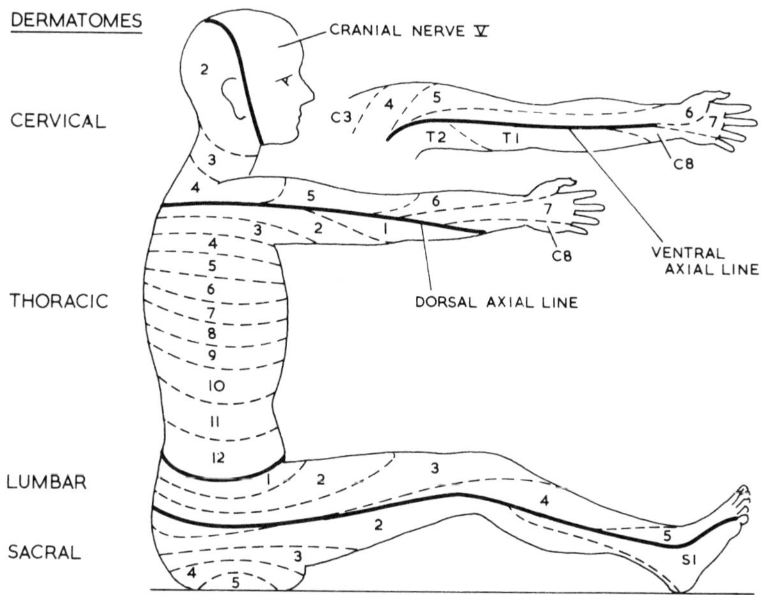

Fig. 13/1 Plan of dermatomes of body and segmental cutaneous distribution of upper limb

spasm with a reduction in spinal movement or a complete loss of movement associated with a torticollis. Involvement of the motor root results in muscle weakness and diminution or absence of arm reflexes. The muscles supplied by the most commonly involved roots are listed below:

Deltoid	C5, (6)
Biceps	C(5), 6
Triceps	C(6), 7, (8)
Wrist and fingers extensors and flexors	C7, 8
Thumb abductors and extensors	C(7), 8
Intrinsic hand muscles	C8, T1

Involvement of the sensory root may produce paraesthesiae and subsequently impairment of all modalities of sensation in the affected dermatome. In the early stages, nerve root irritation may produce increased and unpleasant sensation – hyperaesthesia. Skin dermatomes are shown in Fig. 13/1, but caution must be exercised in attributing symptoms to a specific root on the basis of such diagrams, as there is marked individual variation.

CERVICAL SPINAL CORD COMPRESSION

Cervical spinal cord compression is a very serious condition which occurs most commonly at the C5–6 level. Although there is a variety of presentations, the most usual involves upper motor neurone lesion findings in one or both legs with lower motor neurone lesion findings in the upper limbs. In addition there will be a variety of sensory abnormalities in both arms and legs.

VERTEBRAL ARTERY COMPRESSION

Vertebral artery compression can lead, particularly in the elderly, to brain stem ischaemia and the production of vertigo, tinnitus, visual disturbances, difficulty with speech and swallowing, and ataxia and other signs of cerebellar dysfunction.

Involvement of individual spinal joints or muscle and ligamentous damage in the neck, may produce both local and referred pain often associated with secondary muscle spasm, reduced movement and torticollis. Such symptoms are the usual result of 'whiplash' injuries incurred in road traffic accidents. The particular problems associated with disease of the atlanto-axial joints has been described elsewhere (see Chapter 5).

INVESTIGATION AND TREATMENT OF CERVICAL SPINE LESIONS

The physiotherapist has an important role in the assessment of patients with cervical spinal disease. An accurate history will often pinpoint the lesion and diagnosis, and an assessment of the patient's response to pain and disability will provide useful information in judging the severity of the symptoms and the patient's likely response to treatment. In particular, if a patient's reaction is not to be misjudged, it must be remembered that symptoms bear little or no relationship to radiographic features.

It is vital that the physiotherapist undertakes a careful examination of the neck and that the cervical spine is put through a full range of active and passive movement to try and determine the precise level and extent of the lesion. It may be necessary to hold each spinal position for 10 to 15 seconds to reproduce symptoms. A hurried examination must not be carried out.

Investigations

Plain X-rays including obliques, although useful, must be interpreted with caution. A myelogram or vertebral angiogram may rarely be needed for more precise localization of the lesion. Other investigations such as erythrocyte sedimentation rates and examination of the cerebrospinal fluid will not help except in excluding other diseases. Nerve conduction studies and electromyography may help to decide which nerve roots are involved.

Treatment

Acute symptoms, which are very painful, require rest for the neck and strong analgesics, even opiates (Chapter 14). A collar or neck traction is usually required and in most patients will lead to a resolution of symptoms. Very rarely surgical decompression will be necessary. Occasionally in such cases, myelography may be followed by a deterioration in the patient's condition and such investigations should not be undertaken unless operating theatre facilities are available.

Characteristically *chronic symptoms* tend to come and go and require the use of mild analgesics, a restriction in activity, attention to neck posture and usually the use of a *cervical collar*. Many patients, either on their own or their doctor's advice become martyrs to the use of a collar. In general, the majority of patients will do well with the intermittent use of a soft felt, Sorbo-rubber or Plastazote collar at night. This should be used in conjunction with a single soft pillow. Such management relieves the early morning symptoms of which most patients complain, sets the patient up well for the day ahead and avoids the cosmetic problems of wearing a collar during the day. Patients may need encouragement and even a sedative to acquire this collar-wearing habit. A small proportion of patients will require the use of firmer collars by day and night. It is important that such collars are made in a position of comfort, usually in slight flexion, and that localized pressure areas do not develop.

In this group of patients a programme of *neck traction* may be useful, once the optimum position for relief of pain has been found. Modest weights (up to 5 kg or 10 lb) are usually employed although some advocate much larger weights. Great care must be taken with traction in patients with unstable necks and in those with rheumatoid arthritis, and very small weights should be used.

Spinal manipulation has its advocates. Such treatment is always potentially dangerous in inexperienced hands, particularly in the presence of an acute lesion. Those who are interested in such treatment should attend the specialized courses.

Caution should be used in interpreting the results of the above-mentioned treatment, or indeed of persisting unduly with time-consuming programmes of treatment, as studies show that most patients improve within three months whatever treatment is given.

In some cases *surgical fusion* of adjacent vertebrae may be required or rarely decompression. Such treatment is often technically difficult and may lead to increased demands (and the possibility of increased symptoms) upon the remainder of the spine.

Muscle and ligamentous symptoms will respond to simple analgesics, accurate local injections of anaesthetic and corticosteroids, to relaxing measures such as heat, and muscle-relaxing drugs (e.g. Valium) and to simple exercise programmes. Indeed, when symptoms from whatever cause have been relieved, a suitable *exercise programme* should strengthen muscles and this will afford a protective influence.

Symptoms due to *vertebral artery compression* are helped by reducing neck movements by the use of a collar, although neck traction and exercise programmes must be avoided. Surgical decompression of the vessel may be required.

DIFFERENTIAL DIAGNOSIS OF CERVICAL SPINAL DISEASE

Acute disc lesions, particularly if due to trauma, may be confused with vertebral fracture or compression. The symptoms of chronic disc protrusion associated with cord compression must be distinguished from multiple sclerosis, cord tumours, motor neurone disease, syringomyelia and sub-acute degeneration of the cord due to Vitamin B_{12} deficiency.

The spinal apophyseal joints may be involved in a variety of inflammatory diseases which will require anti-inflammatory drugs (Chapter 14). Such diseases include rheumatoid arthritis, ankylosing spondylitis, psoriatic arthritis and Reiter's disease (Chapter 6). A variety of cardiovascular diseases may impair vertebral artery blood flow including atherosclerosis, cardiac valvular disease, thrombosis and embolism.

Spinal tumour or infective lesions (tuberculosis, staphylococcus, etc.) may cause nerve root symptoms. Herpes zoster (shingles) may cause similar nerve root symptoms and diagnostic confusion until the typical vesicular rash appears. Involvement of more than one or two nerve roots suggests damage to the brachial plexus, as with viral radiculitis, thoracic outlet syndromes and drooping of the shoulders with marked downward movement of the outer end of the clavicle, often found in middle-aged women.

DORSAL SPINE

Although dorsal spinal abnormalities are found commonly in radiographic studies of the general population, the incidence of symptoms is low. Nerve root symptoms are the commonest with pain radiating to the front of the chest or abdomen. The pain may simulate that arising from thoracic or abdominal viscera.

Treatment may include use of analgesics, a firm bed, extension and rotation exercises, weight reduction, the use of a firm brassière for those with heavy or pendulous breasts, a full posterior spinal support, and occasionally nerve root blocks.

LUMBAR SPINE

Clinical features

There are some differences between the type and causes of symptoms in the lumbar spine compared with the cervical spine. In particular, there are no vascular symptoms. Ninety per cent of symptoms affect the L5 or S1 roots. The symptoms in order of frequency are:

(a) Symptoms due to trauma or degenerative changes in the intervertebral discs or spinal joints producing pain and muscle spasm in the associated spinal dermatome (see Plate 13/6 and Fig. 13/2).

(b) Symptoms due to damage in muscles and ligaments produced by trauma, abnormal loading or bad posture. If close to the skin surface the signs may be localized but are usually similar to (a).

(c) Symptoms due to pressure of osteophytes or postero-lateral disc protrusion on the spinal nerves.

(d) Symptoms due to pressure of osteophytes or central disc protrusion on the cauda equina. The spinal cord terminates at the level of the second lumbar vertebra.

SYMPTOMS (A) AND (B)

Changes which fall short of actual nerve compression cause local pain and produce an area of referred pain, often called lumbago, which is listed in Table I, page 152. The pain is deep-seated and nagging, and may be associated with muscle spasm and reduced spinal motion.

SYMPTOMS (C)

Nerve compression produces similar or more severe pain but in addition there are motor effects which are listed in Table I and altered, reduced or absent sensation in the areas shown in Fig. 13/2. There is muscle spasm, often with reduction in lumbar lordosis and mild lumbar scoliosis. It must be appreciated that there are individual variations in nerve distribution and the listed effects must be interpreted with caution.

Nerve compression is associated with nerve irritation detected by reduced straight-leg raising with a positive Lasègue's sign or hip extension with the knee flexed (sciatic and femoral nerve stretch tests). Nerve compression symptoms in the distribution of the sciatic nerve, constitutes sciatica, a term often abused by medical and lay people. The symptoms

Table I: Lumbar nerve root symptoms and signs

Spinal segment and root involved	*Area of referred deep pain*	*Muscle weakness and wasting*	*Reduced or absent reflexes*
L2	Upper buttock, groin	Hip flexors, adductors	
L3	Mid-buttock, anterior aspect of thigh	Hip flexors, adductors Quadriceps	Knee
L4	Lower buttock, round lateral aspect of thigh to anterior aspect of knee	Quadriceps Tibialis anterior	Knee
L5	Lower buttock, lateral aspect of thigh and calf	Tibialis posterior Peronei Toe extensors	Ankle
S1	Posterior aspect of thigh and calf	Calf and toe flexors Hamstrings, glutei	Ankle

from a prolapsed disc are usually aggravated by straightening up from a stooping position far more than bending, lifting weights, coughing, sneezing and straining at defaecation. The pain is eased by rest, each patient having a preferred position.

SYMPTOMS (D)

Cauda equina compression is a most serious condition. Involvement of all the nerves may occur with profound motor and sensory changes in the legs. Further, involvement of the sacral nerves will produce additional motor and sensory changes but, more importantly, sphincter disturbances with retention of urine and faeces. Similar cauda equina symptoms may appear slowly with a spinal tumour or with spinal stenosis. In spinal stenosis, which is due to developmental or bony changes reducing the space available for the spinal cord, the compression symptoms may be exercise-related and may improve with rest, suggesting a vascular component to the symptoms which is not present.

Involvement of individual spinal joints, ligaments and muscles in inflammatory or traumatic processes will give rise to muscle spasm and pain in the distributions listed in Table I.

INVESTIGATION AND TREATMENT OF LUMBAR SPINE LESIONS

The physiotherapist must assess the lumbar spine in the manner described for the cervical spine. However, in the lumbar spine, psychological factors are probably more important as almost everyone has had

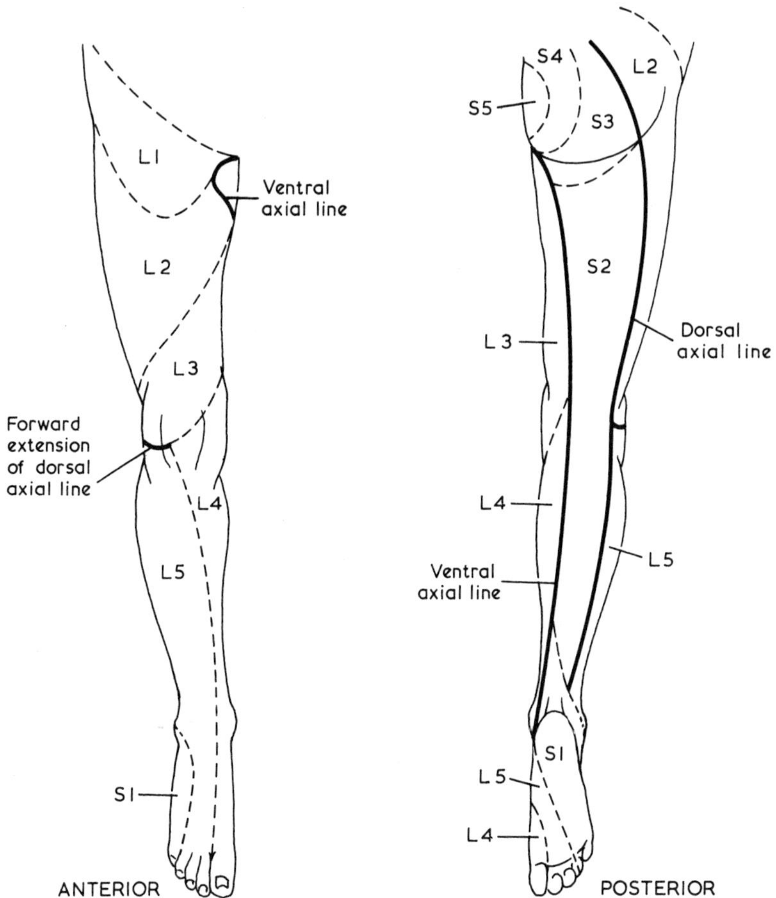

Fig. 13/2 Plan of dermatomes of lower limb

backache at some time, and most people feel that backache is an inevitable result of the stresses of modern living. Backache is a major cause of loss of work but not all cases have significant pathological lesions in their spines. In other cases the backache may be related to an injury for which the patient is claiming compensation and in most cases this will complicate assessment. In many of these patients symptoms will not finally clear until adequate compensation has been received, usually three to four years later.

Investigations

Plain radiographs must be interpreted with caution as changes in the lumbar spine are very common with increasing age and bear little relation to symptoms. Oblique rather than lateral radiographs are required to demonstrate the apophyseal joints. A myelogram may be required to localize both root and cauda equina lesions (Plate 13/7). Examination of the cerebrospinal fluid and other investigations are of little value except in excluding other conditions (Table II, p. 156). In some cases nerve conduction studies and electromyography may help to decide which nerves and muscles are involved.

Treatment

Most patients experience relief of pain with clearing of the neurological symptoms and signs if a basic programme of treatment is followed.

DRUGS

The use of full dosage of a simple analgesic (see Chapter 14), often supplemented by a muscle relaxant such as Valium. In severe cases opiates may be required.

REST

Ideally the patient should have complete bed rest, with no pillows, on a firm mattress supported by boards for a period of up to three weeks. After an acute attack, patients should be encouraged to persist with such arrangements for sleeping each night; if necessary for ever. Most patients prefer a firm bed, once they have tried it.

In most patients it is unnecessary to proceed further, since symptoms will settle after a few days of the above-mentioned treatment.

TRACTION

For patients who do not settle quickly with rest, light traction may be required. Although 1.5–2 kg (3–4 lb) is usually sufficient, some recommend much heavier traction.

MANIPULATION

Some advocate spinal manipulation. Such treatment, when undertaken by properly trained experts, is often beneficial and in sequential radiographs has been shown to reduce disc protrusion. In the face of massive central disc protrusion such manipulation can be very dangerous. Patients must be X-rayed before manipulation and it should be avoided if there is substantial root pain, bilateral root pain, possible bladder involvement, severe osteoporosis or inflammatory joint disease.

SPINAL SUPPORTS

For those patients who cannot afford the time for bed rest, a plaster jacket may produce the same results in an acute attack. It needs to be worn for at least four weeks and often for longer. Symptoms which are unchanged after two to four weeks in such a jacket must be re-assessed carefully. Such treatment should reduce the symptoms and failure to do so suggests other causes or perhaps psychological factors. In the recovery phase use of some spinal support, preferably a properly made surgical corset, is important. Many patients require to use such support intermittently over many years.

PHYSIOTHERAPY

Patients may find simple local heating a useful adjunct to an exercise programme as muscle spasm and pain will be reduced. Patients need to be taught a simple regime of spinal exercises that they can carry out not only for a few weeks while symptoms persist but also for many years in an attempt to reduce the relapse rate. At the same time patients must be taught how to lift, and to be conscious of their posture at all times.

WEIGHT REDUCTION

This may be vital if repeated attacks are to be avoided, and the physiotherapist can do much to reinforce this information.

SURGERY

Surgical decompression must be undertaken quickly in patients with cauda equina compression. This will require laminectomy and removal of the prolapsed material. In those with more chronic symptoms due to disc protrusion or osteophytes, unresponsive to other treatment, surgical removal of the compressing material may be required. In patients with very persistent symptoms, particularly if these are arising from the apophyseal joints, spinal fusion may be required. Some surgeons recommend spinal fusion as a primary procedure at the time of removal of the prolapsed material. However, these major operations must only be undertaken after careful assessment of the patient, as a disturbing number of patients continue to have symptoms despite apparently successful surgical treatment.

DIFFERENTIAL DIAGNOSIS OF BACKACHE

Although the conditions described above are the commonest causes of backache, the complaint is so frequently encountered in the general practitioner's surgery and in the orthopaedic clinic that other conditions must be remembered. It is easy for both patients and medical personnel to dismiss low backache as an inevitable consequence of the human race

Table II: Commoner causes of low backache

	Cause	*Investigations*	
		Radiological	*Other*
Congenital	Short leg		
	Sacralized L5	Diagnosis	
	Lumbarized S1	,,	
	Spondylolysis	,,	
	Spondylolisthesis	,,	
Traumatic	Prolapsed disc	Myelogram	
	Ligamentous tear		
	Fracture	Diagnosis	
Degenerative	Osteoarthrosis	Diagnosis	
	Hyperostosis	,,	
Inflammatory	Ankylosing spondylitis	Sacro-iliitis	ESR
	Reiter's disease	,,	,,
	Colitic arthritis	,,	,,
	Psoriatic arthritis	,,	,,
	Pyogenic osteomyelitis	Helpful	,, , white cell count
	Tuberculosis	,,	,, , white cell count
	Osteochondritis	Diagnosis	
Neoplastic	Secondary deposit	Helpful	Bone scan, Alkaline phosphatase
	Myeloma	,,	ESR, bone marrow
	Spinal cord tumour	Myelogram	
	Primary bone tumour	Helpful	Bone scan, Alkaline phosphatase
Metabolic	Osteoporosis	Changes	} Calcium, Phosphorus,
	Osteomalacia	often Diagnosis	} Alkaline phosphatase
	Paget's disease	Diagnosis	Alkaline phosphatase
	Pyrophosphate arthritis	,,	
Postural	Pregnancy		
	Obesity		
	Occupational		
	Hip disease	Diagnosis	
	Scoliosis	,,	
Other system disease	Gynaecological		} Local
	Renal	IVP	} Examination
	Rectal	Barium enema	}

having adopted an upright posture. Table II, above, lists some of the conditions which may cause low backache.

Vertebral fracture due to trauma, osteoporosis or neoplastic deposit is the only common cause of acute symptoms apart from acute disc protrusion and muscle or ligamentous tears. Further, there are age-related diseases in that osteochondritis (Scheuermann's disease) affects those under 15 years and neoplastic disease, osteoporosis and Paget's disease are uncommon in those under 50 years.

Assessment of low backache requires a full examination of the spine with the patient undressed, examination of the sacro-iliac and hip joints, measurement of leg length, a neurological examination and sufficient general examination to exclude the possibility of tumour (myeloma and secondary deposits from primary tumours in the lung, breast, kidney, prostate and thyroid glands are the commonest). Bowel and gynaecological diseases may cause backache and appropriate examination including rectal and vaginal examination will be required. The minimum radiographic requirements are an antero-posterior view of the lumbar spine and pelvis, a lateral view of the lumbar spine and a coned view of the lumbo-sacral junction. All patients over the age of 40 years should have a chest X-ray. The other relevant tests are shown in Table II.

Chapter 14

Drug Treatment of Joint Disease

by ALASTAIR G. MOWAT, MB, FRCP(ED)

Since the cause of most rheumatic conditions remains unknown, specific drug treatment is only available for a few diseases. These include gout, for which suitable drugs exist, and also various forms of septic arthritis in which antibiotic therapy is very effective. However, for most diseases a range of non-specific drugs can be employed, such treatment merely suppressing the symptoms and having little or no effect upon the course of the disease. It is important, therefore, to use such drugs with care and to ensure that the effects of treatment do not exceed the effects of the disease.

Patients with inflammatory joint disease complain of pain, of stiffness, particularly in the mornings and after periods of inactivity, and of aching due to muscle spasm. Drug therapy should be directed towards the cause of these symptoms, inflammation. It is rarely necessary to give muscle relaxants and the following simple analgesics are rarely helpful alone.

ANALGESICS WITH NO ANTI-INFLAMMATORY EFFECT

(paracetamol; phenacetin; codeine and dihydrocodeine; dextro-propoxyphene; pentazocine)

This group of drugs is excellent for relief of pain in osteoarthrosis and is, in general, remarkably free of side-effects, especially the gastro-intestinal side-effects which are so common with anti-inflammatory drugs. Massive overdosage of paracetamol may cause liver necrosis. The relationship between phenacetin and an important type of renal damage, renal papillary necrosis and interstitial nephritis, is suspected but has not been proved. Indeed, other drugs may be involved in this 'analgesic nephropathy', but since phenacetin is at best a poor analgesic drug it seems wisest to avoid its use. The codeine group of drugs causes constipation, which may add further discomfort and disability to the elderly arthritic. Many preparations contain two or more of these drugs in combination and several are available as soluble tablets or mixtures.

ANTI-INFLAMMATORY ANALGESIC DRUGS

Basic drug therapy of inflammatory joint disease should include an adequate dose of one of this group of drugs. It is helpful to consider them as either minor anti-inflammatory drugs, propionic acids, or major drugs, salicylates, indomethacin, pyrazoles.

Propionic acids

This group of drugs, many of which have been introduced recently, includes fenoprofen, ibuprofen, ketoprofen and naproxen. They combine minor anti-inflammatory properties with a striking absence of side-effects, particularly those associated with the gastro-intestinal tract, and are thus well tolerated by most patients, a claim which cannot be made for salicylates. They are worth trying in full dosage in most patients with inflammatory conditions. A response to treatment can be expected in one week. Since patients, perhaps surprisingly, can respond quite differently to each of these chemically similar drugs, a failure to respond to one should not lead to the immediate dismissal of the whole group. However, genuine failure to respond means that one of the major anti-inflammatory drugs must be used.

Salicylates

The dose must be adequate (3 to 5 g per day) in divided doses every three to four hours. Blood levels of salicylate of 20 to 30 mg per cent are satisfactory, higher levels being associated with tinnitus, nausea and vomiting. The main problem with aspirin is indigestion. The availability of the drug in soluble form (Solprin), combined with antacid (aloxiprin) and enteric coated avoids this problem in many patients. Other preparations combine aspirin and paracetamol to reduce indigestion (Safapryn) and benorylate has further advantages in being available as a mixture only requiring twice daily dosage. Many associate the indigestion with peptic ulceration and gastric bleeding. There is little evidence that aspirin causes peptic ulceration but it may exacerbate the symptoms of pre-existing ulceration. There is certainly a moderate increase in gastro-intestinal blood loss with aspirin but this is not associated with anaemia in most patients. However, a very small number of patients are hypersensitive to aspirin and in them the drug may produce massive gastro-intestinal bleeding.

Indomethacin

A dose of 100 to 150 mg per day is usually required but to avoid or reduce the side-effects of headache, dizziness, confusion and indigestion, initial dosage should be 75 mg per day. The dose can be increased at the rate of 25 mg (one capsule) each week. A large bedtime dose (100 mg) given either orally or by suppository is very effective in reducing morning stiffness. Interestingly, the suppository route rarely reduces indigestion and thus has little advantage over oral treatment, particularly in those whose disability makes insertion of the suppository difficult.

Pyrazoles

Phenylbutazone is effective in oral doses of 300 to 400 mg per day. However, to the usual side-effect of indigestion is added fluid retention and bone marrow suppression. The marrow damage may lead to a serious reduction in the number of granulocytes and red cells, and occasional blood tests and a careful watch for intercurrent infection are necessary. Because of fluid retention the drug should be used carefully in the elderly and in those with heart and renal disease. Oxyphenbutazone and other metabolites have no advantage over phenylbutazone.

Although many drugs in this group cause indigestion, it must be remembered that it does not follow that an individual patient will react to every drug in this way.

New preparations are appearing regularly, the aim of the pharmaceutical companies being to produce a drug as effective as aspirin but without side-effects, preferably with a twice daily dose.

In using the anti-inflammatory drugs it is important to ensure that an adequate dosage is being given and that the patient is taking the prescribed dose. Further, patients often ask for different and more effective drugs as a means of introducing other problems. Such problems usually reflect the patients' concern about the effect of the disease upon their lives. It is wise to remember that many patients may require a lifetime of treatment and with few drugs available, good reasons are needed to change treatment.

GOLD AND CHLOROQUINE COMPOUNDS

The use of these anti-inflammatory drugs with no specific analgesic effect is usually confined to rheumatoid arthritis and they are considered to have some suppressive effect upon the disease. They should not replace an adequate dose of one of the aforementioned drugs and should not be used together.

Gold

Gold is given as a soluble salt by intramuscular injection. The usual dose is 50 mg per week and little effect will be shown until 500 mg have been given. If the patient has side-effects or fails to respond to a total dose of one gram, treatment should be abandoned. However, if a clear response occurs, either the dose may be reduced or the interval between injections increased, usually to one month. At present such treatment is continued indefinitely. The side-effects include:

(1) albuminuria occasionally leading to serious renal damage;

(2) skin rash;

(3) mouth ulceration and gastro-enteritis;

(4) bone marrow suppression with serious reduction in numbers of granulocytes, platelets or all marrow elements.

With such side-effects, detected by questioning the patient and testing the urine and blood at each injection, the drug must be stopped. It may be necessary to accelerate its excretion with dimercaprol or penicillamine.

Chloroquine

The response to an oral dose of 300 mg per day of a chloroquine compound is delayed four to eight weeks. The serious toxic effects occur in the eye, where corneal deposits will cause irreversible blurring of vision, but the rare retinal damage is difficult to detect. Intermittent treatment reduces the risk of these ocular side-effects.

Physicians tend to favour either gold or chloroquine, and each has advantages over the other.

CORTICOSTEROIDS

The effectiveness of these drugs has been rather forgotten in the concern about their very real side-effects. However, the drugs have marked anti-inflammatory activity, even if the daily dose is kept below 7.5 mg of prednisolone or its equivalent in other preparations, and the side-effects are then much less severe and longer delayed than many imagine.

The indications for the use of these drugs must always be carefully considered, and the diseases in which they may be needed are indicated in Chapters 5, 6 and 7. The smallest effective dose should be used and every opportunity taken to review the dose. There are four clear indications for the use of corticosteroids in rheumatoid arthritis.

(1) In older patients with acute disease, since the benign disease can be rapidly controlled without resorting to complicated treatment programmes.

(2) In patients of any age who must keep active for a year or 18 months

because of work or examination commitments. However, both patient and physician must understand that it may be difficult to reduce or stop the drug after the planned course of treatment.

(3) Severe morning stiffness can be controlled by 5 mg of prednisolone at bedtime.

(4) In patients with severe and unremitting disease. Difficulties arise over the individual interpretation of severe, unremitting disease, and at least one period of in-patient treatment should be tried before resorting to increasing doses of these drugs.

Side-effects of corticosteroids

These include:

(1) Peptic ulceration with dyspepsia, perforation and haemorrhage. The dyspepsia may be reduced by using enteric coated or soluble preparations.

(2) Osteoporosis leading to vertebral collapse and bone fracture.

(3) Salt retention with oedema, moon face and hypertension.

(4) Liability to infection.

(5) Skin thinning and bruising.

(6) Muscle wasting and avascular necrosis of bone, particularly the femoral heads.

(7) Inability to respond to stress since the normal hormonal balance of the pituitary-adrenal axis has been upset.

Corticotrophin

(ACTH and Synacthen)

These preparations, which are usually given by daily intramuscular injection, have the advantage of fewer gastric side-effects and in addition they do not impair the ability to respond to stress. The injections usually prove inconvenient to any but in-patients.

LOCAL CORTICOSTEROID THERAPY

Local injections of a corticosteroid preparation into joints or surrounding soft tissues can be helpful in controlling inflammation. Such injections carry the risk of superinfection, a crystal reaction and bone necrosis, but these risks are minimized if a simple, clean, non-touch technique is employed and clear indications for their use are recognized. These include:

(1) Intra-articular injections for the patient with one or two inflamed joints.

(2) Tendinitis or tendon nodules, although the benefit with nodules may be transitory and surgical clearance eventually required (see also Chapter 15).

(3) Capsular and ligamentous involvement (see also Chapter 15).

(4) As a temporary measure in the treatment of median or other nerve compression syndromes (see also Chapter 15).

Contra-indications to the use of local corticosteroids include:

(1) Uncertain diagnosis.

(2) Proven or possible infection in the joint.

(3) Severe joint damage, since they will be ineffective and may increase joint damage.

(4) Severe local osteoporosis since this may be exaggerated.

(5) A neurological deficit: because there is a risk of producing Charcot-type arthropathy (page 73).

IMMUNOSUPPRESSIVE DRUGS

Although it is convenient to group such drugs as azathioprine, chlorambucil, cyclophosphamide, methotrexate and penicillamine under one heading, they probably act in very different ways. The effect of these drugs in rheumatoid arthritis and other connective tissue diseases is being carefully studied in several centres. The exact mode of action of these drugs is unknown, but the studies show that the drugs can reduce the activity of the disease and often enable steroid dosage to be reduced to safer levels. Penicillamine may prove to be the most effective drug in the treatment of vasculitis. The side-effects of these drugs are serious, the most common being bone marrow suppression. At present these drugs should be used with caution and only in those patients with severe unremitting disease.

ANTIDEPRESSANTS

Although any chronic disease can be expected to produce depression, the extent of the depression reflects the patient's understanding of the disease and its likely effects upon his employment, domestic and social life. Thus antidepressants are rarely required if the medical team has done its work properly. It is not considered that there is any particular psychological state (e.g. rheumatoid personality) either as a cause or effect of joint disease.

Chapter 15

Non-Articular Pain

by CHRISTINE M. MARSHALL, MCSP, DIP.TP

The most common reason people seek medical aid is for the relief of certain symptoms, but it should be borne in mind that there are sometimes other reasons as well – such as the need for help with a disability, reassurance, sympathy or the desire for compensation following some specific incident. The source of their symptoms may be articular or non-articular. For the purposes of this chapter,. structures which are not of bone or cartilage will be assumed to be non-articular. Therefore, pure articular conditions such as arthritis, arthroses and fractures will not be considered, but rather some of the more common non-articular lesions which are the cause of the patient's chief symptom, pain.

EXAMINATION OF THE PATIENT

In this scientific age it is the duty of all physiotherapists to examine their patients thoroughly so that a clear picture is obtained of the symptoms, which is then matched with comparable signs. There can be no substitute for this routine accurate examination, for without it there is no means of applying treatment to the faulty structures, except on a 'hit or miss' basis, or of assessing progress, be it improvement or deterioration. The same basic pattern should be used for the extremities as for the spine – namely subjective and objective (see Appendix, p. 176).

When the patient is first referred for treatment it is often easiest to seek a clear picture of his present symptoms prior to the overall history of the condition. The precise area and behaviour of pain being known, the irritability of the condition can be estimated, so that during the objective examination there is neither over- nor under-examination of relevant structures and exacerbation of pain is thus minimized, but comparable signs are not overlooked. The character of the pain described by the patient can also be helpful. True muscle pain is always diffuse and is often referred, with distribution following a spinal segmental pattern and associated with referred tenderness of the deep structures, while periosteum, fascia, tendon sheaths and skin give accurately localized pain. Functional limitations of the patient should be ascertained and the dominance of pain or stiffness imposing them noted.

The objective examination should be subdivided into active and passive movements. Initially general posture is observed and obvious muscle wasting looked for. Then all muscles and joints underlying, or able to refer pain to the area of pain complained of, and therefore previously ascertained by questioning the patient, must be examined. Movements that reproduce or alter the symptoms are noted. If movements are found to be limited the range obtainable should be measured and recorded; if they appear to be full and painless then a moderate degree of pressure is applied at the limit of range in order to confirm that this is so. During active movement both contractile structures (muscle) and inert structures (joint capsule, ligaments, bursae) move, whereas true passive movement is produced by an outside force so that no muscle contraction occurs. Pain from contractile structures occurs on contraction so that it may be necessary to confirm a muscle lesion by strongly resisted isometric contractions – thus eliminating inert structures. Pain from inert structures occurs on stretching or pressure and it must be decided from the pattern of painful passive movement obtained whether all the inert structures limiting movement at a joint are involved (i.e. a diffuse capsular lesion) or only a small part of them (e.g. a ligament). The examination should not be limited to passive physiological movements but should also include the accessory movements obtainable in the joints under consideration. For a fuller account of this, reference should be made to *Peripheral Manipulation* by G. D. Maitland. Any muscle weakness should be noted, as should any alteration of normal tone. Palpation will reveal any localized warmth which will indicate an active lesion, and any areas of localized tenderness, thickening or swelling.

THE SHOULDER AREA

There are a vast number of causes of pain in the shoulder. The origins may be due to intrinsic disease of the gleno-humeral joint, pathology in the periarticular structures or distant spine, chest or visceral sources. Initial examination including mapping out the area of pain, as already suggested, will give a useful guide as to where the source lies. When the patient is complaining of predominantly shoulder pain rather than neck-shoulder-radiating pains, it is usually indicative of pathology in the gleno-humeral joint or its periarticular structures.

Although the shoulder should be regarded clinically as an area rather than a single joint, due to the number of patients whose pain does arise from some distant structure, only the most common local non-articular causes will be considered here.

Apart from acute traumatic lesions, 90 per cent of painful disabilities of the shoulder are due to acute or chronic tendinitis and bursitis, lesions of the musculo-tendinous cuff and adhesive capsulitis. Arthritis of the shoulder joint causes less than 5 per cent of painful shoulders, apart from patients suffering from generalized arthropathies (Zanca). The reason for this is due to the anatomical arrangement, in that the gleno-humeral joint depends for stability largely on the tendons that surround it rather than the shallow glenoid cavity and remarkably loose joint capsule. The long head of biceps tends to hold the humeral head into the glenoid cavity while the capsule is strengthened by the flattened expansions superiorly of supraspinatus, anteriorly of subscapularis and posteriorly by infraspinatus and teres minor, or in other words, the rotator cuff. It is also strengthened below by the long head of triceps – although not so closely as in other parts of the rotator cuff, as here capsule and muscle are separated by the axillary nerve and posterior circumflex humeral vessels. Therefore, this inferior part of the capsule, which on abduction of the arm is tightly stretched over the head of the humerus, may be subjected to the greatest strain.

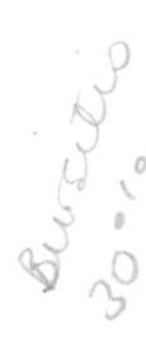

Degenerative tendinitis

Progressive degenerative changes in the structure of the rotator cuff have been noted, even in people with no symptoms, particularly after middle age. The supraspinatus tendon is most frequently affected, probably due to the position of its insertion on the highest part of the tuberosity of the humerus. This renders it particularly subject to minor trauma as it impinges on the acromion and coraco-acromial ligament during abduction with the arm medially rotated. Due to this mechanical stress and strain, and consequent low-grade inflammation, degeneration becomes more marked, the tendon shows signs of thinning and weakness and it becomes stretched – thus being more likely to be caught as the humerus swings under the coraco-acromial arch. The subacromial (subdeltoid) bursa, because of its situation, is also frequently involved in this type of lesion and may shrink with varying degrees of fibrosis. Bony changes may develop later due to the gradual degenerative process. These may take the form of sclerosis, eburnation or minute cyst formation seen in the head of the humerus (Bateman).

The patient complains initially of a catching type of discomfort in the shoulder, of insidious onset with no precipitating incident, particularly on lifting the arm. Limitation of movement gradually occurs. The pain grows into a persistent gnawing ache radiating down the outside of the arm and forearm, which causes difficulty in sleeping and from which he can gain no relief. On examination about 70° active abduction is possible without pain. When looked at more closely there is often found to be a painful arc of movement between 70 and 120° abduction (similarly in adduction) and usually more pronounced on active than passive movement. Obviously some structure must be pinched in this position, the supraspinatus tendon being the most common but also the sub-acromial bursa, and tendons of infraspinatus or subscapularis being other possibilities. In order to differentiate, it will be found that resisted abduction is painful if supraspinatus is the cause, resisted lateral rotation if infraspinatus and resisted medial rotation if subscapularis. Should the bursa be the inflamed area, then the painful arc is often the only sign found, isometric contractions proving painless. The longer the lesion has been neglected, the more likely the shoulder to have become frozen, probably due to general disinclination to use the painful arm, and thus limitation of movements may be found.

AIMS OF TREATMENT

These should be the relief of pain and preservation of joint movement so that 'freezing' is avoided. In order to relieve pain the affected tendon or bursa may be injected with local anaesthetic and/or corticosteroids, and appropriate drugs may be prescribed (Chapter 14). The physiotherapist may apply ice to the whole of the painful shoulder and shoulder girdle area by means of an ice pack, or frequently changed damp towels with ice fragments clinging to them, in order both to relieve pain and to obtain muscle relaxation. It should be remembered that in order to be effective the ice must cover the affected muscles from origin to insertion. This should be done prior to careful exercise designed to maintain and improve range, but avoiding movements that are known to cause pain. Pendular movements with a weight of approximately 1 kg tied to the wrist and the patient comfortably positioned so that the trunk is horizontal (i.e. either prone lying or forward leaning) are often found helpful at first, especially if the patient is given time to relax in this position prior to any attempt at movement. Pure gleno-humeral movement with a minimum of effort is thus obtained. Progression is by way of free active movements and then, if possible, resisted work in order to build up general strength in unaffected muscles, but all the time avoiding as far as possible that part of the range which causes pain. Localized ultrasound, pulsed in order to avoid any heating effect, to the site of the lesion is sometimes found to be of value.

If the condition is at the early stage of localized tendinitis with no limitation of movement, massage in the form of deep transverse frictions to the offending portion of tendon should be accurately applied and the previously described treatments will be unnecessary. Treatment for frozen shoulder is described separately (see page 170).

Calcific tendinitis

Calcified deposits may occur in the tendon substance of supraspinatus and less frequently in that of infraspinatus, subscapularis and teres minor. The reason for the change in tendon substance is still not established although it is possible that abnormal ageing of collagen fibres may initiate the calcification mechanism. Deposits may be present for years, remaining within the tendon, under no tension and without causing trouble, so that if discovered by chance on X-ray for some unrelated condition, they should be ignored. However, symptoms are caused if the tendon is irritated so that the deposit enlarges under pressure within the tendon and so impinges under the coraco-acromial arch during abduction. This may occur as an acute episode of rapid onset, with constant acute pain inhibiting sleep and accentuated by any arm movement, so that there is gross apparent limitation of movement due to pain and muscle spasm. During this stage the shoulder may be warm and swollen. When subacute, the pain is referred to the area of deltoid insertion and the limitation will be found to be an arc of about 70 to 100° abduction. There is little relation between the size of the deposit and the severity of symptoms. Inflammatory changes may also develop in the subacromial bursa. Occasionally spontaneous rupture of the deposit into the bursa may occur, relieving the tension in the tendon and so the symptoms.

TREATMENT

In the acute stage this is initially conservative, aiming to relieve pain by the use of pain-killing drugs and resting the arm in a sling. However, even at this stage, joint range should be maintained as far as possible by the use of ice prior to daily assisted active movements in lying. With improvement (i.e. less pain) exercises may be progressed by frequency and change of starting position and finally by the use of resistance. If improvement does not occur rapidly, the continuing acute pain predisposes to frozen shoulder, so that surgical removal of the deposit, which provides dramatic relief, becomes the treatment of choice. Following this, movement should be begun as soon as pain allows and exercises continued until normal range and power is achieved in the shoulder.

Ruptures of the rotator cuff

It has already been stated that progressive degenerative changes are known to occur in the rotator cuff structures. This may lead to gradual thinning of the cuff, which eventually wears through, or some minor incident such as a fall on the outstretched hand may precipitate it. Alternatively rupture may occur following dislocation of the shoulder. The patient experiences an initial sharp pain in the shoulder and the arm feels limp and useless. This is followed by dull aching of the joint area which steadily increases so that interference with sleep occurs. Pain is usually the predominant complaint and it may be referred down the arm and to the neck. Joint stiffness develops gradually due to continued inability to lift the arm. If the rupture is only partial, then the signs are less definite; pain is less but there is some loss of power and range of abduction.

TREATMENT

Surgical repair may be considered if the tear is very large but the majority of patients obtain satisfactory use of the arm with good conservative treatment. The pain is mainly due to the inflammatory reaction in the torn cuff and subacromial bursa, and for this reason the arm should be rested at the beginning of treatment. However, finger, wrist and elbow exercises together with isometric work for deltoid and non-painful muscles of the cuff, should be commenced immediately, followed by pendular movements as soon as possible. As the pain subsides assisted active movements are introduced and gradually progressed to resisted exercises using normal patterns of movement. It is important to strengthen the accessory muscles of the shoulder, such as biceps and triceps, in order to replace the now inefficient cuff. It is thought that in some patients good range of movement in the shoulder is due to adhesions between the deltoid muscle and thickened subacromial bursa which is also adherent to the rotator cuff especially about the site of rupture (Meviaser).

The biceps tendon

The long head of biceps arises by a long tendon from the supraglenoid tubercle within the capsule of the shoulder joint. It arches over the head of the humerus and emerges from the joint by passing behind the transverse humeral ligament. It is this ligament that is responsible for retaining it in the bicipital groove, and should it rupture, usually due to injury, the tendon will slip in and out of the groove during movement and a painful snapping sensation will be felt. There will also be an associated capsular tear. Inflammatory changes and therefore pain are thus initiated and the patient becomes unwilling to use the arm, the capsule contracts and limitation of movement occurs. On palpation the tendon is usually tender, particularly over the bicipital groove. Conservative treatment should consist of avoiding movements where the tendon is under strong tension, particularly in abduction and external rotation. Pure gleno-humeral movement may be retained by pendular movements of the weighted arm as previously described, first taking care to obtain good relaxation of the arm and shoulder girdle by allowing it to hang in the dependent position for at least ten minutes. As pain subsides, so muscle power of the arm may be built up with progressive resistance exercises, but still avoiding those movements that put the tendon under stong tension.

Degenerative changes may occur during middle age similar to those of the rotator cuff. The tendon frays and the synovial sheath becomes inflamed. On examination there is often pain on resisted flexion of the elbow with supination and tenderness to palpation over the tendon. Symptoms may be precipitated by jerky lifting with outstretched arms or unaccustomed exercises such as the first game of tennis of the season.

Treatment should aim at reducing the inflammation of the sheath, preventing adhesion formation and maintaining full range of shoulder movements. Thus the tendon may be injected with local anaesthetic and/or corticosteroids (see also Chapter 14) and then gentle active exercises should be instituted. Alternatively localized transverse frictions are often beneficial.

Complete rupture of the biceps tendon may occur following trauma. A bulge is noticed in the front of the arm and pressure over the bicipital groove is painful. Elbow flexion is only slightly weak, but the biceps is noted to be ineffective. In most cases, general strengthening of the arm will give good functional use. However, if the patient is young and needs the arm specifically to earn his living, then surgery may be necessary.

Frozen shoulder (adhesive capsulitis)

This is a term that is widely used to describe a syndrome resulting from many diverse pathologies. Although there is a small group where the cause is idiopathic, a frozen shoulder generally results as a reaction to immobility of the arm due to pain, fear or abnormal muscle tone. It is noticed that disuse of the arm in a tense, over-anxious patient with a low pain threshold predisposes to this syndrome, and that older patients are more susceptible. It can thus be appreciated that any of the previously described conditions could initiate a frozen shoulder, as well as referred pain from cardiac, gall bladder, diaphragm or cervical spine lesions.

The patient will complain of pain in the shoulder region which may radiate up to the neck and down the arm. The shoulder is stiff, usually progressively so, and movement is limited in all ranges although this may vary according to the aetiology. The normally loose glenohumeral joint capsule becomes thickened and contracted, losing its folds inferiorly as they become glued together. The synovial membrane becomes stuck to the articular cartilage, the subacromial bursa may shrink and surrounding muscles show protective spasm due to pain, and therefore waste.

TREATMENT

There is no doubt that the most important part of treatment is preventive by discovering and effectively treating the primary cause as early as possible, and explaining to the patient the importance of maintaining the range of movement. In the small group of patients where the cause is idiopathic, fortunately, the condition usually recovers spontaneously although this may take up to two years.

However, a large number of patients with frozen shoulders of varying degrees from varying causes are referred for physiotherapy. The *aim of treatment* must be to relieve pain and improve the range of movement so that they have as good and functional an arm as possible. One effective method of treatment is that suggested by G. D. Maitland using the appropriate grade and combination of accessory and physiological passive movements according to whether pain or stiffness dominate. Alternatively, there are many advocates for a regime using ice and relaxation techniques, which may be by means of suspension or pendular exercises, or those of proprioceptive neuromuscular facilitation techniques. Once pain is subsiding and range of movement improving then appropriate muscle strengthening techniques may be incorporated in the treatment, remembering that they should only be used in the pain-free range available. Sometimes manipulation under anaesthetic is undertaken in the later stages and when this procedure is used it is important that the physiotherapist should be in the theatre to observe the range of movement achieved, for it will be her job to encourage and assist the patient to maintain it afterwards, despite initial soreness.

For use of analgesics and/or local injections of anaesthetic and corticosteroid, see also Chapter 14.

THE ELBOW AREA

Tennis elbow

This is probably one of the most common causes of pain at the lateral side of the elbow. Differential diagnosis must be made from referred pain from cervical spondylosis. The condition is usually found in people over 30 years of age and it is caused by repetitive movements at the elbow region, especially pronation and supination or forced extension, not necessarily by playing tennis.

The onset of pain is usually gradual, accentuated by the use of the arm and improved with rest. Radiation of pain to the muscles of the forearm may occur and, if severe, will inhibit gripping. On examination there is pain over the lateral epicondylar area of the humerus on active wrist extension, particularly with radial deviation and with the elbow in extension. Passive elbow extension, especially in adduction, is limited in the last few degrees if examined carefully, with an end feel of elastic resistance. An area of tenderness can usually be accurately located, the most common site being over the lateral ligament or slightly anterior to it.

There have been many different views expressed as to the pathology of this lesion. Mostly it is thought to be due to minor strain in the region of the common extensor origin and, many authorities now say, of extensor carpi radialis brevis in particular. It has been suggested that a small number of resistant cases could be due to an entrapment neuropathy of the radial nerve as it passes over the fibrous edge of extensor carpi radialis brevis and then goes deep into the supinator muscle. When the extensor origin tightens it can compress the radial nerve and thus the symptoms are reproduced by extension and radial deviation of the wrist with elbow extension.

TREATMENT

Initially treatment is usually by injection of corticosteroid mixed with local anaesthetic, into the site of maximum tenderness (see also Chapter 14). Repeated injections may be required. Patients referred for physiotherapy are most effectively treated by deep transverse frictions localized to the most painful part of the tendon, usually for 15 to 20 minutes twice weekly. Ultrasonics, again to the appropriate area, have sometimes been found to be of value. All these measures should be accompanied by rest of the extensor muscles of the forearm. Heat and other forms of massage give only transitory relief. Should these conservative measures fail, surgical treatment may be required.

Golfer's elbow

This is a less common but comparable condition to tennis elbow occurring at the medial epicondylar region of the humerus. The lesion occurs at the common flexor tendon origin at the medial epicondyle and on examination the pain can be reproduced by resisted flexion of the wrist with the elbow in extension. *Treatment* is by local injection of corticosteroid or localized deep transverse frictions to the affected area (see also Chapter 14).

PERIPHERAL ENTRAPMENT NEUROPATHIES

Pressure exerted upon a peripheral nerve gives rise to certain well-known symptoms, namely pins and needles which is then followed by pain, numbness and muscle weakness if the pressure is constant and unrelieved. This may be due to mechanical irritation, trauma, or some indeterminate cause which leads to local inflammation and therefore swelling and thus compression.

Carpal tunnel syndrome

This common condition is due to compression of the median nerve as it passes with the flexor tendons between the flexor retinaculum and the bones of the carpus. Often there is no apparent cause but it may be associated with trauma, such as a Colles' fracture; or any condition which reduces the size of the carpal tunnel such as arthritis or fluid retention in connective tissue as sometimes occurs, for example, in pregnancy.

The characteristic history is of gradual onset of tingling and pain, followed by numbness of the first three fingers, which may spread up the arm. In advanced cases there is slight weakness of the muscles of the thenar eminence, appropriate median sensory impairment and sometimes some autonomic symptoms in the form of painful swelling of the fingers, discoloration and alteration in sweating. The symptoms are often worse at night, disturbing sleep, and the patient may state that some relief is gained by hanging the arm over the side of the bed. Diagnostically the symptoms can often be reproduced by firmly flexing the wrist for one minute (wrist extension may also be used but the results are not so reliable) or pressure over the flexor retinaculum, thus distinguishing it from referred pain from other causes such as cervical spondylosis and thoracic outlet syndrome. If electrodiagnosis is used there is conduction delay in the median nerve.

TREATMENT

This is aimed at reducing the inflammatory reaction and the physiotherapist may be asked to make a splint to rest the wrist in the neutral position at night – this is often diagnostic in the relief it provides. Injection of a suitable corticosteroid preparation is also often successful (see also Chapter 14). Should these measures fail the flexor retinaculum is divided surgically and the nerve decompressed.

Morton's metatarsalgia

This is due to pinching of one of the digital nerves just before it divides to supply the adjacent sides of two toes, most commonly the third and fourth. With continued pressure the nerve becomes oedematous and fibrous thickening, or a neuroma, occurs. There may be a primary acute traumatic cause or it may be due to abnormal hyperextension at the metatarsophalangeal joint due to rheumatoid arthritis, congenital deformity or constant wearing of high-heeled shoes that incline the forefoot down and force hyperextension of the toes. The latter may account for the fact that it is found more commonly in women than men. The patient complains of episodic acute pain in the toes on walking, necessitating removal of the shoe and rubbing the foot. At first there are no symptoms between episodes but with continued pressure dull pain in the metatarsal area may develop. On palpation between the appropriate metatarsal heads, acute pain may be elicited.

TREATMENT

Conservative treatment consists of choosing correctly fitting shoes and wearing a metatarsal pad to prevent hyperextension of the metatarsophalangeal joint. A metatarsal bar may be attached to the sole of the shoe. Faradic footbaths and exercises do not usually help. If no relief is gained from conservative measures then surgical excision of the neuroma is performed.

Other less frequently encountered entrapment neuropathies occur, such as compression of the posterior tibial nerve beneath the flexor retinaculum below the medial malleolus of the ankle (tarsal tunnel syndrome) and of the anterior interosseous nerve at the point where it is given off from the median nerve as it passes into the forearm between the two heads of pronator teres (pronator syndrome). Treatment is either conservative by corticosteroid injection or surgical decompression. (See also Chapter 14.)

'FIBROSITIS'

Many patients complain of pain at sites of tendon insertion, bony prominences or in major muscle masses, and while in most instances careful examination will reveal the source, there are some in whom exhaustive investigation may fail to show any cause. 'Fibrositis' is a vague term describing a condition of pain and stiffness in myofascial structures which is often temporary. The areas involved are usually related to some moving part under stress. There seems little doubt that there are times in a person's life such as bereavement, the menopause, or depression when the threshold of complaint about such pains is lowered. Contributory causes are legion, but common irritants are fatigue, worry, chronic illness and under-nourishment, and these are often augmented by damp, cold or draught. It has been said that these patients keep their muscles as tense as their minds and it may be that this is reaction to chronic strain, poor posture or repeated occupational stress. The most common regions complained of are the neck and shoulders, lumbar and gluteal regions.

On palpation, particularly if the condition is acute, there is usually some muscle spasm as well as general tenderness with certain painful trigger points. These may be nodules which are fibro-fatty or fibrous tissue, and sometimes herniate through the superficial fascia. The reason for the nodules is obscure. The muscles may feel thickened, though exploration has shown little pathological change, but if the condition is of long standing the muscles are more likely to feel stringy and atonic.

TREATMENT

This is aimed at relieving pain, improving the circulation, obtaining muscular relaxation and then strengthening the appropriate muscle groups and good physiotherapy plays an important part. The patient should be fully supported in a comfortable position while some form of superficial heat (such as infra-red irradiation or hot pad) is applied. This should be followed by massage and then isometric postural exercises which may be progressed to resisted exercises later. The actual course of treatment should be short but the patient should be carefully instructed as to the value of home heat (hot bath, shower or lamp) and continuing the exercises. For use of analgesic drugs see Chapter 14.

APPENDIX

Examination for Non-Articular Pain in the Shoulder Region

A. SUBJECTIVE EXAMINATION
(by questioning)

(1) Map out on body chart precise areas of pain complained of. Indicate types of pain and worst area(s). Show any areas of altered sensation.

(2) Note factors exacerbating and relieving pain. For how long?

(3) Is sleep interfered with? Can the arm be slept on at night? State of symptoms on rising in morning.

(4) Do symptoms impose any functional limitations?

(5) Have recent X-rays been taken? Which areas?

(6) Is general health good? (So eliminate cardiac, gall bladder or diaphragmatic causes.)

(7) What tablets are being taken for this or any other condition?

(8) History, i.e. onset and course followed. Now improving, deteriorating or static? Previous history?

(9) Any past history of similar symptoms? How treated and result?

B. OBJECTIVE EXAMINATION
(by testing and observation)

(1) Posture – head on neck, spine, shoulder levels. Wasting of arm. Localized thickening or swelling.

(2) Routine check of all neck movements.

(3) Active shoulder movements. Note limitations and range/pain relationships.

(4) Resisted isometric contractions of all muscles underlying areas of pain charted or able to refer pain to these areas.

(5) Muscle power of above muscles.

(6) Passive physiological shoulder movements – pure movement (e.g. abduction of shoulder joint with scapula fixed). Note range/pain relationship.

(7) Passive accessory gleno-humeral movements. Check those of the sterno-clavicular and acromio-clavicular joints.

(8) Check elbow movements.

(9) Check 'case notes' for reports and relevant tests.

C. PLAN APPROPRIATE TREATMENT

REFERENCES

Bateman, J. E. *The Shoulder and Neck.* W. B. Saunders (London), 1972.

Boyle, J. A. and Buchanan, W. W. *Clinical Rheumatology.* Blackwell (Oxford), 1971.

Cailliet, R. *Shoulder Pain.* F. A. Davis Co. (Philadelphia), 1966.

Copeman, W. S. C. (ed.) *Textbook of the Rheumatic Diseases.* Churchill Livingstone (London), 4th ed. 1969.

Cyriax, J. *Textbook of Orthopaedic Medicine Vol. I.* Baillière Tindall (London), 5th ed. 1969.

Gray's Anatomy (ed. Warwick, R.). Longman (London), 35th ed. 1973.

Johnson, E. W., Hughes, A. C. and Haase, K. H. 'Carpal Tunnel Syndrome – A Review.' *Archives of Physical Medicine & Rehabilitation*, **43**, 420–5, 1962.

Kapell, H. P. and Thompson, W. A. L. *Peripheral Entrapment Neuropathies.* William & Wilkins Co. (Baltimore), 1963.

Kellgren, J. H. 'Observations on Referred Pain Arising from Muscle.' *Clinical Science*, **3**, 175, 1938.

Kellgren, J. H. 'Preliminary Account of Referred Pains Arising from Muscle.' *British Medical Journal*, **1**, 325, 1938.

Lewis, Sir T. 'Suggestions Relating to the Study of Somatic Pain.' *British Medical Journal*, **1**, 321, 1938.

Maitland, G. D. *Peripheral Manipulation.* Butterworth (London), 1970.

Mason, M. and Currey, H. L. F. (eds.) *An Introduction to Clinical Rheumatology.* Lippincott (Philadelphia), 1970.

Melville, I. D. 'The Differential Diagnosis of Nerve Compression Syndrome in the Hand and Arm.' *The Hand*, **4** (2), 1972.

Mennell, J. McM. *Joint Pain.* Little Brown & Co. (Boston), 1964.

Meviaser, J. S. 'Ruptures of the Rotator Cuff of the Shoulder.' *Archives Surgery*, **102**, 483–5, 1971.

Roles, N. C. and Maudsley, R. H. 'Radial Tunnel Syndrome.' *Journal of Bone and Joint Surgery*, **54B** (3), 1972.

Stewart, I. M. 'Nerve Entrapment in the Upper Limb.' *The Hand*, **4** (2), 1972.

Stoddard, A. *Manual of Osteopathic Practice.* Hutchinson (London), 1969.

Wiles, P. and Sweetman, R. *Essentials of Orthopaedics.* Churchill Livingstone (London), 1965.

Zanca, P. 'Shoulder Pain – Involvement of the Acromio-clavicular Joint.' *American Journal of Roentgenology*, **112**, 493, 1971.

PART III

Physiotherapy for Children

BARBARA KENNEDY, MCSP

Chapter 16

Physiotherapy For Children – I

development – the importance of play – physiotherapy

In working with children the physiotherapist can expect a wide and varied case-load. The range includes neurological, respiratory, orthopaedic and rheumatic conditions as well as mental subnormality and multiple handicaps. That paediatrics has become a specialty of physiotherapy is due more to the differences between children and adults than to the actual conditions, some of which are specific to childhood, while others closely resemble the adult forms. It is the study of the child's basic development, his patterns of learning and behaviour which provide the necessary framework on which to build up physical treatment for any particular condition. Observation of normal children of all ages will reveal a wealth of information which can be utilized when dealing with those less fortunate.

One natural advantage which the physiotherapist can put to good use is the child's enjoyment of movement. This is apparent from the earliest days when the baby learns to move his arms and legs, to play with his hands, and to kick off his blankets. It is seen in the toddler who is never still, and quite tireless in practising his new-found skill of walking. In the playground children can be seen running and jumping and twirling for no other purpose than the pleasure it gives them.

The first part of this Section will be devoted to outlining the principles on which the treatment is based, under the headings of: (i) Early development; (ii) the Importance of play; (iii) Physiotherapy, including the introduction of child and parents to the physiotherapy department, general management, and the role of parents in treatment.

The second part of this Section (Chapter 17) describes some specific conditions. These are: (i) Congenital abnormalities – talipes, congenital dislocation of hip, torticollis; (ii) Scoliosis; (iii) the Brachial Palsies; (iv) Respiratory conditions in babies and young children – bronchiolitis, pneumonia, bronchiectasis and cystic fibrosis, asthma; (v) Mental Subnormality (Chapter 18) – some of the more common causes with suggestions for giving physical help.

Other conditions seen in the Paediatric Department but not included here are: (i) Cerebral Palsy; (ii) Spina Bifida; (iii) Still's Disease. The former two conditions are described in detail in *Neurology for Physiotherapists* edited by J. E. Cash, and therefore they have only been mentioned in general terms in this Section. In view of the importance of early handling and stimulation of all physically handicapped children, the sections on early development and play are particularly relevant to this subject. Some suggestions for stimulation and the provision of equipment for the multiply handicapped child (see Chapter 18, p. 220) may also provide a useful starting point in some cases.

Still's disease or juvenile rheumatism is far less common than either cerebral palsy or spina bifida. The aetiology and principles of treatment are very similar to rheumatoid arthritis (see Chapter 5, p. 49).

EARLY DEVELOPMENT

As the greatest changes in growth and development of the central nervous system, and therefore in the general activity of the child, take place in its first year of life, the study of this period is of the utmost importance. Probably for parents, the major milestones are smiling, sitting, standing, walking and talking. Between and around these achievements, there are a host of others – less spectacular but of equal or even greater importance in providing the total framework from which all activity springs. Physical and mental activity develop side by side, and up to a point are interdependent.

In early life, all movements are reflex. Later these reflexes are modified by 'higher', more complex ones, e.g. righting reflexes, balance reactions, and by willed movements. It is important to bear in mind the fact that the later willed or voluntary movements depend on the variety and quality of the earlier ones. Even the simplest voluntary movement depends on: (i) an adequate stimulus; (ii) the integration of the stimulus at conscious or unconscious levels; (iii) the resulting motor response.

Interference for whatever reason with any of these functions will result not only in limiting the immediate response. Because the pathways are not working to their full capacity the sensory feedback will also be inaccurate, and there will be a deficiency of stored experience which, in its turn, will affect any future response. In this way, learning is affected.

Thus a baby who is backward in development may be so for a number of reasons.

LACK OF ADEQUATE STIMULATION

Baby may be deprived of human contact from being left in his cot or pram all day, away from the rest of the family, with no toys or rattles and nothing to watch. He may even be fed without being picked up.

Therefore, he suffers from the loss of tactile, auditory and visual stimulation, and has no opportunity to learn. These are the deprived babies from poor homes, of inadequate parents, or disinterested 'daily minders'. Sometimes, physically handicapped children, those who have prolonged hospitalization or immobilization are also in danger of being deprived, unless special care is taken to ensure that they have the opportunity to see and hear and touch those things which they would experience in normal circumstances.

LOSS OF SPECIAL SENSES

Blind or deaf babies will obviously be behind in activities requiring sight or hearing – though later they may partially compensate for this. There may be sensory loss in children with neuromotor defects, either because they cannot move, and therefore cannot appreciate movement, or because sensation itself is deficient.

BRAIN DAMAGE

Depending on the area affected, brain damage may result in impairment of the appreciation of sensation, of integration, or of the motor response.

MILESTONES OF DEVELOPMENT

It is more satisfactory to regard these rather as a related sequence than as isolated events which must be achieved in a certain number of weeks or months. Babies vary greatly and there is a wide age-span covering the rate at which a normal child develops. The following plan should be read only as a guide to the sequence of normal development:

(1) Head control.
(2) Hands.
(3) Rolling.
(4) Sitting.
(5) Creeping, crawling and bottom shuffling.
(6) Standing and walking.
(7) Gait.

These headings have been arranged to show the sequence in which the beginnings of control are acquired, but it is stressed that all these activities overlap and are related one to another.

Head control

At birth the baby's head lolls when unsupported. If placed on his tummy he will turn his head to the side. In supine it is also generally turned to one side.

At six to eight weeks, when his eyes begin to focus, he starts to turn his head to look and will survey things in mid-line in the supine position. In the prone position he is beginning to lift his head off the bed.

At about three months he has full control of head rotation in supine, is getting good extension in prone, and is less wobbly when sitting on mother's knee. Quite soon he can lift his head in prone to look round from side to side.

By six to seven months he holds his head high in prone, and is beginning to raise it in supine. Although unable to maintain a sitting position, he can control his head if his trunk is supported.

With practice, head control and sitting balance improve. Head raising in supine develops together with increasing trunk and arm movements. Independent sitting and the ability to sit up from supine are both achieved by nine to ten months.

THE PULL TO SITTING TEST

This test is often used to demonstrate the degree of head control. The examiner takes hold of the baby's hands and pulls him into a sitting position. At birth and for a few weeks after, the head falls back with no attempt to right itself. By three months there is less head lag and by five or six months it will compensate throughout the movement, and it may even actively flex as the child tries to sit up as soon as he grasps the examiner's fingers.

Hands

At birth the baby shows predominant flexor tone throughout the body, and his hands are mainly fisted with the thumb held across the palm, though there is occasional extension of the fingers. By stretching the flexors of the fingers anything pressed into the palm elicits the grasp reflex, which in the first month or two is strong enough to lift the baby up by holding on to the examiner's fingers. The grasp reflex gradually fades in three to four months, and is replaced by voluntary grasping.

At four months, when eyes and head have gained some control, he is able to grab and hold a rattle and take it to his mouth for further investigation. Later he learns that it is fun to hold and release, to grab and throw. Also at about four months, he begins to play with his own hands, watching them move in front of his face. He also holds toys in his two hands, and transfers from one hand to the other at six to seven months. Early grasp is a simple flexion of the hand and fingers, the little and ring fingers playing the major part. This is known as palmar grasp.

By about nine months, the action of the hand has changed, the index finger has become the dominant feature, and is used for poking, and, with the thumb in a pincer grasp, to pick up quite tiny objects. This is the beginning of fine manipulation which will continue to develop over many more months as all the fingers become independent and fine skills are acquired by practice.

PARACHUTE REACTION

This test is often performed when screening children for cerebral palsy or other conditions where there is brain damage. The child is held under his chest, and moved rapidly forwards and downwards towards the bed – from six months onwards he should extend his arms and open his fingers as if to save himself – flexion or retraction of one or both arms indicate some neurological abnormality.

Rolling

This is an important part of development requiring co-ordination of most parts of the body. The earliest rolling is from side to supine or side to prone, depending on which position the baby prefers. This in its turn may well depend on how the baby was nursed in his early days. Rolling from prone to supine occurs at about five months, i.e. when he can lift and rotate his head and upper trunk while the lower trunk and legs flex. Here is the beginning of trunk control and rotation. Rolling from supine to prone generally follows about one month later (head flexion in supine occurring later than head extension in prone), and about the same time as progress is being made in sitting.

Sitting

Baby starts to sit between six and nine months. At first he leans on his hands for support, initially with his arms forwards, then at his sides. As balance is acquired, one arm becomes free for play, and then both, so that baby sits unsupported. During this time, head and trunk control have improved in all positions and he is able to sit up from supine, rolling over on his elbow to do so, and at first pulling himself up with the other hand on the side of the cot. This pattern of sitting up, using trunk rotation, continues until the age of four or five years, when the child is able to sit up symmetrically.

Creeping, crawling and shuffling

These are all valid modes of progression of which a child may use each in turn, one only, or none at all. Unfortunately, there is great confusion about the terms creeping and crawling and in any discussion one must be quite sure that all concerned are using the same terms for the same actions. In this Section, creeping refers to progress in prone with tummy on the floor; crawling refers to progression on hands and knees, moving one arm and one leg alternately.

CREEPING

This may start with pivoting in a circle at about six months. Some babies push up on their extended arms and move backwards, others kick their legs and wriggle forwards. There are many variations and the preference for one is of little significance unless combined with other signs of abnormality, e.g. if a child consistently uses only his arms to creep and has difficulty in sitting one might suspect some neurological abnormality of the legs.

CRAWLING

This occurs at about the same time as sitting balance is acquired, and the child is generally already beginning to pull up to stand. Quite a large number of normal children never crawl, but go straight to standing and walking. Some crawl for only a few days, others for many weeks, but this seems to have little bearing on their general development.

BOTTOM SHUFFLING

This is a self-descriptive method of progress and is sometimes an alternative to crawling. Obviously, the pre-requirement is the ability to sit and balance while moving either one arm and leg, or both legs. Normal and abnormal children may be seen to bottom shuffle, so it is not a diagnostic sign unless associated with similar and consistent patterns in other activities, e.g. the refusal to use the other arm and leg and inability to sit symmetrically would lead one to suspect infantile hemiplegia. It is of interest to note that normal children who bottom shuffle are often late in walking.

Standing and walking

Although the stepping reflex can be demonstrated in the newborn infant, this is only a transitory state which disappears in a week or so. However, at a few weeks he starts alternate kicking, and soon enjoys 'feeling his feet' when held upright with his feet on mother's knee.

By the time he is five months old, he sustains most of his weight, and starts to bounce. Most children start to pull themselves to standing soon after they have learnt to sit. They then enjoy standing at the cot rail; often their first steps are taken moving sideways along it. The actual age at which children stand and walk varies greatly. Some will stand at eight months and walk at ten, others not until eighteen or twenty months. The average is reckoned to be ten months for standing and thirteen months for walking unaided.

Gait

At first the child walks on a wide base in a rather square-set fashion.

He has little balance and no movement of the pelvis. Gradually, with practice, his balance improves and his feet get closer together, and he learns to run. However, not until the age of three or four years does walking resemble adult gait, i.e. with pelvic rotation. Given the opportunity most children start climbing as soon as they get on their feet, but walking up- and downstairs using alternate legs is not achieved until two or three years, neither is the ability to stand on one leg, or jump on two. Hopping on one leg takes another year.

Conclusion

To summarize briefly, it may be seen that there is a definite link between the development of different motor skills. Rolling and sitting both require some head control; sitting also needs the support of the hands and arms; sitting up uses and consolidates the same pattern of movement as rolling and so on. It becomes evident that one must understand this progression of acquired skills in the normal child in order to appreciate and treat effectively the abnormal.

THE IMPORTANCE OF PLAY

The value of play to a child cannot be over-emphasized because this is how he learns. When a mother plays with her baby, he learns to watch her face, listen to her voice, to follow with his eyes, reach with his hand, to localize sound, later to imitate both sound and expression. He touches his mother's face and hair and finds it soft, holds his bottle or rattle, and discovers it is hard. So he learns about texture, and temperature, shape and weight. Then he can learn about the purpose of things, rattles to shake, or punch, or roll, some noisy, some cuddly. He learns to select what is appropriate for his purpose – a soft toy to sleep with, a rattle to bang when he wakes.

Although good toys tend to be expensive, they are a good investment provided they are carefully selected. They may be supplemented by improvisations, using everyday household materials, such as a wooden spoon and saucepan which can be used for a variety of activities, cardboard boxes, particularly large ones, are great fun for climbing in and out and under, and later provide much imaginative play. A plastic bucket also has many uses, as container, seat, table, or just something to carry about (Plate 16/1).

While finding good toys may be relatively easy, what is more difficult is to provide the handicapped child with the right toy at the right time. Both age and ability must be considered as he will quickly tire of a toy which demands too little effort, and reject or become frustrated by one which demands too much. This is particularly difficult with those children whose intellect demands more than they are physically able to accomplish. The parents of such children are often grateful for advice at Christmas and birthdays, and this is often a good way to develop a wider interest in treatment. It is useful to be able to lend out the catalogues of the firms supplying well-made or educational toys, so that the rest of the family can see what has been suggested. Some local authorities have Toy Libraries, which should help to provide variety and progression.

The physiotherapist will also want to give advice on the use and suitability of large toys, such as bouncers, swings, walkers and tricycles. It is, however, much more difficult to give advice once the article in question has been purchased; so it is essential to raise the question of these things at the earliest opportunity. In fact, this makes a good starting point to introduce ideas of management to parents when they first bring their child for treatment. It can be explained to them that baby may well be helped by one or other of these things, but that it would be better to delay buying any of them until his problems have been fully assessed. It is helpful to be able to try out the different types of equipment on the market, and see which is beneficial, and which harmful to each individual. Equipment should never be recommended for home use unless the physiotherapist has seen the child use it, and is certain that it will continue to be used to advantage.

Of this group of equipment, the baby bouncer is perhaps the greatest problem, as everyone has a friend whose baby loves it, and for whom it works wonders! One must be rather wary of recommending these for handicapped children, particularly until one has made a careful assessment, e.g. it is tempting to 'bounce' the lethargic, floppy baby, but one must be sure that it is not in the process of developing extensor spasticity of the legs – which might be increased by the bouncing.

Care must also be taken when treating mentally subnormal children, though they may well benefit from using the bouncer to stimulate activity and build up their muscle tone which is often low; the danger in this case arises from the fact that having learnt the art of bouncing these children will be quite happy if they never do anything else. The danger is even greater at home, where mother is also so happy that she cannot bear to terminate the sessions. This danger must be foreseen, and the length of time spent in the bouncer strictly limited. It should also be discarded when it has served its purpose, and the child is able to progress to a new activity.

Provided they are used with discretion and the contra-indications are recognized, bouncers can provide useful and enjoyable activity to meet specific needs. Occasionally the bouncer may have a more static use as an aid to standing or even sitting by giving trunk support to the very hypotonic child, to whom it is difficult to give the experience of an upright posture in any other way. It gives the physiotherapist a chance to position the child's legs and to encourage it to take some of its weight.

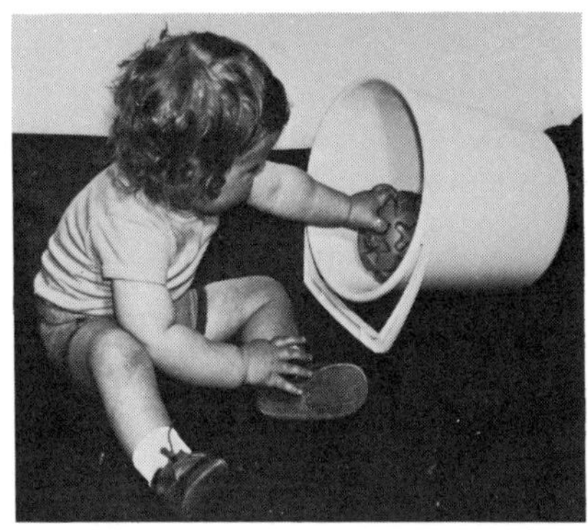

Plate 16/1 A plastic bucket has many uses (*see p. 187*)

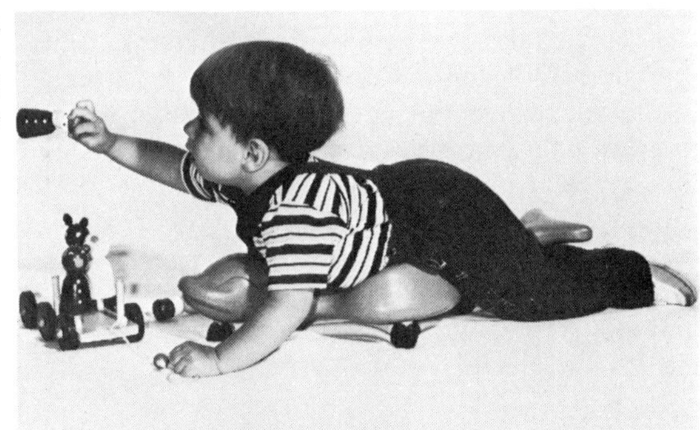

Plate 16/2 Dolphin Crawler gives enjoyment, mobility and arm exercises for boy with spina bifida (*see p. 190*)

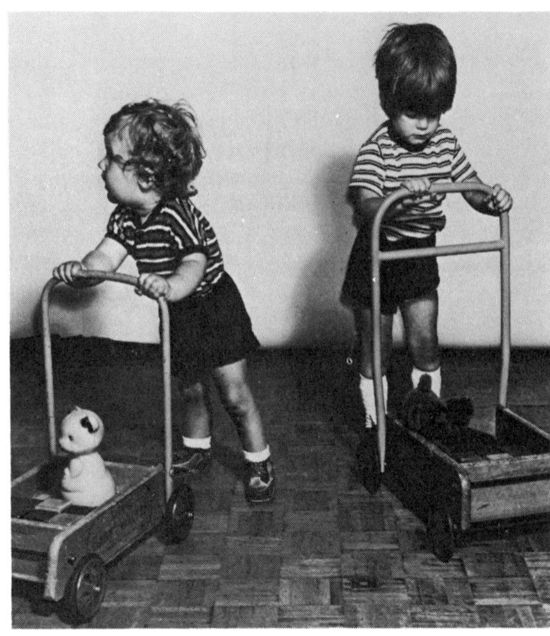

Plate 16/3 Pushing trucks may be a stage in learning to walk. Trucks must be the correct height for the child (*see p. 190*)

Baby walkers are often a useful aid, but must also be used with discretion. There is a variety of these on the market, and each child must be assessed individually for his particular needs. This includes safety. If he is too tall for the model chosen, or too floppy, he may overbalance and fall, overturning the walker as he goes. The older child who is hyperactive but unsteady may try, when no-one is looking, to climb out and may get stuck or fall.

Baby chairs and swings must be similarly considered for fit, safety and function. More will be said about these later.

A toy well worth its place in the children's department is Galt's Dolphin Crawler (Plate 16/2), which provides useful prone activity, and a good means of mobility for children with lower limb paralysis, particularly spina bifida, as it also strengthens the muscles of the arms and shoulders. Other useful toys are those for riding astride with the feet on the floor, cars, tractors, engines of various or adjustable heights. Pushing toys can help young children learning to walk, but it is important that they are of a suitable height and do not tip up or run away. Handles can be raised, trucks or prams weighted to prevent this (Plate 16/3).

Bicycles, tricycles and Go-karts provide exercise and mobility at some stages of treatment. If necessary, they can be adapted with seat backs and foot straps, and can sometimes be provided by the Department of Health and Social Security.

PHYSIOTHERAPY

Because their requirements are so different from adult patients, it is much more satisfactory for children to be treated away from the general department. Not only are the children helped by the more informal atmosphere and the presence of other children, but the parents are also more relaxed, and enjoy meeting each other and discussing their mutual problems.

At the first attendance, it is important to put both child and parents at ease before embarking on any particular techniques. Children hate to be rushed, and mothers are invariably upset if their offspring 'won't do what the lady says', or worse, stamp and scream! (probably because he expects either to be hurt, or left in hospital). One can learn a lot from talking to the mother, and father if he is present, hearing of their difficulties and fears, and what they think is the matter with their child. They will be grateful for a simple explanation of the treatment and what it is hoped to achieve. Progress depends very much on co-operation between parents, child and physiotherapist and each needs to know from the outset what is expected from him or her. For babies and for the under-fives, work must be presented as play; even so, it is quite within their powers to understand that treatment time is purposeful.

A quiet and unhurried approach is essential for all young children, particularly for babies who easily become upset by sudden movements or noises. They in their turn can move very quickly, wriggling and rolling into dangerous situations unless precautions are taken to protect them. A baby must not be left in any place from which he can fall. In the ward, cot sides must be left raised and locked.

Powers of concentration vary, not only between one child and another, but in the same child from day to day. It is necessary to recognize the 'off' days and adjust the treatment accordingly, thus avoiding frustration and preserving a good working relationship for next time.

A few children in the under-five age group will respond to a direct approach and can be taught straightforward exercises. Others need the incentive provided by toys and games for longer. At all stages it is important to maintain the child's interest and to change the activity before he becomes bored. Encouragement is the greatest spur; even a dull child will work for praise, whereas threats or bribes provide only another distraction. Praise, of course, must not be given indiscriminately, but it is usually possible to find some simple achievement to provide a starting point.

Games and toys must be chosen to provide the activity which is required and not merely for their own sake, otherwise valuable time will be wasted. Similarly, older children may enjoy the interest and companionship of classwork but it must be remembered that the aim is treatment of the individual and that each has his own specific needs.

In selecting a child for a class, various aspects must be considered; these include the age, personality and physical needs of the child, as well as the size and nature of the class and the experience of the physiotherapist. Most children begin to enjoy working together at about the age of four or five, but at this age will need considerable individual help, either during or in addition to a group session. Classwork in its generally accepted sense is better delayed until the age of seven or eight.

Schoolchildren attending for specific exercises, e.g. breathing, posture, re-education after injuries, are generally more satisfactorily treated if their parents are not present. Once he has learnt them, the child is pleased to demonstrate the exercises to his parents and feels that he is responsible for his own treatment when it is continued at home.

Younger children, and severely handicapped older ones, are normally treated with mother present, so that she can learn what to encourage in his daily routine, and what to include in her home treatment sessions if these are recommended. Sometimes it is desirable to work entirely through the mother, so that it is she who handles the child throughout the treatment, the physiotherapist giving the instructions and explaining why they are necessary. This is extremely useful in the case of young children in hospital who need tipping, and can be persuaded to do so over mother's knee, possibly while the physiotherapist gives the same treatment to dolly or teddy.

Home treatment

This must be kept as simple as possible, and if it is to continue for a long period, as short as possible. Parents and child should understand the importance of regular treatment, and over-enthusiastic parents restrained from insisting on prolonged sessions in the early stages which can result in exhaustion and frustration for all concerned. It is wise to make a note of the home treatment given at each visit, so that the same exercises can be checked and different ones given to provide variety. It is also wise to ascertain that the treatment prescribed is practicable at home, e.g. that there is enough space to perform the exercises and that any apparatus required is available.

For suppliers of good toys, see p. 223.
For Bibliography see p. 224.

Chapter 17

Physiotherapy for Children – II

congenital abnormalities – scoliosis – brachial palsies – respiratory conditions

---

CONGENITAL ABNORMALITIES

A congenital abnormality may be defined as a defect already present in the infant at the time of birth. Sometimes more than one abnormality may be present, for instance a congenital heart condition may be associated with talipes or congenital dislocation of the hip.

The three main causes of congenital abnormalities are: (i) genetic factors; (ii) intra-uterine pressure; (iii) intra-uterine infection.

The conditions described here are some of those most commonly seen in the physiotherapy department.

TALIPES EQUINOVARUS

As the name suggests, the foot is twisted downwards and inwards. The head of the talus is prominent on the dorsum of the foot, the medial border of which is concave. In severe cases the sole of the foot may face upwards and if untreated, the child walks on the dorsum of the foot. The majority of cases are bilateral (Plate 17/1).

Aetiology

The cause is uncertain, but there is often a genetic element. It has been suggested that the development of the foot is arrested before birth as a result of some unidentified infection of the mother, and that the initial abnormality may be in the bones with secondary changes in soft tissue. Alternatively, it is possible that moulding of the foot occurs when the fetus lies awkwardly in the uterus, and that the primary change is in soft tissue, the bones only becoming misshapen later, if the deformity is not corrected.

There are three components of the deformity:

(i) Plantar flexion at the ankle (equinus). The talus may lie almost vertically instead of in the horizontal position.

(ii) Inversion at the sub-taloid and mid-tarsal joints. The calcaneus faces inwards (varus).

(iii) Adduction of the forefoot at the tarsometatarsal joint. Some cases also have internal rotation of the tibia.

There is shortening of tibialis anterior and posterior, and the long and short flexors of the toes. The calf muscles are wasted and the tendo-calcaneus drawn over to the medial side of the heel.

Similarly, the ligaments and joint capsules on the medial side of the ankle and foot are tight and the plantar fascia forms a tight thickened band on the medial side of the sole. On the lateral side of the leg, the peronei and lateral ligaments and capsules are overstretched and weak.

Treatment

Treatment should be commenced early, on the first day of life if possible, and continued until the child walks. It consists of over-correction of the deformity by manipulation, and maintenance by splinting and active use of all the leg muscles, particularly the peronei. In severe cases open reduction of the deformity may be performed within a few days of birth as an alternative to manipulation.

If conservative treatment fails to correct the deformity, osteotomy of the os calcis must be considered.

MANIPULATION

Manipulation to obtain over-correction may be performed on young babies by the doctor or physiotherapist without anaesthesia. In mild cases where no splinting is necessary, the mother is taught to manipulate the feet each time she changes the nappy.

During manipulation, the baby's knee is flexed and the lower leg firmly held to prevent any strain on the knee. Each part of the deformity is stretched separately.

The *manipulations* are:

(i) To correct the heel: the heel is pulled down and out, stretching the tendo-calcaneus and structures on the medial side. For a good result the heel must be fully corrected in the first two or three weeks of life. After this time an inverted heel is unlikely to respond to manipulative measures.

(ii) To abduct the forefoot: the baby's left heel rests in the palm of the physiotherapist's right hand so that her thumb supports the outer side of his leg, and her index and middle fingers hold his heel. The ball of the thumb acts as a fulcrum as the foot is bent sideways over it, the physiotherapist using her left thumb and index finger to grasp along the base of the toes (see Plate 17/2).

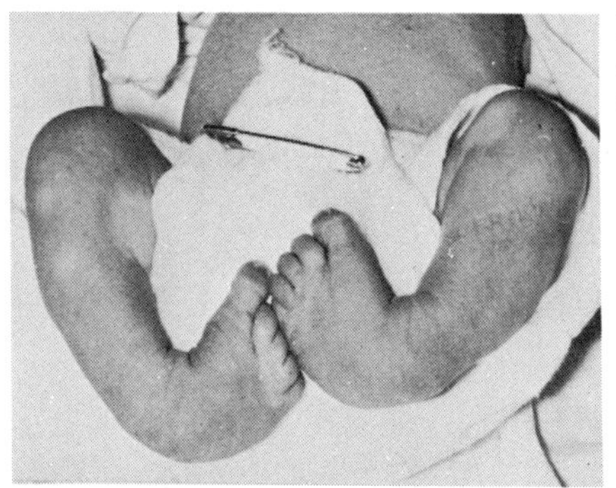

Plate 17/1 Congenital talipes equinovarus, showing severe bilateral deformity (*see p. 193*)

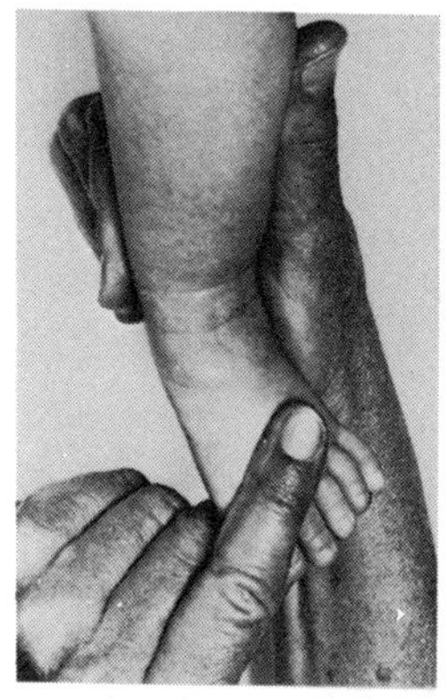

Plate 17/2 Manipulation to abduct the forefoot (*see p. 194*)

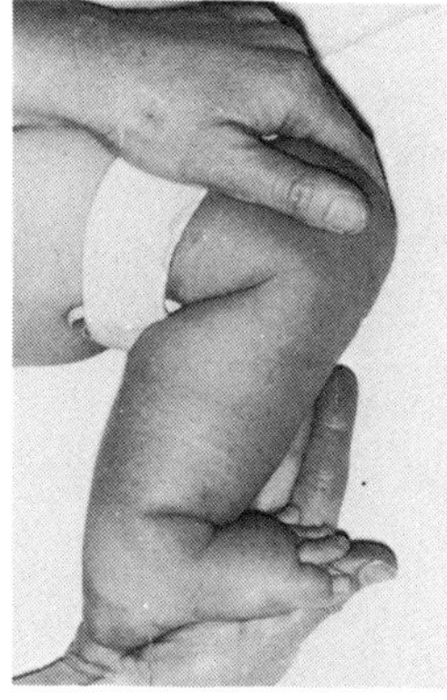

Plate 17/3 Combined eversion and dorsiflexion (*see p. 197*)

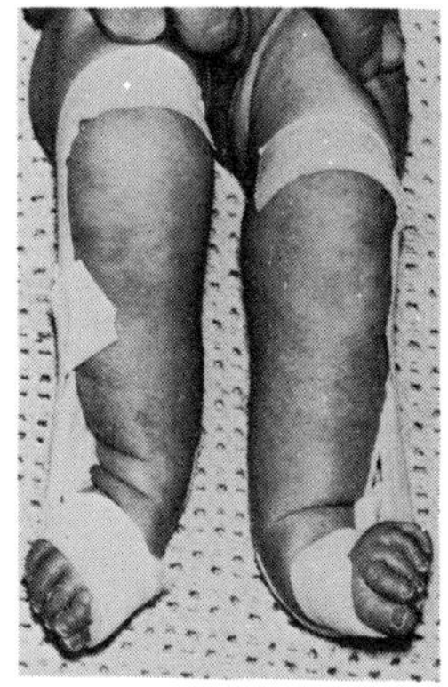

Plate 17/4 Strapping for talipes equinovarus (*see p. 197*)

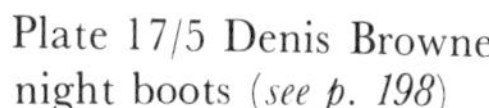

Plate 17/5 Denis Browne night boots (*see p. 198*)

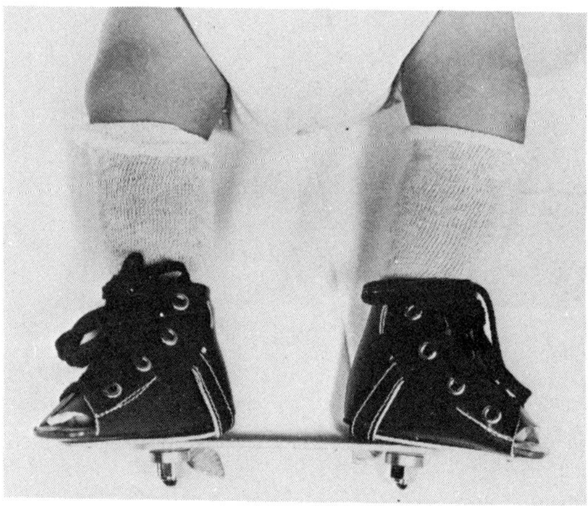

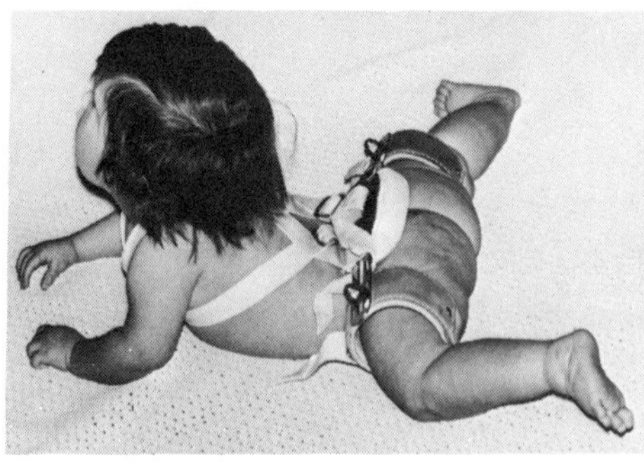

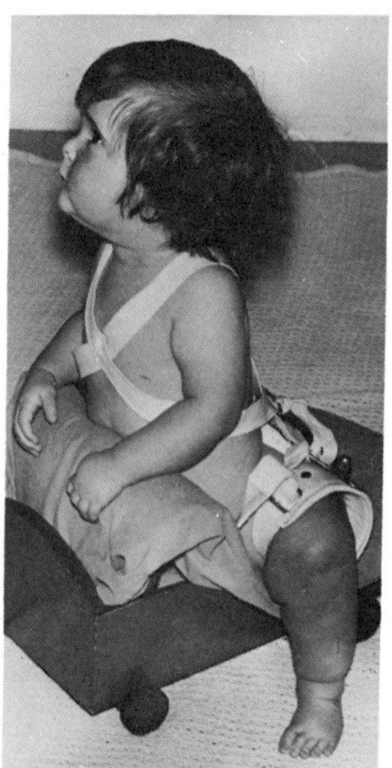

Plate 17/6 Denis Browne splint in C.D.H. maintains hip abduction but allows child to move rest of body freely, above and right (*see p. 200*)

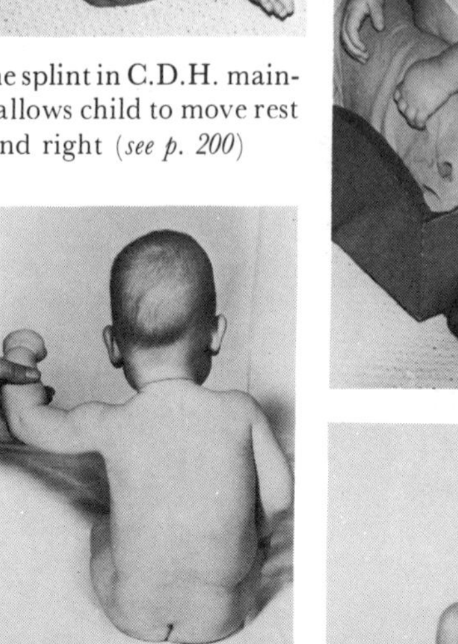

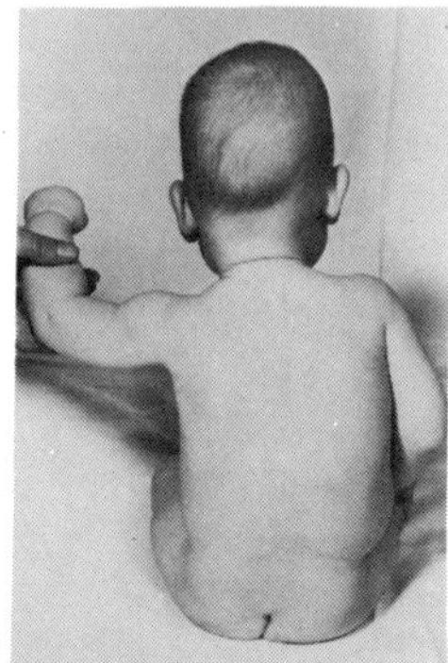

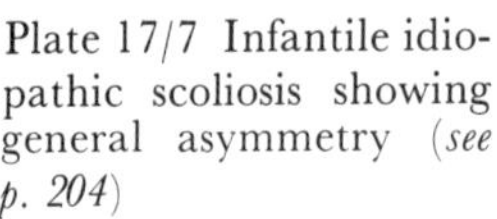

Plate 17/7 Infantile idiopathic scoliosis showing general asymmetry (*see p. 204*)

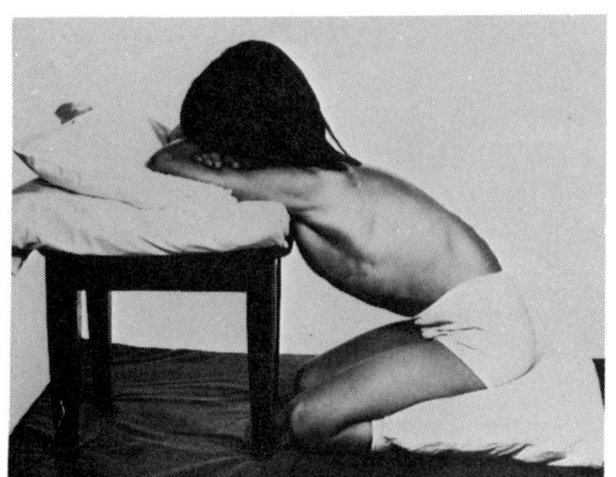

Plate 17/9 Asthma, in a comfortable position relaxation and breathing are easier (*see p. 213*)

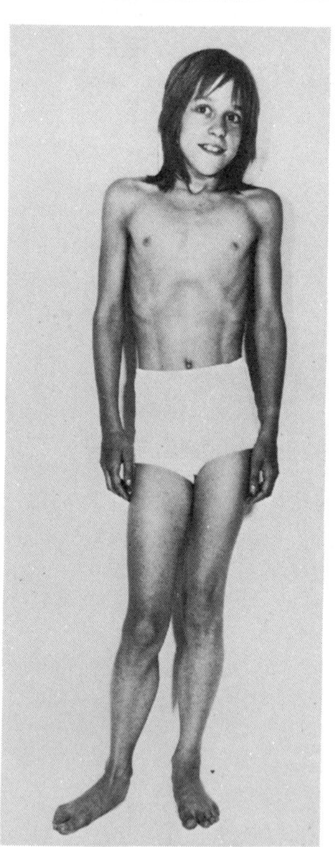

Plate 17/8 Asthma, typical stance (*see p. 212*)

(iii) To combine eversion and dorsiflexion: the fully corrected foot can be pushed up and out so that the dorsum touches the outer side of the leg (see Plate 17/3). Care must be taken to ensure that dorsiflexion occurs in the ankle joint and not in the sole of the foot. This depends on adequate correction of the tightness of the tendo-calcaneus; sometimes a tenotomy is needed to achieve this.

SPLINTING

Splinting may be by strapping, Denis Browne splints or plaster of Paris. The splints or plaster will be applied by the doctor and will maintain the feet in eversion and dorsiflexion. Strapping may be applied by the doctor or by the physiotherapist under his direction.

It is important that treatment should not be interrupted, so every effort must be made to maintain the skin in good condition. Three points are worth noting:

(i) Care of the skin by painting it with Tinc. benz. co. before the strapping is applied. If, in spite of this, the skin becomes wet and soggy, gentian violet may be liberally applied and strapping continued. Very rarely a baby may be allergic to zinc oxide strapping but may tolerate Dermicel or a similar preparation.

(ii) Reinforcement of the corrective straps so as to prevent these from dragging on the skin.

(iii) Padding pressure points with adhesive felt.

STRAPPING

(See Plate 17/4.) The lateral malleolus is protected by a small piece of adhesive felt. Another piece, ½ to 1 inch (1 to 2.5 cm) wide depending on the size of the foot, is wrapped round the medial side of the big toe and under the base of the toes.

Three strips of 1 inch (2.5 cm) wide zinc oxide strapping are used; one to correct each part of the deformity:

(i) The first starts below the medial malleolus, passes under the heel, up the outer side of the leg and over the bent knee.

(ii) The second starts above the medial malleolus and passes across the sole of the foot, around the forefoot (covering the felt). *N.B.* It is important that no tension is applied up to this point. The strap is then pulled upwards and outwards to the lateral side of the leg.

(iii) The third strap maintains dorsiflexion and passes under the sole of the foot and up both sides of the lower leg.

Reinforcement by strips of zinc oxide 2 or 3 inches in length, applied diagonally across the strapping on the lateral side help to prevent these from dragging on the skin. A cotton bandage secured with more strapping is useful protection and can be reapplied if it becomes soiled.

Initially strapping is renewed every two or three days until full over-correction can be maintained without undue circulatory disturbance, generally in two or three weeks if treatment is started early. It is then reapplied weekly or fortnightly. Some form of splinting must be retained until the child is standing when its own body weight acts as a corrective force. Before this time there is a strong tendency for the condition to relapse. In the later stages, Denis Browne night boots (Plate 17/5) may be worn during sleep times and removed for periods of activity. It is important that these should fit well and that the parents know how to apply them and are conscientious in doing so.

EXERCISE

Whatever form of splinting is used, the baby is encouraged to kick at first against his mother's hands, the end of the pram or, when he is old enough, against the floor. This strengthens his muscles and reinforces the correction of the deformity. Each time the strapping is removed, the peronei can be stimulated by stroking over the muscles, or along the outer border of the foot. After a few months, full-time splintage may be replaced by night boots, leaving the baby free to exercise during his waking hours, and the parents are taught to move the foot through its full range, to stimulate the peronei and encourage the child to stand.

Advice to parents

Parents must understand:

(i) The importance of continuous treatment.

(ii) The danger of the feet relapsing if treatment is stopped too soon.

(iii) The necessity of keeping splints or strapping dry. This should not be too difficult if the baby wears plastic pants.

(iv) The importance of inspecting the toes to check the circulation, particularly after splinting has been renewed. The baby should return immediately to hospital if the toes become blue or swollen.

TALIPES CALCANEO-VALGUS

This is much less serious than the equinovarus deformity. It tends to recover spontaneously. The baby is born with the feet in a position of eversion and dorsiflexion. All the anterior tibial muscles are shortened together with the ligaments over the front of the ankle.

Causes

It is probable that the deformity develops shortly before birth due to the awkward position in which the fetus lies.

Treatment

Treatment consists of gentle stretching of the foot into plantar flexion and inversion, and encouraging active movements in the same direction. The mother is taught to do this several times a day. If the condition is severe or persists, a small splint may be made to keep the foot in plantar flexion and inversion.

CONGENITAL DISLOCATION OF THE HIP

Congenital dislocation of the hip (CDH) occurs more often in girls than boys. There are strong familial tendencies, cases occurring in siblings or in different generations of the family.

Dislocation may occur before or at birth, or, in the less severe congenital subluxation, when the child starts to walk. The acetabulum is shallow, its upper rim is deficient and the roof slopes upwards at a greater angle than normal. The neck of the femur may be inclined more forwards than normal, so that the head easily slips upwards and backwards out of the acetabulum. Flattening of the femoral head may occur later, from pressure against the ilium when the child begins to bear weight, or from avascular necrosis after forceful manipulation has replaced the head of the femur in the acetabulum. Fatty tissue may fill the shallow acetabulum, the capsule is stretched and may show hourglass constriction, and the muscles become shortened in their abnormal position. Laxity of the ligaments may be a primary cause of dislocation.

Signs

The most significant signs are limitation of abduction of the flexed hip and shortening of the leg. With the baby's hips flexed to 90° it should be possible to abduct both hips so that the thighs are lying in the same plane. If the dislocation is bilateral the leg shortening may be less apparent though there is often some inequality and abduction is limited on both sides. There is also broadening of the perineum. Sometimes a click is obtained when moving the hips into the flexion abduction position, and this may be due to the head of the femur riding over the rim of the acetabulum, but clicks can also be elicited in normal joints. Diagnosis is confirmed by X-ray.

If the dislocation remains unreduced when the child starts to walk, the mechanical instability of the joint and loss of a fixed point of insertion for the abductors of the hip results in the inability of these muscles to hold the pelvis level when the patient stands on the affected leg (Trendelenburg's sign). Fortunately, this is rarely seen except in older patients. Testing for signs of dislocation of the hips is now part of the routine examination of neonates. Early diagnosis is important, as the prognosis is very much better if treatment is commenced soon after birth.

Treatment

In young babies, simple reduction may be performed without anaesthetic, and maintained by a Denis Browne, Barlow or Von Rosen splint, all of which are designed to keep the hips in flexion and abduction. These splints may also be used for babies whose hips are not dislocated but who have physical or radiological signs of subluxation, while for very mild cases in young babies, the use of double nappies may be sufficient to keep the hips abducted.

If it is not possible to obtain full abduction without the use of forceful manipulation, reduction may be obtained by: (i) traction to both legs with gradually increasing abduction until the legs are at an angle of 180°; (ii) adductor tenotomy followed by gentle manipulation; (iii) open operation if all attempts at closed reduction have failed.

All three procedures are followed by plaster of Paris with the hips in 90° flexion and 90° abduction (the frog position), or in any position in which the reduction is most stable.

Treatment lasts until the head of the femur has been maintained in the acetabulum for at least one year and the acetabular roof has formed satisfactorily. For the last few months plaster may be replaced by a Denis Browne splint (Plate 17/6a). This maintains the hip abduction but allows the child to move the rest of the body freely. At this stage the child is encouraged to move his legs by sitting astride a truck or other suitable toy and paddling himself along (Plate 17/6b). He can also learn to walk and climb in the splint. In this way the rotary movement at the hip joint drives the head of the femur into the acetabulum, so stimulating normal shape and growth.

Following removal of splinting, the child walks on a wide base but gradually the gait becomes normal without further treatment. Exercises to teach the child to walk on a narrow base are contra-indicated as strong adduction too early may cause re-dislocation.

TORTICOLLIS

Wry neck or torticollis is a condition quite frequently seen by the physiotherapist. The child holds his head tilted to one side so that the ear is drawn towards the shoulder on the tight side. At the same time, the face is turned to the opposite side.

Structural torticollis

A cervical hemivertebra may be the cause of torticollis but this is very rare and there is no treatment.

Infantile torticollis

This is the type most commonly seen. It is often associated with sterno-mastoid tumour. A small hard lump consisting of fibrous scar tissue can be felt in the muscle belly at birth or shortly afterwards. The scar tissue contracts, so shortening the muscle. The clavicular head of the muscle may stand out in a tight band and the head is pulled over into the typical position.

CAUSE

The cause is unknown. A fibrous tumour may be present before birth or a haematoma may result from a traction injury during birth. Facial asymmetry and moulding of the head is often a factor, but this slowly improves if the muscle can be stretched and the head held straight. In untreated cases facial asymmetry may persist and after some years it becomes irreversible.

Fetal torticollis

The appearances are similar to the infantile type described above but there is no tumour and little or no limitation of passive movement.

Asymmetric moulding of the head, probably from the position in utero, results in it being held consistently on one side. Active rotation to the other side is made difficult by the shape of the head. The infant frequently prefers to lie on one side only.

The condition often improves spontaneously as the baby grows and gets more active. The moulding of the head disappears more slowly in about a year.

Physiotherapy is sometimes given if the infant is slow to start moving. It follows the pattern given below.

Treatment

Physiotherapy, consisting of stretching, active exercises and general management, should be started early, usually at about four weeks, and is generally successful up to the age of six months. After this time the muscle is more difficult to stretch, and although it is worth while continuing with physiotherapy, tenotomy of the sterno-mastoid may have to be considered at a later date.

STRETCHING

The movements performed in stretching the sterno-mastoid are:

(i) Side flexion of the head and neck away from the tight side;

(ii) rotation of the head so that the face is turned towards the tight side;

(iii) both movements combined, side flexion followed by rotation.

If the baby is small the mother can do the stretching while he lies on her lap. In order to make him feel secure, she must sit on a chair low enough for both feet to rest firmly on the floor. The baby lies across the mother's knee, in the case of a right torticollis his head rests on her right knee. She places her left hand over the point of his right shoulder to hold it down; her left forearm keeps his arms and trunk tucked close in to her own body. She places her right hand on the right side of the baby's head, avoiding his ear, and brings his chin to the mid-line before performing side flexion (bringing the head towards her) and rotation (turning the face away from her).

If the child is too big, a second person must be enlisted to help. The child lies supine on a flat firm surface – a thin sponge bathmat on a table is ideal as it will not slip. The assistant holds the baby's shoulder down, while the mother takes his head between her hands and performs the movements as before.

Each movement should be through the fullest range possible, performed five or six times at each session and repeated two or three times each day. Although the mother must be taught to stretch the neck as soon as possible, the physiotherapist must realize that she is bound to be frightened of doing so, especially as the baby is likely to cry. She should be reassured and gain confidence, by being allowed to practise getting her hands into the correct position without actually stretching. When she is able to do this easily she starts stretching the neck under supervision before doing so at home.

ACTIVE EXERCISE

From about ten weeks old the baby can be encouraged to turn his head through the full range of rotation by attracting his attention with a coloured toy or rattle. At first this is done in supine, later in prone, later still in sitting. It is important to move the rattle slowly, giving the infant time to fix his eyes on it and accommodate to the movement. By changing his position, by holding down one shoulder the movements of flexion, extension and side flexion may be encouraged in a similar fashion.

GENERAL MANAGEMENT

The baby should be encouraged to lie on alternate sides; frequently one side is less used than the other.

The cot or pram should be placed so that the baby is encouraged to look towards the tight side; toys should be hung on this side.

The baby should not be sat up too early or for too long; his head will drop to the tight side if his muscles are weak or tired.

Ocular torticollis

Occasionally children of three or four are sent for treatment because they hold the head on one side. There is full range of passive movement and the child is able to correct the head position actively with help, but resumes the torticollis position as soon as left alone.

The cause lies in weakness of one eye and physiotherapy should be delayed until this has received attention. Usually the head is held straight as soon as the eyes are treated.

SCOLIOSIS

This is such a vast and controversial subject that it is impossible in this context to give more than a brief outline.

Scoliosis is lateral deviation of the spine which, because of the normal antero-posterior curve, is always accompanied by rotation. The primary curve may vary in degree, extent and location and is usually progressive. Secondary or compensatory curves form above and below the primary one so that the child can maintain an upright position.

Rotation is most marked in the thoracic region. As the vertebral bodies rotate to the side of the convexity, the corresponding ribs are projected sharply backwards forming the typical hump on that side. This is matched by a bulge on the anterior aspect of the chest on the opposite side. Complications of progressive deformity include impairment of respiratory function and in very severe cases nerve root pressure.

True scoliosis, even when not progressive, is an irreversible condition and must not be confused with postural scoliosis, which is seen much more often in physiotherapy departments and responds well to treatment.

Congenital scoliosis

This is a structural deformity resulting from maldevelopment of one or more vertebrae (producing hemivertebrae). The ribs may also be malformed and be more or fewer than normal. There is adaptive shortening of muscle and connective tissue. Sometimes the deformity increases with growth, but although no improvement can be expected, the condition often remains static and symptom-free if there are good compensatory curves.

Paralytic scoliosis

This may occur as a result of muscle imbalance. Poliomyelitis was once the major cause of this type, but it may be seen as a complication of any neurological or muscle-wasting disease. Some cases of cerebral palsy, particularly the athetoid types who have an asymmetric distribution of spasm, may develop severe scoliotic deformities.

Treatment of the lower motor neurone types is on similar lines to that for idiopathic scoliosis. Those due to cerebral palsy must be considered in the light of their general treatment and management.

Idiopathic scoliosis

(See Plate 17/7.) *Infantile idiopathic scoliosis* may be noticed when the baby is two or three months old. The majority of cases effect a spontaneous recovery in about a year; a few progress to severe deformity in spite of all forms of treatment.

Adolescent idiopathic scoliosis does not become apparent until the child is three or four years or even older and remains in a fairly mild form until the early teens, when rapid deterioration may take place.

Nothing is known of the cause in either case. Changes occur in bony and soft tissues as the condition advances.

TREATMENT

Mild cases which are not deteriorating must be observed regularly to make sure that the deformity is not increasing.

Treatment of severe and progressive cases is by supportive and corrective splints. If in spite of these the curve increases, spinal fusion or other operative procedures must be considered and will be performed at the age thought by the surgeon to be the most suitable.

PHYSIOTHERAPY

It is not possible either to correct the existing deformity or to influence the progressive tendency of the primary curve, therefore physiotherapy is sometimes thought to be of no value. Bilateral exercises may be ordered to improve muscle tone and the general condition and to maintain mobility in the secondary curves with a view to possible surgical correction later.

Breathing exercises may be given to improve or maintain respiratory function.

Postural scoliosis

This is a much less serious condition, seen frequently in teenage girls. Strictly speaking it is not a true scoliosis as only the normal anatomical rotation accompanies side flexion, hence it can be distinguished from other forms of scoliosis by the fact that the curve disappears on traction or forward flexion of the spine.

CAUSES

The condition usually appears at a time of rapid growth. The child – usually a girl – tends to adopt a consistent asymmetric stance and the general musculature is poor. One leg may be shorter than the other, causing the pelvis to drop on that side.

TREATMENT

More than an inch of leg shortening may be compensated by raising the heel and possibly the sole of the shoe. Gross shortening may require surgical intervention to obtain a better cosmetic appearance than a very high raised shoe.

Successful physiotherapy depends very largely on the patient's co-operation. As most patients are in the older age group, the initial explanation and planning of treatment to include only what is most effective is of even greater importance than usual. Attention should be paid not only to correction of posture in standing and walking, but also in sitting, with reference to school desks and chairs and whether she can see and hear adequately from her place in the classroom.

Correction of posture in front of a long mirror is useful particularly to start with, but this is not always available at home. Bilateral strengthening and balance exercises may be given to develop the feeling of a symmetric posture in movement. Home treatment should be kept to a minimum – one exercise done well is worth ten done in a hurry.

General health, including adequate diet, rest and exercise should not be overlooked.

BRACHIAL PALSIES

These are not very common but sometimes follow a difficult birth. They may be caused by pressure between neck and shoulder or by traction on the arm or head. There is damage to the nerves or nerve roots, resulting in paralysis of the muscles in the arm supplied by them. The prognosis will depend on the degree of damage. This can vary from mild bruising followed by recovery in a few weeks, to severe tearing of the nerves resulting in permanent paralysis and the danger of deformity. Fortunately the latter cases are rare.

Erb's palsy

The fifth and sixth cervical nerve roots are damaged resulting in paralysis of deltoid, supraspinatus, infraspinatus, teres major, biceps and supinator.

SIGNS AND SYMPTOMS

The arm may be completely flaccid at birth but soon assumes the typical position of adduction and internal rotation at the shoulder, with pronation of the forearm and flexion of the wrist and fingers.

TREATMENT

This should be started as soon as possible with the aims of protecting the shoulder joint and preventing deformities.

An aeroplane splint may be used to support the shoulder in abduction and lateral rotation, with the elbow at 90° flexion and the forearm supinated. Suitable splints can also be made quite easily from Plastazote, Orthoplast or similar materials. These are light and comfortable and can be adapted and altered as the baby grows. Pinning the sleeve of the nightdress to the pillow is not recommended because of the danger of straining the shoulder joint if the baby moves.

Passive movements and the encouragement of whatever active movements are possible are started immediately and taught to the mother so that she can continue at home.

In severe cases, where splinting must be continued for several months it is important to see that the infant has opportunities for the activities normal for his age, e.g. in the prone position, rolling over, and sitting himself up, and it is essential to give the help necessary to achieve this.

Klumpke's paralysis

The seventh and eighth cervical and first thoracic nerve roots are affected.

SIGNS AND SYMPTOMS

Paralysis of the extensors of the wrist and fingers results in the wrist being held in the flexed position. The small hand muscles are also affected.

TREATMENT

Small cock-up splints for the wrist can be made from plaster of Paris, Plastazote or Orthoplast.

Passive movements are started early and active use of the hand encouraged as recovery takes place. The use of two hands together should be assisted if necessary, at the appropriate age (six months), so that normal sensory development should not be lost.

RESPIRATORY CONDITIONS

These form a large part of the physiotherapist's work with children. Although the structure and function of the respiratory tract are similar to those of the adult, the fact that the lungs are so small increases the danger of the infant quickly developing severe respiratory distress. Consideration of the size and age of the patient also suggests variations of treatment in presentation and technique, even though basic principles remain the same.

BRONCHIOLITIS

Bronchiolitis is an acute viral infection of the bronchioles occurring in infants, especially in their first year.

It is characterized by bronchiolar obstruction due to oedema and mucus accumulation. This results in coughing, wheezing and dyspnoea. The respiratory rate is greatly increased, often to more than twice normal, which for a sleeping baby is 30 per minute. In severe cases the baby is limp and pale and may be cyanosed. Immediate complications include cardiac failure and bronchopneumonia.

Treatment

The infant is nursed in a tent with oxygen and humidity.

Physiotherapy in the form of postural drainage and vibrations is given three- or four-hourly. If the infant's condition permits it is more satisfactorily treated out of the tent, so that it can lie on a pillow on the physiotherapist's knee; otherwise it must be positioned over pillows inside the tent.

If necessary, mechanical suction may be used to withdraw secretions. This technique requires experience, skill and great care in order to avoid damaging the delicate membranes lining the respiratory passages.

PNEUMONIA

Pneumonia is fairly common in childhood.

Bronchopneumonia

Bronchopneumonia is often preceded by an upper respiratory tract infection and may be a complication of infectious diseases such as measles and whooping cough.

Aspiration pneumonia follows inhalation of food or vomit.

SIGNS AND SYMPTOMS

Cough, fever and a raised respiratory rate are usually found.

Râles (moist sounds, i.e. little bubbling noises) may be heard on listening to the chest.

A plug of mucus may block one of the smaller bronchi, resulting in collapse of the lung tissue beyond. This area of collapse can be seen on the X-ray.

Lobar pneumonia

This is a more acute condition and results from bacterial infection, especially by the *pneumococcus*.

SIGNS AND SYMPTOMS

There is a sharp rise in temperature accompanied by coughing, rapid shallow breathing and often pain in the chest. The chest pain is sometimes referred to the abdomen, simulating appendicitis. Consolidation of the whole or part of the lobe may follow the inflammatory reaction to infection. The consolidated area may be easily recognized on the chest X-ray.

Treatment of pneumonia

In the *acute stage* the treatment is by drugs and, if necessary, the administration of oxygen.

In the *sub-acute* and *chronic stages*, where there is obstruction of the bronchi, collapse or consolidation, postural drainage and breathing exercises are given: (i) to assist expectoration and so clear the bronchial passages; (ii) to increase air entry.

In older children postural and mobility exercises may help to improve their general condition where this is poor following prolonged illness.

INHALATION OF A FOREIGN BODY

Inhalation of a foreign body is a common cause of collapse of lung tissue in children. One commonly inhaled object is a peanut, which because of its oily texture is not only difficult to shift, but causes irritation of the lung tissue. Other items include small beads, bits of plastic toys, as well as teeth or fragments of tonsil following operation for their removal.

SIGNS AND SYMPTOMS

These may follow a specific incident when the child was seen to choke and cough. Alternatively, there may be no known history and the symptoms are noticed over a period. The child may appear quite well, but has a persistent cough and is often breathless on exertion. There may be obvious diminution of movement on one side of the chest, and a dull note on percussion indicating diminished air entry.

X-rays are always a necessary part of diagnosis in chest conditions. In this case they will demonstrate the area of collapse and/or indicate the position of the foreign body.

Treatment

Foreign bodies must be removed by bronchoscopy. Often no further treatment is necessary. If the affected area does not re-expand spontaneously, physiotherapy may be given as for lobe collapse.

BRONCHIECTASIS

CAUSES

This chronic condition of dilatation of the smaller bronchi may follow any prolonged or repeated chest infection, particularly if there has been blocking of one of the larger bronchi by a plug of mucus or a foreign body. A congenital weakness of the walls of the bronchi may be a predisposing factor. The small bronchi become over-stretched by the accumulation of secretions, which become thicker and more infected. The elasticity of their walls is lost as well as the sensitivity of the tissues lining them. Eventually the walls of the bronchi collapse, forming cavities filled with thick sticky purulent material.

SIGNS AND SYMPTOMS

Bouts of coughing occur, often, but not always, producing purulent sputum, greenish in colour and foul-smelling. These may be precipitated by a change of posture which causes the secretions in the lungs to move into contact with healthy tissue and stimulate the cough reflex. This is often apparent when the child goes to bed or when he wakes in the morning.

In the long-standing cases there may be clubbing of the fingers and even of the toes.

The child is often thin and small for his age.

Diagnosis is confirmed by a bronchogram which demonstrates the dilatation of the bronchi.

Treatment

MEDICAL TREATMENT

This includes the control of infection by antibiotic drugs and investigation into the cause of the condition, e.g. the exclusion of cystic fibrosis.

SURGICAL TREATMENT

If the condition is limited to a well-defined area, lobectomy or partial lobectomy offers a good prognosis. The healthy remainder of the lung quickly expands to fill the space created by removal of the infected part and normal function is restored.

PHYSIOTHERAPY

The principal aim of treatment is drainage of the affected area. Therefore the physiotherapist must know: (i) the exact site of the lesion; (ii) the appropriate drainage positions. These are shown in Fig. 17/1 on page 214.

Postural drainage, percussion, shaking and vibrations, and breathing exercises are used to facilitate coughing and expectoration. Sputum should be collected and measured each day. If there has been little or no sputum prior to treatment the amount may increase in the first day or two, but should then gradually decrease in quantity, becoming thinner, clearer and less purulent.

Some adaptations of treatment for babies is given on page 213.

CYSTIC FIBROSIS

Cystic fibrosis is a disorder of the exocrine glands. The mucous secretions are abnormally viscid and tend to block the ducts of the glands, thus preventing the proper function of the organ as a whole. Lungs and pancreas are affected as well as the sweat glands, which secrete an excessive amount of salt.

CAUSE

The condition is inherited by an autosomal recessive gene, which if carried by both parents gives a one in four chance of a child being affected.

SIGNS AND SYMPTOMS

In its early months the baby may suffer from malabsorption, due to the lack of pancreatic secretions, and fail to thrive.

He is underweight and may pass a large number of pale, bulky and unpleasant smelling stools.

He is particularly prone to chest infections which do not resolve and frequently progress to a condition similar to bronchiectasis. Formerly these chest infections would prove fatal before the child reached his teens.

DIAGNOSIS

Diagnosis is made from analysis of sweat which contains an abnormally high proportion of chloride and sodium.

Treatment

Early diagnosis and treatment with the administration of pancreatin and other drugs, and attention to diet now makes the prognosis less gloomy. Particular care is needed to avoid respiratory infections and to provide immediate treatment when they do occur.

Chest physiotherapy plays a vital part and should be started in infancy. All areas of the lungs should be drained and coughing encouraged in order to clear the respiratory passages. This must be done two or three times a day and continued regularly, whether the child is at home or in hospital. It is therefore important to teach the parents to carry out the technique, and for older children to learn to perform their own postural drainage and breathing exercises.

ASTHMA

Unfortunately asthma is a common condition among children. It is characterized by spasmodic episodes of wheezing and shortness of breath which may last anything from a few minutes to several days.

CAUSES

A large proportion of cases have a family history of asthma or hay fever. Boys are more often affected than girls. Psychological and physical factors both play a part and it is not always easy to draw a clear line between these.

The psychological aspect may be seen in the child with an unstable home background and/or excessive emotional pressures from one or both parents. Often there is an anxious, over-protective and continually fussing or nagging parent with a frustrated and secretly rebellious child whose asthma may become a weapon as well as a defence.

Allergy is a common cause. The child may be sensitive to one or to a whole series of items, e.g. house dust, dust in the coats of various animals, feathers, pollens and some foods. Attacks can be precipitated by upper respiratory tract infections. In many cases even when a physical cause is evident there is a strong emotional overlay, some apparently minor incident or anticipated event being sufficient to start an attack.

SIGNS AND SYMPTOMS

During the asthmatic attack expiration is made difficult by the narrowing of the smaller bronchi. This is due either to spasm of their muscular walls or to oedema of the mucous membrane lining them. The child feels he is unable to breathe and makes greater efforts to take air into his chest, using his accessory muscles of respiration to do so. This results in a stiff hyper-inflated chest with tension in the muscles of neck, shoulders and abdomen. The first sign of an attack may be wheezing, or a hard dry cough. Later coughing becomes easier and produces varying quantities of sputum as breathing gradually returns to normal. Attacks often occur at night or in the small hours of the morning.

Initially no permanent changes occur, the chest returning to normal between attacks. In time the lungs tend to remain hyper-inflated and the chest wall becomes rigid in the position of inspiration, with high shoulders and kyphosis of the dorsal spine (Plate 17/8). There is a close link between asthma and eczema; both conditions are frequently found in the same patient, one deteriorating as the other improves. Appetite and general health are often poor. The child looks pale, undersized and underweight for his age, but is often of high intelligence.

Treatment

MEDICAL TREATMENT

Various drugs will be prescribed by the doctor in charge, but it is useful for the physiotherapist to know what they are and how often they should be given. Parents tend to get confused, to forget and need reassurance. Bronchodilators and sometimes sedatives are given at the onset of an attack. A smaller maintenance dose may be given in the intervening periods. Steroids are occasionally used as a long-term treatment if all else fails to bring about improvement.

Allergies may be isolated by skin tests and treated by desensitizing injections. If the child is sensitive to house dust or feathers it is obviously important that these should as far as possible be eliminated, at least at home. Pillows and bedding should be of synthetic materials; if possible floors should be carpeted and vacuum-cleaned frequently.

MANAGEMENT

Because of the distressing nature of attacks parents often panic because they feel they are unable to help, and this is quickly communicated to the child, making him even more tense and breathless than before. Stemming from this situation he tends to receive an unhealthy amount of sympathy and to be treated as an invalid. This focuses attention on his symptoms and makes them more likely to recur. It is important that the asthmatic child should be treated as normal, participating as far as possible in all the activities of his age group.

Physiotherapy

The physiotherapist can contribute a great deal by teaching the child to control his attacks and showing his parents how best to help him.

Treatment should commence when the child is relatively fit, i.e. between attacks.

First priority is to find a comfortable relaxed position which can be adopted during attacks, so that the child can breathe more freely.

(i) *Side lying* is usually the easiest position to start with, using one or more pillows as necessary. In order to relax the abdominal muscles and give the diaphragm room to move, the top leg should be well flexed and across the body so that the position is halfway between side lying and prone. The arm on the under side is flexed and drawn back so that the hand rests on the abdomen.

(ii) *Kneel sitting* with forward support. The child sits on his heels, or on a cushion placed over them, and leans forward to rest forearms and head on pillows or a stool. In this position the abdominal, pectoral and neck muscles can relax and breathing becomes easier and quieter (Plate 17/9).

(iii) *Forward sitting*. The child sits on a low stool so that the feet are firmly on the floor, and leans forward with his elbows on his knees. Relaxation of the head, neck and shoulders is taught in the treatment session and practised in the home.

BREATHING

The child is encouraged to breathe out quietly and to feel the tightening of the abdominal muscles under his hand. No command is given to breathe in, but attention is drawn to the movement of the diaphragm as the abdominals relax. Forced movements, hissing or whistling are discouraged as they produce tension in the muscles of the throat and upper chest.

The positions and breathing must be practised when the child is well, so that they become almost automatic and are more easily adopted when an attack threatens.

Secondary to this part of treatment, attention may need to be directed to posture and general mobility. In respect of the latter, the parents are often amazed to see how much their child can do in the way of climbing, jumping and ball games. This also provides a chance to practise the breathing exercise when breathless after activity.

SUGGESTIONS FOR CHEST PHYSIOTHERAPY FOR BABIES AND YOUNG CHILDREN

Postural drainage

This is most easily done with the baby lying on a pillow on the physiotherapist's lap (see Fig. 17/1, p. 214). The baby feels comfortable and secure and can lie in the prone, supine, side- or half-side-lying positions with additional support provided by the physiotherapist's hands on his chest. The physiotherapist should sit on a low chair so that she can regulate the degree of tip by moving her knees. In Fig. 17/1D she achieves this by having her right foot on a low platform; in Fig. 17/1C she produces the same effect by extending her left knee.

Thus, all areas of the lung can be drained with minimum disturbance. If possible, the baby should be positioned so that his face can be seen, so that his colour can be checked frequently. A toy unbreakable mirror can be useful if arranged so that the physiotherapist, and the baby, can see his reflection, particularly when draining the posterior segments of lower lobes. Other toys, mobiles, or musical boxes may also be arranged

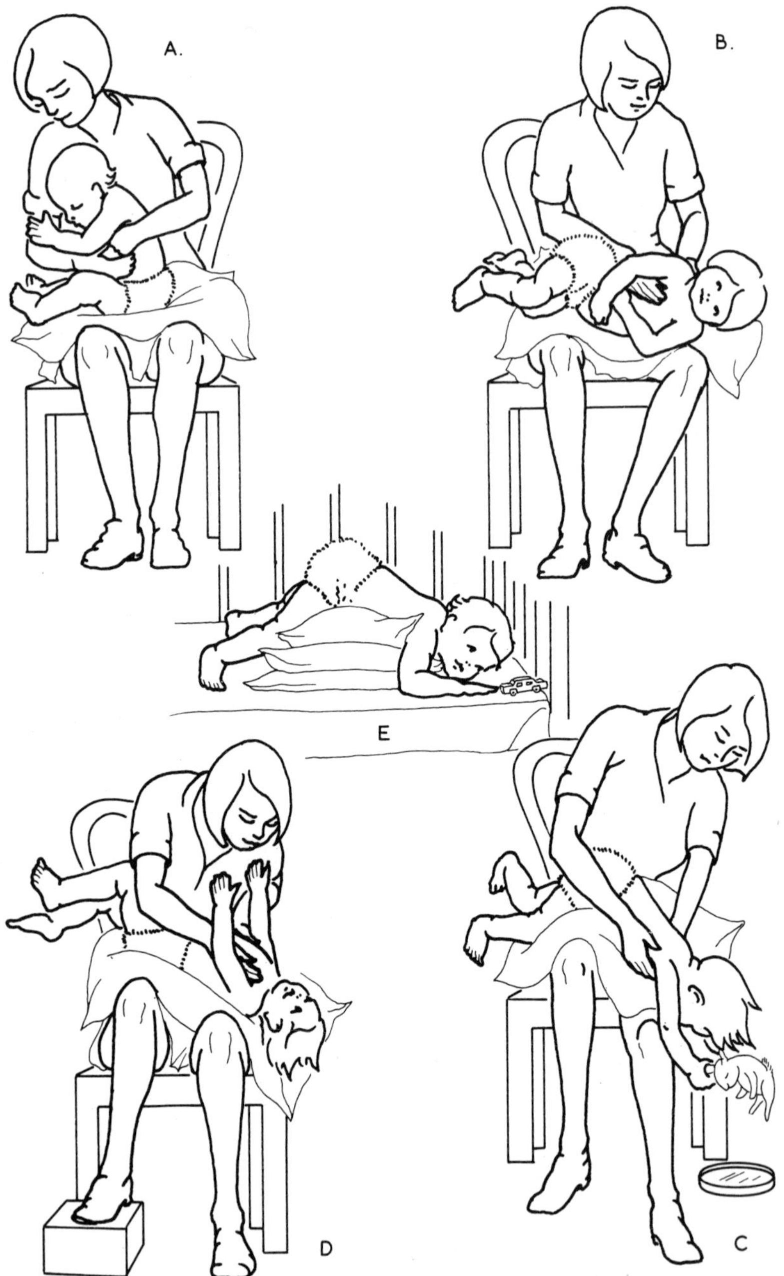

Fig. 17/1 Some positions used for postural drainage for babies. A. Upper lobes, apices. B. Right middle lobe. C. Lower lobe, posterior segment. D. Lower lobe, anterior segment. E. Over pillows in cot – lower lobes, posterior segments to hold the attention of toddlers who are often happier treated on the lap, but still tend to get restless. They can, of course, also be tipped over pillows and are often found afterwards administering the treatment they have received to their favourite doll or teddy.

Details of the correct drainage positions for each area of the lungs are shown in the diagrams.

'Exercises'

It is quite easy to give vibrations and shaking in time with the baby's natural expiration. Toddlers will often imitate sounds and may 'sing' Ah-Ah-Ah while their chests are gently clapped or vibrated. Laughing is good exercise and if not too ill, most babies enjoy being tickled and encouraged to use their arms, by grasping the physiotherapist's thumbs while she performs 'circles' or 'hugging and stretching'. They quickly learn to participate; and so help to maintain mobility of chest and shoulder girdle, which can become quite stiff even in very young children.

All children love bubbles and blowing them is often a good introduction to the very young as well as helping to overcome the fears of many slightly older children, who may be away from home for the first time and view any new face or treatment with apprehension. Bubble-blowing requires little effort and therefore does not cause tension in the muscles of the throat or chest – even if the child does not blow them he enjoys watching and will reach out to catch them and a great deal of activity can be stimulated in this way.

Fat, lethargic babies are sometimes 'chesty' and may benefit from a spell in the baby bouncer. The activity improves their general musculature as well as increasing the rate and depth of respiration.

Simple direct breathing exercises should be commenced as soon as it is possible to get the child's co-operation. This varies from about the age of two years to four or even five years. The easiest starting positions are side lying or supine with knees bent. The child's hands rest over his diaphragm and he feels his 'tummy get smaller as the air goes away' and larger as he fills up again with air. This can then be repeated with hands on the lower ribs.

For Bibliography see p. 224.

Chapter 18

Physiotherapy for Children – III

mental subnormality

It is becoming recognized that some groups of mentally subnormal children can benefit from the services of physiotherapists willing to specialize in this field. Two categories of subnormality are recognized, the educationally subnormal (ESN), and the ESN (Severe).

The ESN child is one of limited intelligence who would not benefit from education in a normal school, but is able to receive some education in a school for the educationally subnormal. Here he can be taught to read and write and is prepared to become an independent member of the community.

The ESN (Severe) child is not capable of benefiting from any formal education. A large number can be trained to a moderate degree of self-care and to perform simple tasks. They will always need constant supervision and help, and eventually it will be necessary for most of such children to have institutional care.

Education authorities are obliged to provide schools for the severely subnormal of school age.

Because no other provision is made for them, a third group of children are frequently found in schools for ESN (Severe). These are the multiply handicapped whose combination of mental, physical and social difficulties make both management and training appear a formidable task; one which nevertheless can sometimes have its rewards.

Causes

Mental subnormality may result from cerebral malformation, injury or degenerative disease. Some conditions are genetically determined, others may be due to maternal infections during critical periods of pregnancy. There is sometimes a familial link but often no known cause is discovered.

MICROCEPHALY

The brain is small and lacks the normal number of convolutions.

Although the face grows to normal size the skull barely grows after birth and the head circumference rarely exceeds seventeen inches. The child is nearly always severely mentally subnormal and in addition often has motor disabilities. Sometimes there is a familial tendency; there may also be a connection with infections during pregnancy.

HYDROCEPHALUS

There is increased pressure in the ventricles due to an excess of cerebrospinal fluid. The condition may be present at birth or occur spontaneously later; it is also frequently associated with spina bifida. Treatment by the insertion of a Spitz-Holter or Pudenz valve is sometimes successful in stabilizing the condition; but unless performed early some brain cells will remain permanently damaged. In untreated cases the head grows very large to accommodate the increased fluid, thus adding to the physical problems of management and training.

DOWN'S SYNDROME (MONGOLISM)

This is perhaps the commonest of genetically determined conditions causing mental subnormality. The defect is due to an extra chromosome which increases the normal number of 46 to 47. The child is often the youngest of several and there are seldom more than one in the same family. Mongols are easily recognized at birth by their typical facial appearance, broad and flattened with small nose and slanting eyes; the tongue may appear too large for the rather small mouth. Hands and feet are broad and short; frequently the terminal phalanx of the little finger is in-curved and a single deep crease runs right across the palm (Simian crease).

There is generalized hypotonia with hypermobility of the joints. Milestones are always delayed and speech may remain infantile and difficult to understand. A large number suffer from congenital heart defects and a high proportion of these do not survive early childhood; usually they succumb to repeated respiratory infections. In general they are happy, sociable children, fond of music and anxious to join in all that goes on. The higher grade mongol can be trained to do easy repetitive work.

Metabolic disorders

CRETINISM

This is the result of under-secretion of the thyroid gland and may be diagnosed at a few weeks of age. Although the baby appears normal at birth it quickly becomes dull, listless and unresponsive; the skin feels cold and is coarse and dry, the complexion sallow and the lips thickened. Early treatment with thyroxine will prevent progressive brain damage which would lead to subnormality.

PHENYLKETONURIA

This is a condition of defective amino-acid metabolism. It can be diagnosed by a Guthrie test carried out when the child is one week old. Treatment is by a special diet from which most of the usual proteins are excluded because of their phenylalanine content. If this is started early and vigorously adhered to, the child should develop normally. The children affected are fair-haired and blue-eyed; if untreated their growth is stunted and they become physically retarded and severely mentally subnormal.

Brain damage

Injury to a potentially normal brain may be incurred at birth, e.g. by anoxia or kernicterus; or later as the result of meningitis, encephalitis, hypoglycaemia, severe dehydration, metallic poisoning or fractures of the skull.

EARLY SIGNS AND SYMPTOMS

Some of the clinical signs of specific conditions have already been described. Many babies appear normal until they start to fall behind in their physical development. Smiling is frequently delayed. These children are often poor feeders, making little effort to suck, and in due course resisting the introduction of solid foods. The general muscle tone is often low and they lie passively in their cots, taking little notice of their surroundings. Alternatively some are irritable and restless with a high-pitched cry which is difficult to calm.

Most subnormal children lag behind because they lack the drive and inquisitiveness to investigate and try out new channels of activity; thus they never experience those things normal to a child of their age and so they fall even further behind. As they get older they have a strong tendency to repeat the same action, or sound, or word, over and over again (perseveration). They dislike change and easily develop set patterns of behaviour which are hard to break, like sitting and rocking, or various mannerisms of the hands. Drooling is also common even when there appears to be no physical reason for it.

Initially it may be difficult to distinguish between mental and physical handicaps (cerebral palsy, deafness, defects of vision). An accurate diagnosis may only be possible after prolonged observation. Delay in social responses and motor behaviour and the exclusion of other handicaps indicates the likelihood of mental subnormality.

FITS

Fits are neither a cause nor a sign of subnormality but a great number of mentally subnormal children have fits of either the grand mal or petit mal variety. Although not causing subnormality in the first instance, continuing, uncontrolled fits can result in further cerebral deterioration. The most common drugs used to control fits are phenobarbitone and phenytoin.

TREATMENT

Treatment starts with the parents, for it is they who will have to care for the child and to teach him all the things a normal baby learns automatically. This can be a long and difficult task and the parents will need all the support one can give. Contact between the doctor and physiotherapist is extremely important and it is helpful if the physiotherapist can be present at the consultation. Anxious parents are liable to forget or even not hear what is said to them at a time of stress; the physiotherapist should know what has been advised in order to reinforce it later. One of the most difficult things for parents to accept is the fact that it is often impossible to forecast exactly how far their child will develop. It is also sometimes difficult to explain that although there is no cure for the basic condition, it is still possible to help the child to develop more fully by special attention to early handling, play and management. Parents need the help of all members of the paediatric team, doctors, therapists, social workers, to achieve a realistic approach, and to persevere in training their child.

Treatment should start as soon as possible so that the months of infancy are not wasted. A constant factor in subnormal children is their inability to initiate anything on their own. They may have sight, hearing and feeling; they may be able to move; but they are unable to link the two. Therefore an important part of treatment is to find a way to bridge the gap, to motivate, and eventually to teach independence. Another characteristic, following from the lack of motivation, is resistance to change. Subnormal children do not move much and are quite happy to be left alone. So it is essential that they should be moved, so as to change their positions and their activities at regular intervals. It is also important to progress from one activity to the next as soon as the first is becoming established. A daily timetable including all the possible activities may be useful at home or in hospital so that nothing is forgotten.

As a normal baby learns from the people and things around him, it is important that the handicapped baby should have not less but more opportunities to learn in this way. Mothers (and fathers) are often afraid to disturb their baby because they know there is 'something wrong with him' and need to be reassured that he needs to be picked up and played with like any other baby. It is important to talk to these children even when they are too young to understand so that they become aware of the shades of expression in the voice and in the face. It also helps the mother to relax and thus makes a better relationship between her and her child.

Many subnormal children do not present for treatment until they are two years old or more, when they are placed in Special Care nurseries. The suggestions put forward may be adapted by therapists or nurses for use with these older children.

Some suggestions for play

(i) Take baby on your lap and encourage him to hold up his head and look at you and to look around.

(ii) Put him on his tummy across your knee; try to increase the length of time he stays there each day. As he gets used to the position see that he has something to watch.

(iii) Handle his arms and legs, hands and feet. Talk to him about them, calling them by their proper names, so that he learns the proper names straight away and is not confused by things having more than one title.

(iv) Hold his hands and take them to touch his mouth, eyes and ears.

(v) Play Pat-a-cake and Peep-bo.

(vi) Show him his toes, help him to feel them with his hands.

(vii) Put a rattle in his hand, if necessary keep your own hand round his; shake the rattle. Then take your hand away and see if he will do it on his own.

(viii) Dangle a bright toy in front of him. Move it slowly until he fixes his eyes on it. Teach him to follow with his eyes and head from side to side and then up and down.

Obviously it is not desirable (or possible) for baby to have someone playing with him all day. He needs time to be alone and opportunity to try out his own play. To encourage this a 'play bar', a length of wood fixed across the cot, can be used to suspend a selection of rattles and toys (Plate 18/1). These should be at a suitable height so that they can be seen and touched. Toys, however nice, are of little value if they are out of reach or even out of sight of the child for whom they are intended. Different toys should be chosen to give a variety of colour, shape and texture and should be changed frequently.

All babies and all physically retarded children should spend several periods each day in prone, to develop head control and strengthen their back muscles. Untreated older children may be quite helpless and miserable in this position which they have never known. Plastic foam wedges are of great value in this situation; the child is more comfortable and finds it easier to lift his head and play with toys on the floor in front of him (Plate 18/2). For smaller children a 'roller' made of the same material often fulfils the same purpose. It may also be difficult to con-

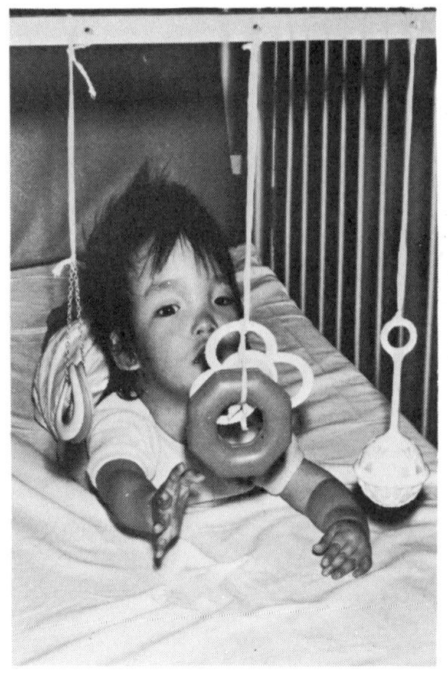

Plate 18/1 The Playbar in use in a hospital cot (*see p. 220*)

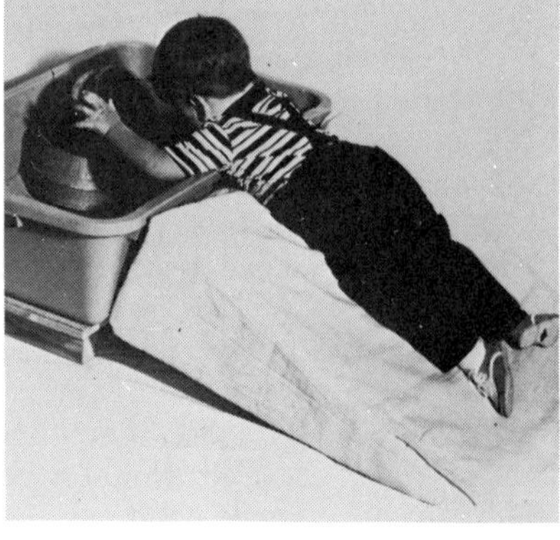

Plate 18/2 A wedge pillow encourages head control while the hands are free to play (*see p. 220*)

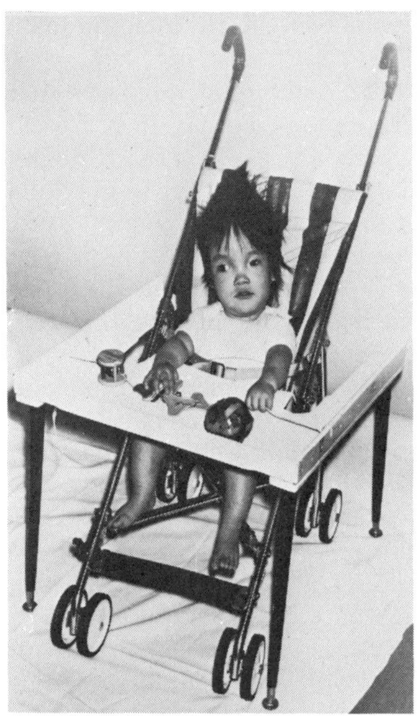

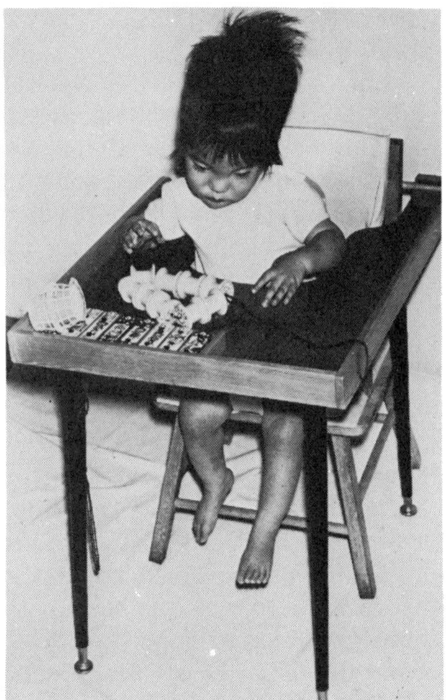

Plate 18/3 A one-year-old hydrocephalic boy starts to sit in a baby buggy push-chair but soon progresses to an adapted nursery chair with no head support. He needs a cut-out table with rim to which his toys are attached (*see p. 222*)

vince the parents of the necessity for their child to play on the floor in this position when he is able to look more socially acceptable propped in a chair. But floor play must be encouraged so that the child learns to move. Rolling is important but should not be accepted indefinitely as the only means of progression. Efforts must be made to persuade the child to an alternative method, either on knees, seat or feet. Sometimes the Dolphin Crawler is appropriate at this stage (Plate 16/2).

At the same time it is desirable that the child should be sat up fairly early so that he can see what is going on. The selection of a suitable chair demands careful assessment of his needs and abilities, particularly where there is a physical as well as a mental handicap. Consideration must be given to fit, comfort, support and safety. The chair should be arranged so as to provide something to watch, thus encouraging head control. A cut-out table should be provided with a rim to prevent toys rolling off, so that the child can use his hands. A series of holes along the side of the rim enable toys to be threaded on to a string running across the table (Plate 18/3).

The type of chair should be reviewed regularly with reference to the child's growth and physical progress.

Although at first he may need full support he should fairly soon acquire some head control and should then start sitting for short periods in a chair only extending to shoulder level; the first chair is then gradually withdrawn.

Many 'special' chairs are available but a plain wooden nursery chair makes a good basis for a variety of adaptations. Plastazote is a useful material for making inset linings for chairs and pushchairs. If desired it can be covered in some suitable material and is effective in providing a comfortable fit and support which can be altered or removed as the requirements change. Insets can also be made of wood or plastic foam rubber. For the multiply handicapped child, the Britax Star Rider car seat makes a useful first chair, giving maximum support in a good posture. Fixing it securely, at the correct angle, sometimes presents a problem, but it can be strapped on to a wooden kitchen chair or in an old-type pushchair which has no front bar. It may be found more satisfactory in use if the harness is replaced by webbing and Velcro straps fastening through a central ring.

Kneeling and standing can both be started relatively early so as to provide as much different experience as possible. Support from the physiotherapist or a helper will be necessary at first. Both positions are best introduced with the child playing at a table of suitable height. If there are sufficient helpers children may benefit from playing together round the table. Occasionally standing splints are useful for very subnormal and hypotonic children. These can be made of Orthoplast, Plastazote or plaster of Paris, and are used initially to give the child an idea of the standing position. He will soon begin to enjoy the experience and try to help himself. As soon as he begins to support himself the splints are no longer necessary.

Some multiply handicapped children will unfortunately never be able to stand and walk alone, but the difficulties of management will be greatly eased if they can be left to stand holding on, and walk with help. Although this appears to be more important when they are older and bigger, it is better to start when they are still young. Less disabled children enjoy all the normal nursery apparatus, and water play, painting, swings, slides and climbing frames, all of which provide an incentive to exercise and exploration. They also like moving to music and action songs; these can be used to help overcome any specific physical difficulties, but the greatest benefit is in learning to do things with others and become independent. These activities may appear closer to the work of the playleader or nursery teacher than the physiotherapist; the ideal situation is one in which the two work together.

SUPPLIERS OF GOOD TOYS

Educational Supply Association and Abatt Toys
P.O. Box 22 The Pinnacles
Harlow
Essex

Fisher Price Toys made by Mettoy Playcraft Ltd.
14 Harlstone Road
Northampton
and available in many good toy shops

James Galt & Co. Ltd.
P.O. Box No. 2
Cheadle
Cheshire
and branches in large towns

Mothercare Shops in most big towns

Reeves & Sons
Lincoln Road
Enfield
Middlesex

Thomas Hope Ltd.
St Philips Drive
Royton
Oldham
Lancashire

BIBLIOGRAPHY

Ellis, R. W. B. and Mitchell, R. G. *Disease in Infancy and Childhood.* Churchill Livingstone, 7th ed. 1973.

Finnie, N. R. *Handling the Young Cerebral Palsied Child at Home.* Heinemann, 2nd ed. 1974.

Griffiths, R. *The Abilities of Babies.* University of London Press, 3rd Impression, 1964.

Hutchison, J. H. *Practical Paediatric Problems.* Lloyd Luke, 3rd ed. 1972.

Jolly, H. *Diseases of Children.* Blackwell, 2nd ed. 1968.

Lloyd-Roberts, G. C. *Orthopaedics in Infancy and Childhood.* Butterworth, 1971.

Wiles, P. and Sweetman, R. *Essentials of Orthopaedics.* Churchill Livingstone, 1965.

PART IV

Disorders of Skin

Chapter 19

Skin Diseases

by DOREEN CANEY, MCSP, DIP.TP

Few patients are referred to physiotherapy departments for the treatment of skin disease. The range and efficacy of other methods of treatment (drugs and dressings) have reduced the need for physiotherapists to spend their time in treating these conditions. However, a small number of patients are still referred. This usually occurs where drug treatment alone has proved inadequate to alleviate the condition, or where drug treatment is more effective if combined with ultraviolet irradiation.

In order to treat these patients effectively, the physiotherapist needs to have an appreciation of the methods of treatment available to her and a knowledge of the skin conditions concerned. She should also appreciate that the skin is frequently a mirror of the mental state of the patient. As in all other conditions she should therefore treat the patient as a whole rather than confining her attention exclusively to a localized area.

METHODS OF TREATMENT

Relaxation

If the patient is being treated by tranquillizing drugs, instruction in relaxation techniques may be of great benefit as an adjunct to treatment. Many physicians now believe that the ability of the patient to relax without recourse to sedative drugs (which may become addictive) is of prime importance. Because of this more patients who find it difficult to relax may be referred for instruction in the future. Physiotherapists should ensure that they are skilled in communicating the art of relaxation and should use this in the treatment of skin conditions, if the condition is related to mental stress. Training in relaxation is also important where the skin condition causes itching (for example, eczema). The patient's natural desire to scratch will cause further skin irritation and the ability to relax will be of great benefit in controlling this.

Ultraviolet irradiation

The beneficial effect of natural sunlight and the improvement seen in many skin diseases during the summer months, is sufficient indication of the value of ultraviolet light. Physiotherapists have traditionally used artificial sources of ultraviolet rays in the treatment of skin diseases. Dosage can be varied from the sub-erythemal dose (75% of an E1) through all the degrees of erythema according to the desired effect. In clinical practice the effect aimed for is most likely to be increased cell production leading to thickening of the skin, increased desquamation, increased blood supply to the skin or increased pigmentation. Irradiation of the whole body is said to have a tonic effect. The usefulness of ultraviolet irradiation on areas denuded of skin, e.g. infected wounds, is doubted by many. It seems to be more logical and effective to culture the bacteria and apply the appropriate antibiotic. However, in a few cases, use of the abiotic rays of the spectrum may be appropriate.

When applying treatment the most appropriate ultraviolet source must be used. Treatment given in contact must be from a water-cooled lamp. Treatment given with an air-cooled source may either be from a mercury vapour lamp or fluorescent source. The spectra of these differ. The mercury vapour lamp gives rays from 1849 Å to 3900 Å, while the fluorescent tube gives rays from 2800 Å to 3900 Å. It will thus be seen that the fluorescent source has a higher proportion of longer rays. The longer rays penetrate more deeply and wave bands at about 2500 Å and 2900 Å are responsible for the production of erythema. It therefore follows that where an erythema is aimed for, irradiation from a fluorescent source will probably be the best choice. The initial choice of source is important as the same lamp must be used at subsequent treatments.

Heat

The physiotherapist may also find that the application of mild heat has beneficial effects in the treatment of localized skin infections, such as boils, carbuncles or infected wounds. Heat may be applied superficially using infra-red rays or more deeply by short-wave diathermy or microwave diathermy. The rationale underlying the use of heat is that increased metabolic activity and increased blood supply will aid the local tissues to combat the infection. The heat should be directed to the area of blood supply rather than towards the infection, so that the rate of bacterial growth is not stimulated (for example, heat could be applied to the forearm in the case of an infection of the hand). This type of treatment should be given in association with localized and systemic antibiotics.

Cold

An effective erythema can be obtained by massaging the local area with an ice-cube. This may be preferable to the use of dry heat and is useful in the treatment of an area of skin which threatens to break down into a pressure sore.

Tissue mobilizing techniques

Where the skin condition has led to fibrosis and thickening of the tissues, with the possibility of contracture and deformity, the mobility of the tissues must be maintained, and deep localized massage, with active movements and possibly passive stretchings, may be appropriate.

ASSESSMENT AND RECORDING

In this field no less than in other areas of physiotherapy, the preliminary assessment of the patient's condition is essential. Careful observation of the affected skin area should be made and the extent, type and severity of the eruption should be noted. Standard diagrams of the anterior and posterior aspect of the body are useful, so that the affected areas can be outlined and the pre-treatment record kept with the patient's treatment card.

A careful scrunity of the patient's notes will be made in order to determine relevant points in the history of the condition, especially so that the type of medicaments being given can be known. Some of these may be sensitizers, e.g. coal tar, which will alter the patient's reaction to ultraviolet radiation. The patient's skin reaction to sunlight should be tested if the treatment prescribed includes ultraviolet irradiation. The result of this test and the other findings should be carefully recorded on the patient's treatment card. A special note should be made concerning the extent of the area treated so that at subsequent treatments the possibility of overdose because of altered screening is avoided.

In the treatment of most skin conditions re-assessment of the affected area should be made at each attendance, and the treatment should be based on the findings. A careful recording of the day-to-day condition and the consequent modifications to treatment is therefore of prime importance. Objective evidence such as a tracing of a wound, or the extent of an active area of acne, should be recorded rather than subjective assessments such as 'patient improved'. The physiotherapist should be in a position to base her reports to the dermatologist on factual evidence rather than optimism.

SKIN CONDITIONS REFERRED FOR PHYSIOTHERAPY TREATMENT

Acne vulgaris

This is a chronic inflammatory disease of the sebaceous glands. The condition most commonly affects those parts where the glands are large, i.e. the face, chest and upper back, and is seen in adolescents and young adults primarily, though very occasionally, the condition may persist into later life. The essential lesion of the condition is the blackhead, or comedo, a firm mass of keratin which blocks the follicular pore. This may cause inflammation of the surrounding tissues or it may become secondarily infected with eventual fibrous tissue formation and unsightly scarring.

In mild cases no treatment other than careful skin toilet is required. Severe cases respond well to a prolonged course of a tetracycline antibiotic. The few patients who are referred for physiotherapists to treat are those who have severe acne which is not responding well to other forms of therapy. The rationale underlying this referral is that cases of acne improve in the summer months and therefore ultraviolet irradiation from an artificial source can be used to supplement the effects of natural sunlight. Exceptions to this are patients who have fair or sensitive skins, as they are often made worse by local ultraviolet radiation.

The affected skin area should be washed with soap and water prior to treatment and then irradiated by a general ultraviolet source, in order to obtain desquamation. A second degree erythema should be aimed at and repeated when the effect of the initial dose has died down. Some consultants request that a comedo expressor should be used prior to treatment. The technique of ultraviolet irradiation will vary with the area being treated. The physiotherapist must ensure that her screening techniques are such that there is no possibility of 'overlap' dosage. In the interests of the patient it is as well to screen to the natural bony features of the body, such as the jaw line or the clavicular line. A more acceptable cosmetic effect can be obtained by allowing a natural fade-off of irradiation, but this can only be done where screening is not essential. The maximum size of the irradiated area should not exceed one-sixth of the body's surface area.

Psoriasis

This condition affects approximately one to two per cent of people with white skin. The cause is unknown but the abnormality results in unduly rapid cell division within the epidermis. Normally the cells reproduce at such a rate that the epidermal turnover takes approximately 28 days.

In psoriasis the turnover rate is seven times as fast, i.e. every four days. The amount of skin area affected varies from trivial to extensive. Characteristically, initial lesions are on the extensor aspects of elbows and knees and in the scalp, or over the sacral area. Severe cases may have total skin involvement, although the face is usually spared. The condition appears to be adversely affected by mental stress, although the course of the condition is typically unpredictable and exacerbations cannot always be attributed to this factor.

The affected area shows a slightly raised red plaque, with a sharp margin between it and healthy skin. The plaque is surmounted by dry silvery grey scales. If the scales are removed the underlying skin bleeds easily.

Medical treatment for psoriasis is usually by the administration of local or, very occasionally, systemic agents which contain a toxic substance to slow down the rate of cell division. Where these fail, or in the case of a patient whose condition is becoming rapidly worse, admission to hospital may be advised. It is in the intensive treatment of patients with psoriasis that the physiotherapist is most likely to become involved. The usual treatment is a modification of the Ingram regime. The patient bathes first thing in the morning in a tar bath and scrubs off his psoriatic scales. He then attends the physiotherapy department for general ultraviolet irradiation from a fluorescent source. As the irradiation is given daily, no more than a first degree erythema should be achieved and some authorities believe that a sub-erythemal dose only should be given. The lesions are then covered with Dithranol paste and with a suitable dressing until removal the next day prior to bathing. Removal of the paste can be facilitated by the use of liquid paraffin. This treatment is effective in nearly all cases though many relapse again.

Alopecia areata

This is a relatively common condition in which patches of baldness appear spontaneously. There is no evidence to suggest that any type of physiotherapy will increase the rate of regrowth of hair in the affected areas, although high frequency stimulation and ultraviolet irradiation have been tried. Complete recovery of the affected patches usually occurs but may take from three months to two years. If ultraviolet irradiation is requested, a second degree erythema should be given to the affected area of scalp after careful cleansing with spirit to remove grease. Subsequent treatment would be given when the erythema of the previous dose has died down. The new growth of hair frequently lacks pigment but this is gradually developed.

Vitiligo

This is a condition in which there is a patchy loss of melanin pigmentation. Areas of the body show irregular patches of skin lacking in pigment. The cause of the condition is unknown but it is sufficiently widespread to affect one per cent of the population. Recent advances in the treatment of this condition have shown some success in re-pigmentation after treatment of the affected areas with trimethylpsoralen lotion followed by exposure to sunlight. The drug should be applied to the skin or alternatively taken by mouth approximately two hours before ultraviolet irradiation. The dose should be sub-erythemal and repeated not more often than every five days. The course should be prolonged, extending over a period of three to four months. During this time the affected patches should show evidence of re-pigmentation. If there is no response in this time the treatment is discontinued. However, if improvement is occurring treatment is continued for many months. Unfortunately the re-pigmentation may not be permanent and relapses occur frequently.

SKIN INFECTIONS

Furuncle

A furuncle or boil is an acute staphylococcal infection of the hair follicle. The infection discharges through the hair follicle after a series of inflammatory changes in which necrotic tissue is broken down into liquid pus. Any area of the body can be the site for a boil but areas of friction such as the back of the neck are the most likely. A series of boils affecting different parts of the body is known as a furunculosis. The detailed changes in the development of a boil are identical to those already discussed in Chapter 1 under suppuration (p. 7).

The patient is first aware of pain and an area of redness is visible over the site of the infection. This becomes a raised area which quickly shows a yellow centre. After a short while the skin over this central core breaks down and pus is discharged onto the surface. Frequently a solid core of unliquefied pus is also discharged. The affected area is quickly repaired by fibrous tissue and a scar is left to mark the place where the boil existed.

A single boil is very often left to run its own course. Patients who are obviously prone to this kind of skin infection may be treated with appropriate antibiotics, such as penicillin. Only a few patients will ever find their way to a physiotherapy department. The treatment for those who do will depend upon the stage in which the boil presents itself. In the early stage before the boil has started to discharge mild co-planar shortwave diathermy should be given. This aims at providing heat to the base of the boil, and the electrodes should be positioned so that the field passes deep to the boil. The treatment by heat accelerates the metabolic processes and encourages discharge of pus. Once discharge has occurred, the localized area may be treated by a more superficial type of heat such as infra-red radiation in order to aid the healing process. Boils which do not drain freely or do not discharge their contents completely may be treated by local ultraviolet irradiation using the sinus applicator.

Carbuncle

If the infection spreads subcutaneously to affect a group of hair follicles a large area of skin may break down to reveal a deep slough which may take a long time to heal. This kind of skin infection requires the administration of antibiotics. The patient may be referred to the physiotherapy department when the objects of physical treatment will be to aid the rapid breakdown of slough and assist in the healing of the affected area.

Treatment will be along the lines already indicated for a boil except that initially there is a wider breakdown of the skin and the area of infected tissue thus revealed should be treated by ultraviolet irradiation using a fourth degree erythema or double-fourth degree erythema to the affected area. The surrounding tissue should of course be carefully screened. Following irradiation the site may be dressed using a proteolytic enzyme such as Trypure. Both the irradiation and the enzyme will aid the breakdown of slough. When the area is clean the aim is to stimulate rapid re-epithelization and this may be done by the administration of heat, or a first or second degree erythema dose of ultraviolet irradiation to the wound and surrounding area.

Hidradenitis axillae

The apocrine sweat glands of the axilla are occasionally the site of a severe chronic bacterial infection which may be confused with furunculosis. The condition is more severe and may run a chronic course over ten to fifteen years, during which time there is severe scarring with possible contracture of the fibrous tissue.

The condition appears first as multiple red tender nodules which eventually break down and suppurate. Spread of infection occurs with increasing involvement of all the apocrine glands until these are ultimately destroyed.

Treatment is by local and systemic antibiotics and in order to encourage free drainage surgical interference may be necessary. Scrupulous cleanliness of the area is essential in order to combat the superficial spread of the infection. The patient may be referred to the physiotherapist for mild short-wave diathermy to the axillary region in order to encourage the free evacuation of the infected material by the application of heat. It is also important to ensure that the patient understands the need to maintain a full active range of movement in the shoulder joint to prevent contracture of the axillary tissue.

PHYSIOTHERAPY AS AN AID TO DIAGNOSIS IN SKIN CONDITIONS

Occasionally physiotherapists are asked to assist in the diagnosis of skin conditions. By using a Wood's filter in association with a Kromayer ultraviolet light source, certain types of tinea of the scalp (ringworm) can be shown as a bright blue-green fluorescence. Similarly, erythrasma gives a coral red fluorescence. This condition usually affects the groins, toe webs and the perianal region.

Photosensitivity and photopatch testing are used in the diagnosis of conditions where the skin has become hypersensitive to light. Such conditions may arise as the result of systemic or local exposure to a sensitizing substance. There is a wide range of possible sensitizers including drugs (sulphonamides, chlorpromazine, tetracycline), soaps, antiseptics, and silver and gold salts. In other cases no direct cause for the hypersensitivity can be found. Because the tests require the use of an ultraviolet light source, physiotherapists may be asked to assist with them. A Kromayer lamp with a filter of ordinary window glass is used for the test. This eliminates rays below 3200 Å. The minimal erythema dose (MED) for the lamp without the filter is calculated using a normal skin.

Photopatch testing is carried out in the following way. Patch tests of the suspected sensitizer are applied to both sides of the back or other suitable skin surface (one side then acts as a control). The patches are removed and the skin cleaned after 24 hours. The control areas are then covered with black paper to obscure the light. The test areas are irradiated by the Kromayer lamp with the filter using the minimal erythema dose. The areas are inspected 24 hours later. A positive reaction is shown by a reproduction of the photo allergy and the sensitizing substance can then be identified. A comparison with the control side will show the degree of photosensitivity.

BIBLIOGRAPHY

Epstein. *Archives of Dermatology*, 93–216, 1966.

Pillsbury, D. M., Shelley and Kligman. *Cutaneous Medicine*. Saunders, 1961.

Rook, A., Wilkinson, D. S. and Ebling, F. J. G. *Textbook of Dermatology*. Blackwell, 2nd ed. 1972.

Sneddon, I. B. and Church, R. E. *Nursing Skin Disease*. Arnold, 1968.

Wilkinson, D. S. *The Nursing and Management of Skin Diseases*. Faber and Faber, 3rd ed. 1969.

Chapter 20

Leg Ulcers

by C. R. BANNISTER, MCSP

Definition

Leg ulcers are essentially chronic lesions of the skin and connective tissues, but deeper structures are also often involved. Caused by abnormalities of the circulatory system, ulcers rarely occur upon a normal limb.

They are designated venous or arterial types according to the vessels at fault. The first presents the problem of impaired venous return, the second that of diminished arterial supply. Signs, symptoms and treatment fundamentally differ. About 95 per cent of leg ulcers seen in our departments are venous in origin, the remainder being arterial, although cases involving both systems are seen.

ANATOMY OF LOWER LIMB CIRCULATION

The following simple description concentrates upon the practical needs of our study. Anatomy cannot be fully discussed in such a brief chapter and reference should be made to a standard textbook.

The arterial system

Leaving the heart at the left ventricle the aorta passes through the thorax and abdomen where mesenteric, coeliac, renal and other visceral branches form. At the level of the fourth lumbar vertebra it divides to form the right and left common iliac arteries. Opposite the lumbosacral articulation the common iliacs divide into the internal and external iliac arteries. The external iliac runs downwards along the medial border of psoas major muscle and enters the thigh beneath the centre of the inguinal ligament, becoming the femoral artery. Four centimetres below the ligament the arteria profunda femoris branches. The main vessel proceeds along the adductor canal to pass through the opening in adductor magnus muscle where it becomes the popliteal artery.

THE POPLITEAL ARTERY

This distributes the geniculate branches which form part of the anastomosis round the knee, and at the lower border of popliteus muscle divides into anterior and posterior tibial arteries.

THE ANTERIOR TIBIAL ARTERY

This passes between the tibia and fibula, through the upper part of the interosseous membrane, on the anterior surface of which it then runs to the front of the ankle. Proceeding to the dorsum of the foot it becomes the dorsalis pedis artery. It then continues along the medial side of the dorsum of the foot to pass through the proximal end of the first intermetatarsal space to complete the plantar arch. Branches are given off to the muscles on the antero-lateral side of the leg, to the bones and ankle joint as well as to the foot and toes.

THE POSTERIOR TIBIAL ARTERY

This descends from the lower border of popliteus, at which level the peroneal artery emanates, then courses along the back of the leg, lying on the deep muscles and being covered by gastrocnemius and soleus. Becoming superficial, it is palpable below the medial malleolus. Branches are disposed to the muscles on the back of the leg, the peronei, and to the foot and toes.

The venous system

This consists of superficial and deep groups of vessels, connected to each other directly and by the perforating veins.

The superficial veins

These lie within the layers of the superficial fascia and comprise the long and short saphenii and their tributaries.

LONG SAPHENOUS VEIN

This courses upwards along the medial aspect of the leg. From the small veins of the toes and metatarsal region, the dorsal venous arch, and the medial marginal vein, it passes along the inner aspect of the foot to the front of the medial malleolus, along the medial border of the tibia, then postero-medially behind the knee and antero-medially along the inner aspect of the thigh, passing through the saphenous opening in the deep fascia to join the femoral vein approximately three centimetres below the inguinal ligament. It receives tributaries from the superficial veins of the thigh and from the lower part of the abdominal wall. In addition it drains the superficial tissues of the greater part of the leg with the exception of the lateral side of the leg and foot. A small area on the medial side between the tibia and the tendo calcaneus drains directly into the deep veins. *Thus interference with flow in the deep veins of the calf is particularly liable to affect the venous drainage of the lower third of the medial side of the leg – the area where venous ulceration occurs most frequently* (see p. 247).

SHORT SAPHENOUS VEIN

From the lateral marginal veins of the foot, it passes postero-laterally behind the lateral malleolus, along the back of the calf and, piercing the deep fascia, joins the popliteal vein at the back of the knee.

The superficial vessels are connected to each other by a complicated network of small veins.

PERFORATING OR COMMUNICATING VEINS

These are very important vessels connecting the two parts of the venous mechanism and normally allow blood to flow only from superficial to deep veins. They are mainly located in the lower third of the leg, though important vessels are found above and below the knee.

The deep veins

The deep system consists of the anterior and posterior tibial, popliteal and femoral veins and their tributaries. They lie beneath the fibrous inextensible deep fascia and the muscles immediately below this.

ANTERIOR TIBIAL VEINS

These arise from the vena comitantes of the dorsalis pedis artery. Lying deep to the anterior tibial muscle group, they ascend the leg, pass between the tibia and fibula through the upper part of the interosseous membrane and join the posterior tibial vein to form the popliteal vein.

POSTERIOR TIBIAL VEINS

These accompany the artery. In the lower part of their course they are covered only by skin and fascia. Ascending, they lie upon the deep muscles and beneath soleus and gastrocnemius, joining the anterior tibial veins to form the popliteal vein. Perforators are received from the long and short saphenii.

THE POPLITEAL VEIN

This commences at the lower border of the popliteus muscle, ascends behind the knee to the opening in adductor magnus through which it passes to become the femoral vein. The popliteal receives the short saphenous and geniculate veins.

THE FEMORAL VEIN

This progresses upwards in the adductor canal to pass beneath the inguinal ligament near its centre. Its principal tributaries are the vena profunda femoris, one perforator just above the knee, and the long saphenous vein. At the inguinal ligament it becomes the external iliac vein.

EXTERNAL ILIAC VEIN

This passes along the brim of the lesser pelvis and at the level of the sacro-iliac joint receives the internal iliac vein to form the common iliac vein. At the level of the fifth lumbar vertebral body, the common iliacs unite to form the inferior vena cava which, passing through the diaphragm, enters the right atrium of the heart. In the abdomen the inferior vena cava receives tributaries from the abdominal viscera.

Valves

These are bicuspid structures, placed at intervals along the veins. Their function is to prevent venous back-flow. They are especially numerous in the veins of the lower extremities, particularly in the deep veins.

It should be noted that whilst the superficial veins are supported solely by the partially extensible superficial fascia, the deep veins are sustained by both muscle and the inextensible deep fascia. The deep system assists blood return of the weakly supported superficial group by means of musculo-venous pumps.

The principal musculo-venous pump is composed of the following structures: posterior tibial muscles, deep fascia, deep veins of the lower leg, and perforating veins. On contraction of the calf muscles, the posterior tibial veins are closed and emptied, the blood being propelled upwards. On relaxation, the veins are refilled, not only from the deep veins of the foot, but also from the lower part of the long saphenous vein via the perforating veins and directly from the tissues of the lower part of the medial side of the leg between the tibia and the tendo-calcaneus. Thus venous return from the superficial veins is assisted.

AETIOLOGY AND TREATMENT

Normally blood supply and return are in balance. If either is chronically disturbed, tissues may degenerate and the leg become predisposed to ulceration.

THE ARTERIAL OR ISCHAEMIC LIMB

Such diseases as arteriosclerosis or calcification of the arterial walls can, by narrowing the lumen of the vessel and causing loss of elasticity of its wall, result in diminished blood supply. Physiotherapists are not greatly concerned with the primary condition, but it is necessary to recognize it, give such treatment as we can to improve the blood supply and particularly, to decide upon the kind of bandage needed and its tension. Harm may result from the application of too firm or too heavy a support as an already limited blood supply can be still further restricted with disastrous consequences.

Signs and symptoms

OEDEMA

There may be little or no oedema.

COLOUR

This will be pale bluish pink, turning blue in cold weather.

PULSE

Pulse will be absent in dorsalis pedis, and possibly posterior tibial arteries.

TEMPERATURE

The temperature of the limb will be cold.

TYPE OF PATIENT

This is usually the thin, nervous person, but all types may be affected.

Treatment

There are two objects of treatment, to relieve pain and to improve the blood supply if possible.

MEDICAL TREATMENT

Vasodilator drugs such as Hexopal, Opilon, Priscol or Vasculit may be prescribed.

SURGICAL TREATMENT

Lumbar sympathectomy or other surgery such as the various forms of arterial grafts, may be performed.

PHYSIOTHERAPY

In dealing with these cases, the utmost care must be taken not to damage the very friable skin. Badly applied bandages, careless handling and ill-fitting footwear can all cause harm. If giving massage, one must be extremely careful. Heat must never be applied directly to the extremity;

it causes congestion and can easily blister. Reflex heating is used, infra-red to the abdomen or short-wave diathermy to the popliteal vessels at or above the knee, but never under any circumstances at all below this level.

Careful massage may be given to the limb and sometimes Buerger's exercises may be requested.

THE ISCHAEMIC ULCER

SITE

The ischaemic ulcer is usually found on or below the malleolus (see Fig. 20/1).

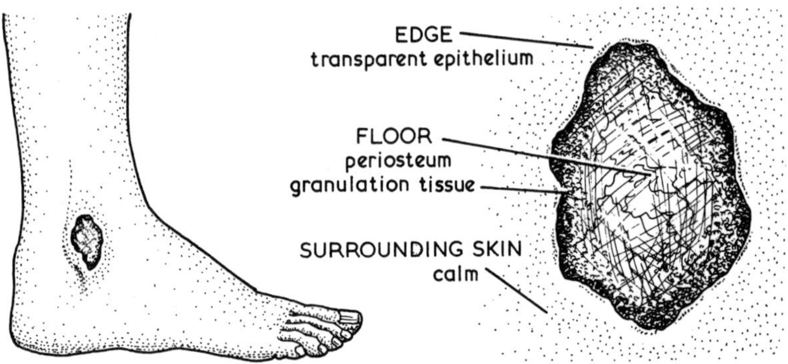

Fig. 20/1 A typical ischaemic ulcer

PAIN

This is often intense, possible causes being infection or anoxia.

The *surrounding skin* is usually calm unless the lesion is infected. The *edge* of the ulcer is of transparent epithelial tissue or, if infected, possibly serpiginous in form. The *floor* often consists only of periosteum with a narrow circumference of granulation tissue.

In such a lesion, the periosteum has little protection and should infection intervene there is a risk of osteomyelitis occurring. Granulation tissue must be stimulated in order to protect the periosteum and initiate healing. Sub-erythema doses of ultraviolet light are indicated, followed by a dressing such as Lassar's paste or paraffin Tulle Gras. In general, a greasy dressing will stimulate granulation tissue growth, but a saline dressing will tend to control this.

Utmost care must be taken in the selection and application of the bandage for, as before stated, compression is harmful because the arteries are already damaged. A crepe bandage may be all that is required.

Briefly, as far as physiotherapists are concerned, all that can be done for these patients is to make the most of such circulation as remains.

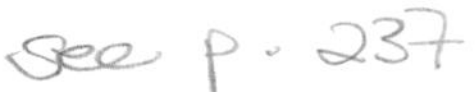

THE VENOUS, OR GRAVITATIONAL LIMB

The major disturbances of the venous system are deep vein thrombosis and varicose veins.

Deep vein thrombosis

This is the clotting of blood in a vein resulting in the occlusion of the vessel. It is the most common cause of leg ulceration and usually occurs in the posterior tibial veins in the calf.

SIGNS AND SYMPTOMS

Before onset the part may be cooler than normal.

ACUTE STAGE

Pain, swelling and inflammation will occur at and below the site of the thrombus.

In the acute and sub-acute stages, treatment is by medical means and the physiotherapist is rarely concerned.

CHRONIC STAGE

The vein may be occluded for almost its whole length, but gradually the clot is absorbed and the vessel re-canalized. During this process, however, valves are destroyed and venous back-flow is then possible. The resulting high intravenous gravitational pressure is reflected upon the perforating veins which gradually distend and render their valves incompetent (Plate 20/1). This pressure is further reflected upon the lower part of the superficial veins, particularly the long saphenous vein, which also becomes varicose.

Venous stasis and oedema follow which, if not controlled, will organize into an indurated mass interfering with free blood flow in superficial tissues. Degeneration of connective tissue and skin may then occur. The leg becomes tense and painful, sometimes inflamed, and predisposed to ulceration. It will regress further unless the process is halted and reversed by effective treatment.

Deep vein thrombosis leads to the breakdown of the musculo-venous pump. Indeed, if valves below the level of the origin of soleus muscle are destroyed, exercise of the posterior tibial muscle group will also propel blood *downwards* in the lower part of the veins, thus increasing tension.

Treatment

The objects of treatment are to control and reverse the changes in structure and mechanics of the limb and to prevent further regression.

MEDICAL TREATMENT

Diuretics may be prescribed.

SCLEROTHERAPY

The doctor may inject at the sites of the junction of perforators with superficial veins, the vessels then being compressed with a firm bandage.

SURGERY

The perforators may be tied and removed (Cockett's operation).

PHYSIOTHERAPY

Physiotherapy is used to reduce the oedema and afford support to tissues as described later.

Varicose veins

Varicose veins occur only in the superficial veins, primarily because of their weak support and the length of the column of blood.

CAUSES

Long standing, constrictive wear, hereditary factors, a scar or a mass causing pressure on a vein at any point along its course, can lead to distension of its walls, gradually rendering the valves incompetent. Venous stasis and swelling may follow and a painful, inflamed area form at the distal end of the affected vessel which, if not adequately supported, will spontaneously ulcerate.

TREATMENT

Long standing should be avoided. Where possible pressure should be removed. Support to the vein and the leg is essential and will relieve symptoms. The condition can only be cured, however, by injection or the surgical removal of the incompetent members, thus allowing efficient return to be re-established by competent veins.

THE VENOUS ULCER (Plates 20/2a, b; Figs. 20/2–20/5)

If preventive measures are not, or cannot be, pursued, the limb slowly regresses and ulcers can easily result. They occur spontaneously or have traumatic origin, and assume one of the following forms:

SPECIFIC INFECTION

(See Fig. 20/2, p. 246.) The *edge* of the ulcer may be serpiginous and possibly undermined. The *floor* of the ulcer may present a thick yellow or black slough or be itself discoloured. It is deep and often uneven and dark. The *base* may or may not be present according to the duration of the ulcer. The *surrounding skin* may be inflamed, an indication of acute infection of even the beginning of cellulitis.

A swab for culture and sensitivity would probably be taken and the dressing prescription based upon this.

Rest is an essential part of treatment.

When inflammation has subsided, an E4 or 2E4 dose of ultraviolet light may be given, this being bactericidal, the skin being protected, usually by sterile paraffin Tulle Gras.

In order to prevent cross-infection of other ulcers, strictest precautions must be observed in dealing with this type.

HEALING

(See Fig. 20/3.) The *edge* of the ulcer is of transparent epithelium, even and calm. The *floor* is clean granulation tissue level with the skin. It is shining and a healthy pink in colour. The *base* is probably non-existent and the *skin* calm.

This stage of ulceration needs only sub-erythema ultraviolet light, a bland dressing and a suitable support.

HYPERGRANULATING

(See Fig. 20/4.) The *edge* of the ulcer is epithelial and even in form. The

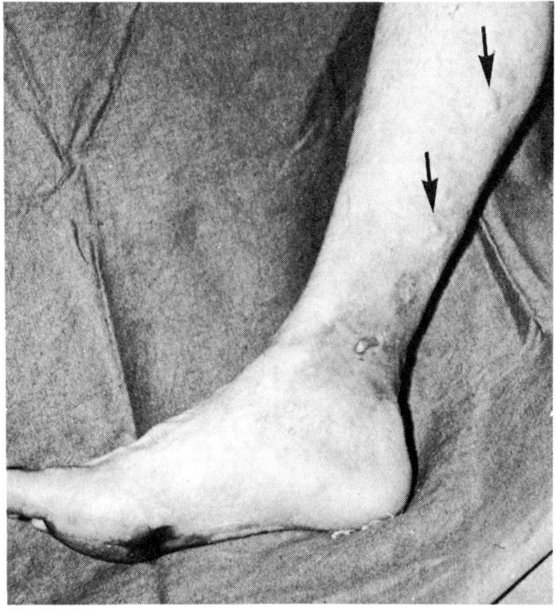

Plate 20/1 Incompetent perforating veins at their junction with long saphenous vein (*see p. 249*)

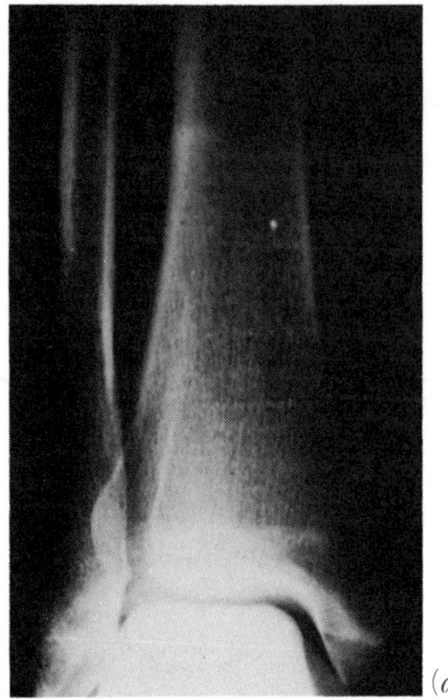

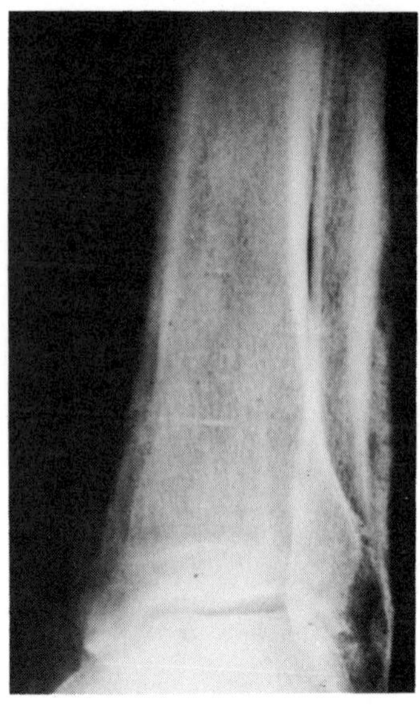

Plate 20/2 Effect of fibrous base of ulcer of 15 years' duration. Compare tibia and fibula of (b) ulcerated left limb and (a) non-ulcerated right limb of same patient. Anterior radiograph taken after surgical excision of ulcer (*see p. 242*)

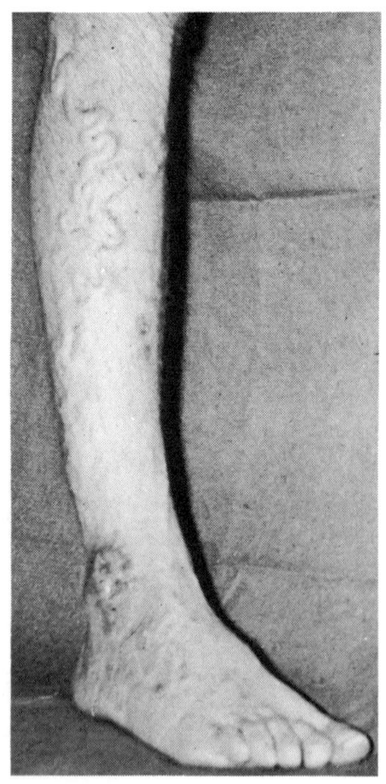

Plate 20/3 Varicose short saphenous vein. Note tortuous and deviated course of the vein (*see p. 247*)

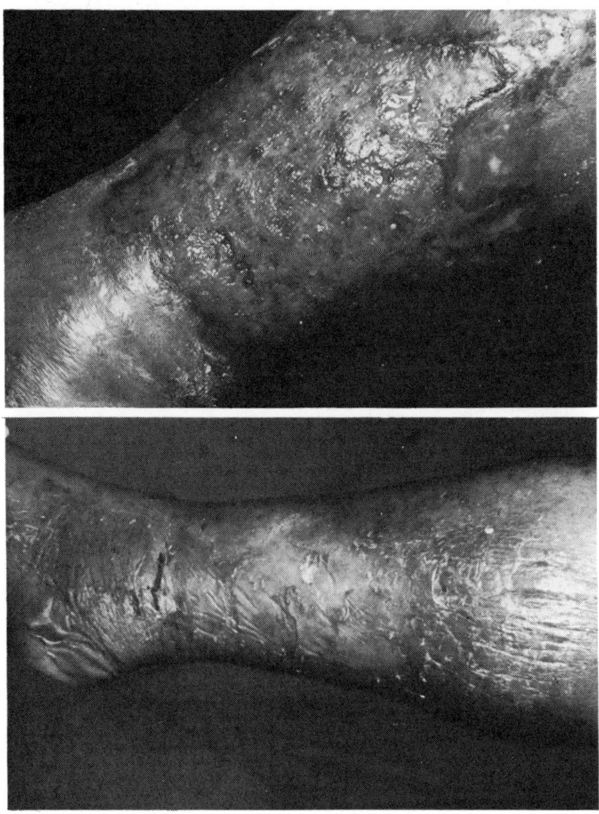

Plate 20/4 *Top:* A chronic gravitational ulcer complicated by congestive cardiac failure, bronchitis and marked obesity. *Bottom:* The same limb after healing by hospitalization, medical care and physiotherapy to ulcer (*see p. 249*)

floor is clean granulation tissue growing above the level of the surrounding skin. The *base* is probably non-existent and the *skin* calm.

In this type the exuberant tissue must be controlled for epithelium will not grow over hypergranulation. A pressure pad over the ulcer dressing is often sufficient but it may be necessary to precede this with a 2E4 dose of ultraviolet light, the skin and non-hypergranulating areas being protected by sterile paraffin Tulle Gras.

CHRONIC

(See Fig. 20/5.) The *edge* of the ulcer is fibrous, thick and vertical. The *floor* is pallid, and deeply set below the skin level. Sometimes low-grade infection is evident. The *base* is a thick, fibrous and almost avascular mass

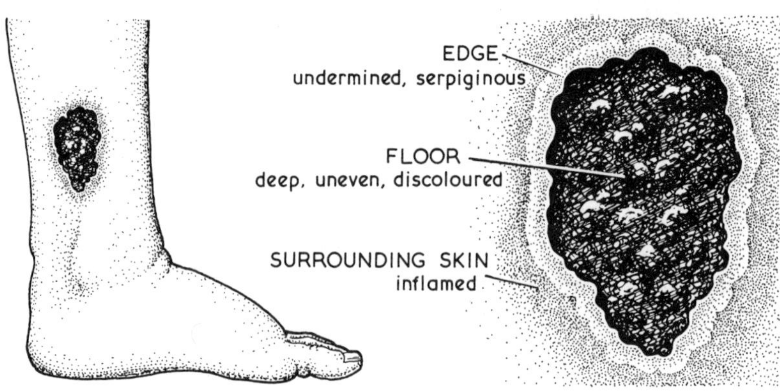

Fig. 20/2 An infected venous ulcer

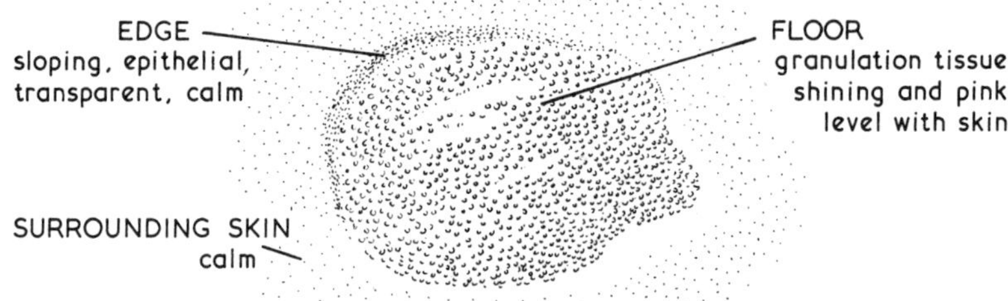

Fig. 20/3 A healing venous ulcer

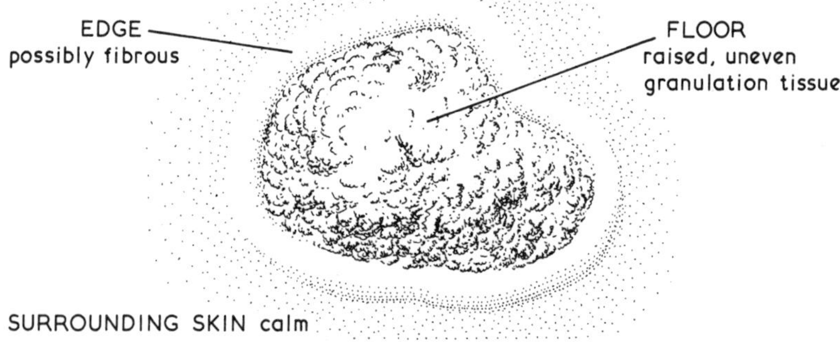

Fig. 20/4 Hypergranulating ulcer

beneath and somewhat larger than the ulcer. Possibly it is mobile but it is probably closely enmeshed in the bone below. The base delays healing and its effect must be removed before an ulcer can heal. The *skin* is calm, but probably thick and indurated.

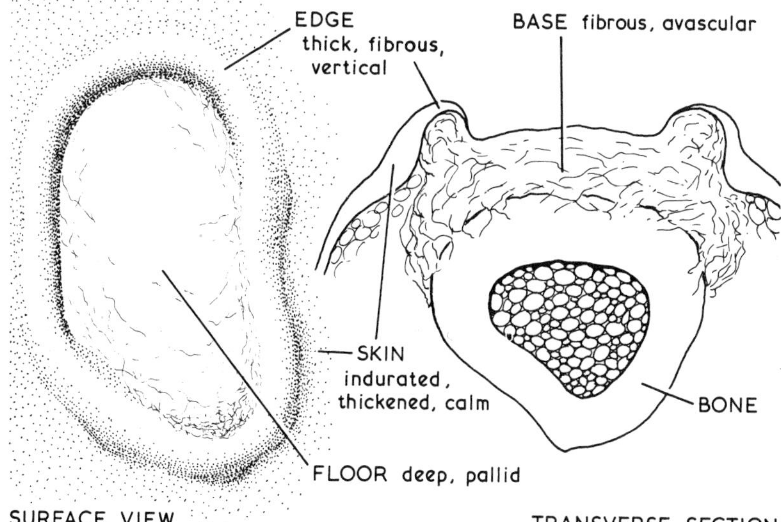

Fig. 20/5 A chronic ulcer

All parts of a chronic ulcer need to be stimulated and mobilized, using massage, ultraviolet light, ultrasound and exercises.

This type is the one most frequently seen in physiotherapy departments.

Site

Venous ulcers occur in the lower third of the limb excluding the foot, more often on the left than on the right leg. There are four commonly seen positions, each with their own characteristics.

MEDIAL LOWER THIRD

This is the most frequent site. Probably a late result of deep vein thrombosis and the consequent incompetent perforators (pp. 237, 241).

LATERAL AND MEDIAL LOWER THIRD

This most often results from varicose veins, the ulcer lying at the lower end of the inefficient vessel distal to the above.

ANTERIOR

This site is frequently at the junction of middle and lower thirds. Always traumatic and infected, the injury usually damages the periosteum and its minute blood vessels. Stumbling when climbing on to a chair or boarding a bus is the usual cause.

POSTERIOR ANKLE

This is a very painful site, often traumatic.

Age

Patients aged from 20 to 93 years have been treated, the greater number being in the 50–70 age-group.

Sex

Approximately 66 per cent of the patients are women and 34 per cent men.

Type

Venous ulcers occur on people of all physiques, but mostly on those of heavier build.

TREATMENT

All regimes are subject to modification according to the general condition of the patient. Many of the subjects have chest, heart or other involvements. Allergic reaction contra-indicates the substance causing it.

In general terms the objects are to re-establish as nearly as possible normal circulation in the limb and to the ulcer site. *Only when efficient blood metabolism is restored can infection be controlled and healing initiated.*

Treatment is based upon the study of predisposing and maintaining causes, and changes in structure such as the fibrous base or induration of connective tissue and skin. It is also dependent upon the type of patient, particularly in regard to the selection of the bandage, i.e. the ability to remove and re-apply this and the extent of activity.

EXAMINATION OF PATIENT

Ascertain the history. Closely examine the limbs and the lesion; compare the size and shape of the legs and the tension and extent of oedema; note areas of induration; determine the range of movements and the reasons for limitation, if any, such as contractures. Examine for varicose veins, signs of phlebitis or thrombosis and incompetent perforators. Note the dorsalis pedis and posterior tibial pulses. Pay particular regard to the incidence of pain and try to elicit the cause. Allergies must be noted.

A tracing of the ulcer may be taken, as follows. A piece of Cellophane is sterilized and laid on the ulcer. This should be covered by a second piece on which is traced the ulcer outline. The first piece of Cellophane is discarded and the tracing is transferred onto the patient's record card with carbon. Fortnightly comparisons may be made and recorded.

Close observation of tissue changes is essential. Although tracings afford useful edge comparisons, the visible progression or regression in all parts actually guides our treatment. Cleansing of the lesion, proliferation of granulation tissue, the filling in of the floor and the formation of a healing edge, are all to be noted.

Objects of treatment

The objects of treatment are six-fold.

REDUCTION OF OEDEMA

Oedema inhibits circulation, healing and phagocytosis. It is itself trauma and will, according to its tension, thrombose minute blood vessels to the skin, connective tissue and fat, causing degeneration of these parts. Oedema limits movement, will become organized, is a culture medium for bacteria, and is a source of pain.

CONTROL OF INFECTION

Infection maintains the lesion and in some specific invasions such as *Proteus*, *Pseudomonas pyocyanea* or *Staphylococcus aureus* will actually enlarge the ulcer by destroying tissue. Infection is also a source of pain. These pathogenic conditions contra-indicate all physiotherapy, with the possible exception of ultraviolet light.

MOBILIZATION OF ALL STRUCTURES and STIMULATION OF ULCER FLOOR AND EDGES

in order to increase vascularity.

ALLEVIATION OF PAIN

INITIATION OF THE HEALING PROCESS

which results from the realization of the above aims of treatment.

Medical

Tests for infection and anaemia would be taken and acted upon. A lesion cannot heal whilst the patient is anaemic.

Diuretics may be prescribed, in order to reduce fluid retention.

Surgical

SCLEROTHERAPY

Incompetent veins (Plate 20/1) may be injected and a compression bandage applied.

LIGATION

A varicose vein too extensive to be controlled by injection therapy would have to be tied and stripped.

Excision and graft of the ulcer, including total removal of the base, would possibly be performed later, when the physiotherapist may be asked to give pre- and postoperative care.

Physiotherapy (Regimes of treatment)

Make the patient comfortable, in elevation if the general condition allows.

Prepare the trolley:

Sterilize the trolley top. Drop out the dressing pack from its outer envelope. Position two pairs of sterile forceps on trolley top, with which the sterile dressing pack will later be opened. Position pair of sterile disposable plastic gloves in wrappers. Position spare paper sterile towel.

On lower shelf place: cleansing solution; dressing solution, cream, etc.; skin barrier; bandages; plastic foam.

Wearing disposable plastic gloves, remove bandages and discard, remove gloves and discard. Place sterile paper towel under limb. Open dressing pack with spare forceps.

Pour out solution (Savlon 1 per cent, Eusol, or sterile normal saline). Scrub up hands. Using 'no touch' technique clean surrounding skin. Clean ulcer and dry with sterile gauze.

Cover lesion with antiseptic pack (toilet solution) and retain this where practicable throughout physiotherapy. Now commence physiotherapy.

Reduction of oedema

The most suitable treatment may be selected from the following.

COMPRESSION FARADISM

In effect, this is the formation of an artificial musculo-venous pump. Pressure localizing pads of plastic foam should be placed on the malleolar hollows, over the ulcer and possibly along the course of varicose veins. Electrodes are placed on the plantar surface of the foot, the antero-lateral tibial muscle group, and possibly the femoral triangle, and the whole held in place by a simple bandage. Pressure is by the blue line, or Bisgaard bandage, applied firmly from toes to knee or above. Comfortable stimulation, enough to elicit a definite contraction is given for two periods of about ten minutes each with a rest between. Faradism is also useful if given without compression.

EXERCISES IN THE BISGAARD BANDAGE

Remedial exercises can be performed whilst the legs are in elevation and firmly bandaged as above.

AIR COMPRESSION

A comparatively recent development has been the design of intermittent pulsating instruments. The principle is that the limb is placed into a double-skinned plastic tube which is alternately filled and emptied of air, both compression and relaxation being sensitively controlled and giving a possible maximum of 100 mm Hg, the usual being 60 to 80 mm Hg for ten minutes. The treatment mechanically reduces the oedema. Simple and quick to apply, this apparatus appears to be a most effective method. It is also indicated for the treatment of contractures of joints, such as the knee.

HIGH ELEVATION

This is a home exercise. For a period of twenty minutes twice daily, the patient lies on the floor with the legs vertical, supported by the wall.

Control of infection

Except in the acute and sub-acute infective stages, all techniques that aid the restoration of the normal blood metabolism assist this aim. Without adequate blood supply, infection cannot be contained. Provided there is no inflammation, the specific physiotherapy treatment for this object is a *bactericidal dose of ultraviolet light.* This is sometimes as high as a 2E4 depending upon the state of the ulcer floor. With an E3 or stronger application it is essential to protect the surround of the ulcer, and this is most easily done by applying sterile paraffin Tulle Gras right up to the edges. Ultraviolet light of this intensity is usually given once, or at the most, twice per week.

Mobilization of skin and connective tissue

Gained primarily by massage, the technique is the rolling of these structures between lightly held fingers and thumb. This can be extremely painful and should not be continued for more than two or three minutes at any one site. This movement should be alternated with kneading. These manipulations may with advantage be preceded by a short treatment of ultrasound, of the order of 1 Wcm^2 pulsed 1 : 1 for 10 minutes.

Massage to ulcer edges is essential in order to regain mobility here and to retain flexibility as the ulcer heals in order to give a free, well-vascularized scar. Cover the lesion with dry sterile gauze. Wearing sterile disposable gloves, feel the ulcer edge and give finger kneading along it, flattening and moving the fibrous wall. Painful areas should be avoided.

Stimulation of ulcer floor and edges

Ultraviolet light is the treatment of choice for this specific object.

At the chronic ulcerative stage using the Kromayer lamp an E2 dose is suggested to the floor and surrounding skin. As the ulcer becomes cleaner and acquires a better colour, the dose should be reduced because intense ultraviolet light deepens a granulating area. At that stage a Sub-E is indicated. *Ultrasonics* may also be used. This treatment is given to the surrounding area and stimulates and mobilizes by increasing the vascularity of a part. It is contra-indicated when an ulcer is maintained by an incompetent vein as this may bleed into the ulcer floor.

Ice is a very convenient method of improving the local circulation.

Alleviation of pain

Pain in a gravitational ulcer is caused by oedema, infection, thrombosis, phlebitis, a varix, or adherent dressings. Relief should follow the treatments indicated, coupled with a thoughtful and carefully applied dressing and support.

THE DRESSING

On completion of physiotherapy, it is necessary to take a fresh dressing pack, and possibly to re-lay the dressing trolley.

Remove the antiseptic pack with which the ulcer has been covered throughout treatment and dry the ulcer. The skin will have to be treated if eczema or maceration are present. A skin barrier such as titanium dioxide paste or zinc and menthol ointment may be used for protection.

The ulcer dressing plays a very important part in infection control and in the healing of an ulcer. This may take the form of a base of tulle, cream, ointment, powder, paste or a solution in which the medication is suspended, or one of the proprietary non-adherent types. The effect of the base on skin and ulcer must be noted.

The simplest effective dressing should always be used. Particularly in the case of tulles or ointment, it must be applied so that the skin is not attacked. The doctor will often prescribe, but if he does not then Lassar's paste, paraffin Tulle Gras, Eusol, lotio rubra, aluminium subacetate are all suitable. The modern proprietary applications are legion. All are effective in various circumstances and it behoves the physiotherapist engaged in this work to study their properties and effects.

If a culture and sensitivity swab indicates a specific infection requiring an antibiotic, the doctor will prescribe or must be consulted. These should be used only under medical instructions, the dangers being allergic reaction in the patient or the raising of a resistant bacterial strain.

The dressing for a painful ulcer or one crossing a joint should be non-adherent, divided horizontally and put on as separate pieces. This may relieve the pain caused by an adherent dressing. An absorbent pad, also divided, is placed over the dressing and the support applied.

THE SUPPORT (Fig. 20/6)

This is the most important single factor in the treatment of venous ulcers. By it we can reduce oedema, simulate the venous pump, and ease pain by giving relief to pendulous and distended veins. Reaction to any support must be watched for.

Where local pressure is required, thin pads of plastic foam or folded gauze may be placed in the malleolar hollows, over the ulcer and along the course of obvious varicose veins. The bandage must be carefully selected according to the needs and abilities of the patient. If the Bisgaard method is chosen, the dressing and pads are held in place by toes-to-knee crepe bandage, this being retained at night, the Bisgaard bandage being removed and then re-applied in the morning before rising. This is a very efficient support, but those most likely to benefit from it are the younger and more active patients. The Bisgaard bandage should not be placed directly on the skin as the sensitive areas could be abraded by its edges.

The most frequently used alternative is the medicated type such as Viscopaste, Calaband, Coltapaste etc., supported by an outer elastic bandage such as crepe, Elastocrepe, Lestreflex, Elastoplast, or Poroplast.

The medicated bandage is non-extensible and must be carefully applied without tension and cut where necessary to conform to the limb. The outer bandage is applied firmly, but never tightly, to the foot and lower third of the leg and eased somewhat as the bandage is progressed upwards. The bandage must extend from the bases of the toes to just below the knee (Fig. 20/6). (If needed the support may be continued above the knee by Tubigrip.) Alternatively, crepe, double-crepe, Tubigrip, Lastonet, Elastocrepe, Elastoplast and Poroplast may be used without a medicated under-bandage.

As the course of treatment progresses, it is necessary frequently to re-assess tension, for blood vessels protected by oedema in the early stages become vulnerable to constriction as that oedema is reduced.

To complete the treatment, simple foot exercises are taught. These must be regularly and frequently repeated at home. They are essential in order to prevent contracture and to maintain the strength of the foot muscles, the long-continued wearing of a bandage being weakening.

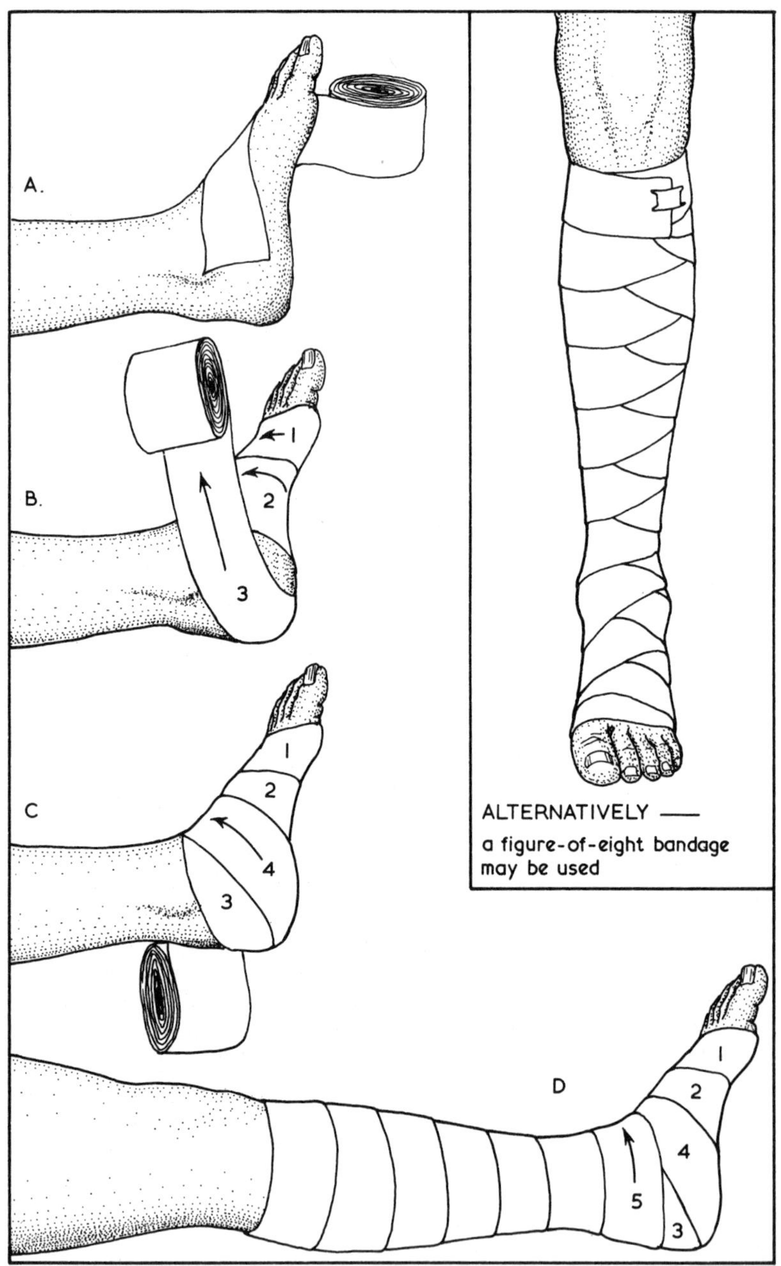

Fig. 20/6 Application of support bandage

Sclerotherapy

The object of intravenous injection is to remove the effect of an incompetent vein in order that competent vessels may re-establish drainage. In this procedure the inner lining of the vessel wall is destroyed. Compression pads are immediately placed over the injection sites by the doctor and a pressure bandage applied. Compression must be maintained for at least six weeks, the venous walls being flattened. Under normal circumstances the condition is reviewed and the bandage changed every two weeks, but if an ulcer is still present this may have to be dressed more frequently. The pads are discarded when the doctor directs.

Re-canalization may take place if intravenous gravitational pressure is allowed. Bandages may only be removed whilst the patient is in elevation or at least half-lying. Except for ultraviolet light, and exercise whilst bandaged, physiotherapy is contra-indicated.

In caring for a post-injection patient, although the doctor usually prefers to do this himself, one must remember that an artificial phlebitis has been induced, as a result of which a thrombus could very easily form. For the injection to be successful, a vein must be kept flat.

Excision and graft

The object of this surgical procedure is to remove the avascular, fibrous base on which the ulcer lies in order to graft the skin on to normally vascularized tissue. Physiotherapists are sometimes asked to provide pre- and postoperative care.

PRE-OPERATIVE CARE

Conservative treatment is given to clean the wound, mobilize joints and stimulate epithelization.

POSTOPERATIVE CARE

The aims at this stage are to aid circulation to the graft and to strengthen, thicken and mobilize it. Surgeons vary in their instructions but the following is a successful postoperative regime.

Ten to fourteen days after the graft, daily sub-erythema doses of ultraviolet light are given. The author believes that five seconds at two inches with the Kromayer lamp is the most effective starting dose. Two or three more treatments are given without progression and then minimal increases are made. This treatment appears to stimulate epithelization, improve the colour and strengthen the grafts.

Wearing sterile gloves, massage may be given above and below the lesion as the graft improves in colour and stability. This is to mobilize soft tissue, particularly near the excised border for this area tends to become fibrous. Mobility is essential, for circulation to the graft would otherwise be impaired.

Progression is made to finger kneading to the excised border and when it is stable, gradually introduce this movement across the graft. Still later, ultrasonics may be given to the area around the graft. Remedial exercises are introduced as soon as possible. Continue in this way until a mobile, well-vascularized graft results.

Physiotherapists should only be called in for the problem cases of leg ulcers – particularly for the extensive but inoperable lesions. Modern medical treatment should be given at the earliest pre-ulcerative stage and is therefore prophylactic. The extensive ulceration that we now see is largely the result of public ignorance of the treatment available. But the work of the great pioneers is being recognized and their methods used. Just as the effects of so many other conditions have been eliminated or minimized, so in the future will the worst of leg ulceration be controlled.

Leg ulceration appears to be a particularly useful study for physiotherapy students because other facets of their work are introduced, viz.:

The behaviour and control of oedema whatever its cause;

Recognition of the fact that swelling is itself traumatic and that wherever it occurs reduction needs to be achieved as quickly as possible;

The care of infected lesions;

The principle of infectious precautions;

The care of skin grafts;

The prevention and treatment of contractures;

The care of unique chronic conditions such as the balance and walking re-education of a patient who has not stood for ten years;

Most important of all is the emphasis on teamwork, for in dealing with the worst of these lesions all disciplines may be called in at one stage or another because, not infrequently, such an ulcer is only a sign of a deeper and much more serious condition requiring the most thorough examination, diagnosis and treatment.

FURTHER READING

Dodd, Harold and Cockett, F. B. *Varicose Veins and the Pathology and Surgery of the Veins of the Lower Limb*. Churchill Livingstone, 1972.

Fegan, W. G. *Varicose Veins, Compression Sclerotherapy*. William Heinemann Medical Books Ltd, 1967.

Fegan, W. G. 'Varicose Feet,' *Nursing Mirror*, August 30 1974.

Tranchell, H. G. and Bannister, C. R. *Circulatory Ulcers: A Physical Approach*. John Wright & Sons, 1960.

Bacterial Skin Infection. British Schering Ltd, Nicholas Laboratories, 1970.

Ulceration of the Leg. British Schering Ltd, Nicholas Laboratories, 1970.

Chapter 21

Burns

by ROSEMARY WOOTTON, MCSP

The skin and its function

It should be remembered that the skin is not just a collection of epithelial cells, but a composite organ of epidermis and dermis.

The epidermis is stratified and made up of five layers of cells, the deepest of these, the stratum germinativum, being the cell-producing layer.

The dermis is made up of two layers. In the upper layer lie the capillary loops, the smallest lymphatics and nerve endings including touch corpuscles, while the deeper layer consists largely of bundles of fibrous tissue with an interlacing of elastic fibres, and this rests directly on the subcutaneous tissue. This latter consists of bundles of connective tissue between which fat cells lie. The glandular parts of some of the several glands and deep hair follicles lie in this area. This subcutaneous layer serves to support blood vessels, lymphatics and nerves and protects underlying structures (see Fig. 21/1).

The skin is the largest organ of the body, representing about 16 per cent of the total weight of the normal adult. It has many functions, but the two most important, when considering extensive skin loss in burns, are protection against invasion by bacteria and prevention of fluid and protein loss from the body.

BURNS

Causes

Burns can be inflicted in many ways, but in each case they result from tissues being subjected to excessive heat.

Flame burns, scalds from steam or boiling water, contact burns or, in some hand cases, electrical burns, are the most common. Flash and chemical burns and indeed friction can all result in similar destruction and provide a Burns Unit with a great variety of cases from a wide cross-section of the population. Burns often result from accidents in the home, during work and play, and of course involve all age groups. Modern warfare accounts for many burns. The pilots who crash in flames, the

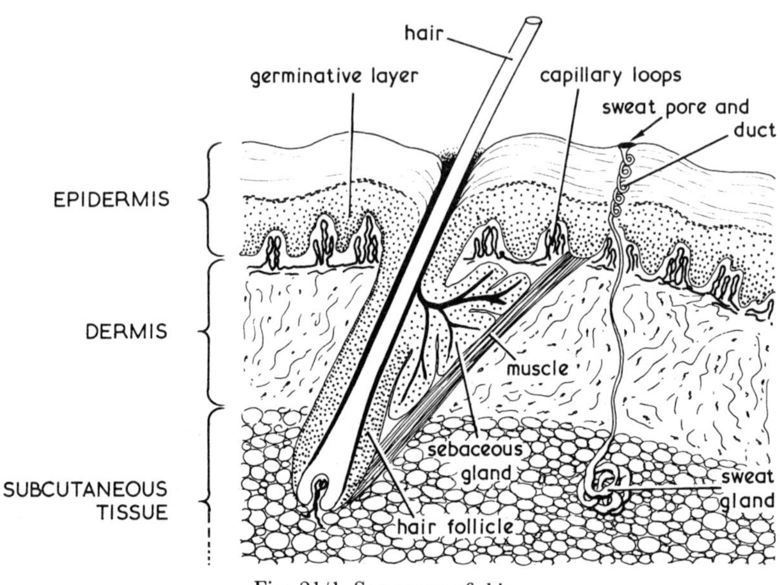

Fig. 21/1 Structure of skin

civilians living in the battle zone, and those subjected to the effects of 'blitzkrieg', more particularly since the introduction of the Napalm (naphthalene) bomb, are all examples of war burns.

Effects

In any burn, particularly if it is extensive, the immediate and serious effects are shock, severe fluid and protein depletion, and the chance of gross infection if every possible care is not taken.

SHOCK

Shock is the first hazard to be combated or, better still, prevented. Crile has stated that 'The best treatment for shock is prevention' and since shock is anticipated in burns it can be counteracted by early treatment. In burns, shock is delayed and results from the fluid and protein loss from the blood due to the increased permeability of the vessel walls. Because of this loss, the viscosity of the blood is increased. The compound effect of decreased circulatory volume and increased viscosity leads to a fall in blood pressure based upon decreased venous return to the heart.

When fluid loss is allowed to continue vasoconstriction takes place, eventually affecting the blood supply to the viscera and alimentary tract, sometimes resulting in kidney and liver damage.

In partial thickness burns, blisters occur due to seepage of fluid between the layers of the epidermis. Together with loss of fluid into the tissues, again due to the increased permeability of vessel walls, this gives rise to gross oedema.

INFECTION

Infection is another serious complication in burns. Organisms embedded in hair follicles and sweat glands can survive the sterilizing effect of excess heat and provide sources of infection. Further infection can occur from contamination from outside sources. This is why the isolation and treatment of these patients are carried out under the strictest conditions. The necrotic skin and constant oozing provide the ideal host for receiving and growth of bacteria, and where this is not adequately combated general toxic effects are produced. Locally infection complicates surgery, for obviously where there is infection there will be an inability to accept grafts and consequent production of scar tissue.

Classification

Under this heading we must consider the depth, the size and the position of the burn in assessing its severity. Burns fall into two categories, partial thickness and full thickness. In the former, the epithelium and superficial layers of the dermis only are involved and healing can occur by first intention. In full thickness burns the dermis is totally destroyed and with it the epithelial lining of the sweat glands and hair follicles so that no regenerative islands are left and healing can occur only from the wound edges, resulting in unstable scarring and underlying contractures.

It must be borne in mind that the assessment of depth of some burns is not easily definable in the first 48 hours, and even then the difference between partial and full thickness burns can by no means be correctly defined. What appears to be deep may prove to be partial, and what is partial thickness may indeed become deep due to further destruction of partly damaged cells by pressure or infection. A special method, infrared photography, is being used to determine burn depth, and the results of this are most helpful.

Partial thickness burns may be acutely painful since the nerve endings are damaged, whereas in full thickness burns the nerve endings are totally destroyed, and therefore the acute pain and immediate systemic effects from it are often less severe. Burn areas, of course, are invariably of mixed partial and full thickness involvement.

The depth of the burn is dependent on the temperature to which the area is exposed and the duration of the exposure.

In assessing *the extent of the area* involved the 'rule of nine' is useful to remember (see Fig. 21/2). The percentages of the total body area in adults are as follows:

head and neck	9%
front of trunk	18%
back of trunk	18%
arms	9% each
legs	18% each
perineum	1%

It is of interest to note that the palm of the hand is 1 per cent. As a rule 20 per cent burns in adults and 15 per cent in children necessitate

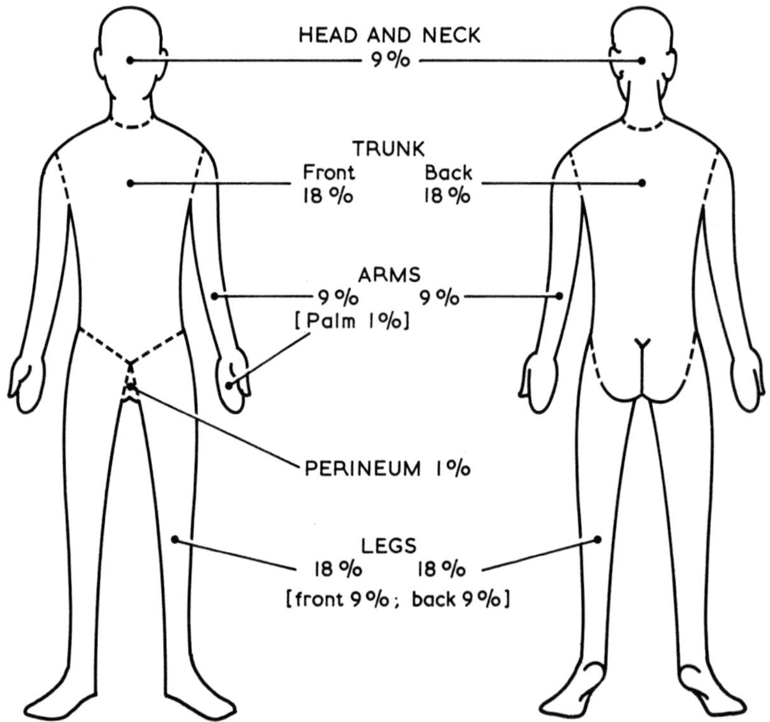

Fig. 21/2 Rule of Nines

intravenous fluid replacement. No one area gives rise to greater fluid loss than another but it is stated that there is greater loss in superficial than in deep burns.

With regard to *the position of burns*, wherever hands, feet, face and joints are involved, these should be regarded as major burns. It is the obvious functional importance of hands and feet that place them in this category. Burns of the feet, because of their weight-bearing function, are major burns. It has been stated that the hands are, next to the brain, man's greatest asset and when they are burnt it must be remembered that man is robbed of a large quota of his independence.

Joints fall into this major burn concept because their flexor surfaces, so often involved, tend to contract, thus producing accompanying ligamentous tightening and if neglected, resultant joint changes. As far as the face is concerned, apart from the cosmetic importance of treating it as a major burn, burns of the eyelids can produce contracture. This in turn, because the result is inadequate coverage of the eyes, can lead to corneal ulceration. It must also be remembered that facial burns are often associated with inhalation burns and involvement of the respiratory tract, when tracheotomy may be necessary.

From the point of view of *infection* some areas are known to be much more prone to *pseudomonas* than others, e.g. the trunk and the inner side of the thighs.

The severity of burns is not estimated only by their extent, depth and position. *The age and general condition* of the patient must also be taken into consideration. The elderly and the very young are at much greater risk than other age groups, the former due often to their lower resistance to infection and their relative immobility resulting from possible secondary disability such as heart and lung conditions or arthritic joint changes. The more elderly the patient, the lower the percentage of burn that may prove fatal.

In children it is generally accepted that they are at great risk because the relationship between their total body surface and their circularized volume is such that they lose comparatively more essential constituents of the body through a burn of given extent than an adult.

General treatment

Ideally severe burns are treated in specialized Units and more and more of these centres are being established. Not only do they provide the immediate specialized care that is urgently required, but, by the very nature of their construction, equipment and running, they are geared to minimize the chance of infection so very prevalent in burns. Infection can be kept to a minimum, if burnt patients are admitted early to such units, by the administration of prophylactic antibiotics on arrival and by treatment with exposure methods under conditions of isolation.

In units where patients are nursed in individual rooms the temperature of these rooms can be controlled and the patient receives all the intensive care that is necessary following such severe trauma.

Compensation for fluid loss is of prime importance and is done in the very early stages intravenously. Plasma, fresh blood, dextrose and saline are used variously in an attempt to replace losses accurately. Anoxia – a condition of lack of oxygen in the blood – is treated by the giving of oxygen by mask.

Pain has to be controlled with small, frequent doses of analgesics since pain only increases shock, but care has to be taken where narcotics are used that the patient's breathing is not affected and indeed that he should not become addicted.

The general systemic condition demands careful attention. There may be secondary anaemia due to damage and destruction of red blood corpuscles. It is essential that a check be kept on the fluid, protein and electrolyte balance. Nutrition plays a very important part in recovery as many of the problems both early and late stem from excessive losses combined with greatly increased energy demands.

Local treatment

It has been recognized for many years that early excision of sloughs – the necrotic skin caused by burning – is ideal, and that new skin cover is the dressing of choice for the raw areas thus created.

At East Grinstead it has been common practice to excise dead tissue at seven to ten days. In the case of burns of the hands, where the burn depth is clearly definable, *slough excision* is undertaken on the third day so that mobility and function can be regained as soon as possible. Blood loss may be great at operation and it must be replaced. In some units three to four weeks are allowed to elapse before operation, during which time natural separation of the slough gives an absolute indication of the depth of the burn.

When possible the defect created by de-sloughing is covered by *autografts* – skin cut from the patient's own body – but some advantages have accrued from covering the defect initially with *lyophilized or freeze-dried skin* for periods of two to five days postoperatively, when this is replaced by autografts taken at the original operation but temporarily stored. There are many advantages in using lyophilized skin. These are usually post mortem homografts taken from cadavers not longer than twelve hours after death.

In those who are extensively burnt the cutting of autografts causes further trauma to an already very sick patient, and it renders more areas prone to possible infection and allows further fluid loss. By using homografts, patients are spared this in the early stages and those who are seriously debilitated and suffering from chest conditions are spared the stresses of unnecessary and prolonged anaesthesia. Their general condition is allowed to improve before surgery is imposed upon them.

Homografts can also stimulate growth of epithelium in partial thickness burns and healing of such areas can thus be achieved in a few days.

When it is difficult to determine the depth of burns homografting may aid differentiation and the partial thickness area will re-epithelize quickly and then reject the homograft by the formation of fluid and pus. On the full thickness site the graft will take, rendering the surface under it clean and ready, at a later date, to receive autografts. The early application of homografts also lessens the incidence of contractures and by giving temporary cover decreases pain and improves the general well-being of the patient.

As previously mentioned the ideal environment for the treatment of burns is one where infection can be most readily controlled. Whereas specialized units were at one time few and far between, there are now several and more are being constructed and others reconstructed along more modern lines. Though, for some, the isolation of single rooms is irksome and a severe psychological strain, it is obviously the best way of preventing cross-infection.

In such an environment treatment *by exposure of the patient* can be easily carried out. Patients lie devoid of cover. Room temperatures can be controlled to individual needs. By this method burnt areas remain dry and unwelcome hosts for bacteria which thrive under moist, warm conditions. Sometimes light sheet cover is permitted, but only when suspended from cradles and kept well away from the burn surfaces. Strict aseptic routine is followed and persons entering the rooms must don mask and gown before attending the patients.

Where burns are circumferential, *rotating beds* are sometimes used to alternate pressure. Positioning of patients is particularly important to prevent contact of burnt surfaces such as the neck, the axillae and the perineum.

Hands are sometimes exposed and supported in elevation with rolls of Sorbo in the palms. Sometimes a boxing glove type of dressing is used. In this the fingers are separated by interdigital dressings of light gauze and the thumb is brought forward into opposition and they are bound down around a pack of dressing in the palm. The wrist is maintained, by splinting, in a position of extension.

After homografting a patient may still be left devoid of dressings, especially on extremities and in places where dressings are not easily applied such as the neck and axilla. This will enable early movement to be started without the risk of friction from dressings.

After autografting light dressings of Tulle Gras – Vaseline impregnated gauze – surmounted by light gauze dressings and firm crepe bandages are applied to maintain good graft position. Whilst this situation lasts, movement within the dressings is contra-indicated.

Dressings may have to be used more extensively in the aged, epileptics and alcoholics, where restlessness might split the eschar and give ample opportunity for bacterial invasion.

SALINE BATH THERAPY

Saline baths used to be employed a great deal for the badly burnt, but in some units their popularity has waned, because of the dangers of cross-infection. However, when they are used, they can be invaluable in facilitating early movement and easing the removal of dressings. Patients can be gently immersed in tanks containing normal saline, diluted 1 in 20, at body temperature. Exercises under these conditions are more comfortably carried out and, once over the initial fear, patients come to look forward to and enjoy their bath and respond well to encouragement to move in the water. Saline baths are generally given every other or every third day.

When saline bath techniques are used it is general practice to discontinue them for at least five days after grafting.

Sometimes before bathing or dressing a light pre-medication is used, but more commonly nowadays analgesia is produced by an intravenous or inhaled agent.

PHYSIOTHERAPY IN THE TREATMENT OF BURNS

Most patients suffering from burns require some physiotherapy. In extensively burnt patients *breathing exercises* are the earliest treatment given. Many of these patients suffer inhalation burns when the mucous membrane linings of the respiratory tract become inflamed and oedematous and because of this tracheostomy may have to be performed. This carries with it, as always, the danger of still further infection if it is not managed, and suction carried out, with the greatest possible care.

If burns involve the trunk and are deep, the patient will be encased in a tight 'armour' of eschar and chest movements are inhibited. The patient must be encouraged to breathe as deeply as this will permit and as long as the area remains dry the physiotherapist can place her hands directly on to the chest, but when the area is moist sterile gloves must be used and when the area is very sore exercises will have to be given by command only, unless of course there is severe respiratory infection; this must then rank as a priority and all the usual methods of posturing and percussion must be employed, covering the chest with sterile towels or using sterile gloves.

Sometimes the eschar or burnt skin is so tight and restricting that longitudinal incisions have to be made in it to facilitate adequate expansion. Incisions may also be necessary in limb burns, when these are circumferential to relieve venous and lymphatic engorgement.

Positioning of the patients is most important and a close watch must be kept on this not only by the physiotherapist, but also by the nursing staff. Most frequently it is burns overlying the flexor aspect of joints which give rise to contracture, and wherever possible these must be prevented and controlled. Splints are obviously advantageous, though with severe burns these are most difficult to apply effectively. Plaster of Paris, Cramer wire, covered with Polyurethane foam, and Plastazote and Orthoplast are all used in an effort to support and maintain good functional positions of joints including the cervical spine. Here it must be stated that some contractures are not completely preventable, but it is still important that every effort is made to minimize them. The use of boards and splints to prevent foot drop are essential and knees should be maintained as straight as possible. The head and neck should be supported in a mid- and extended position. Since oedema is very prevalent in burns, hands in particular should be elevated by fixation to suitable apparatus beside and above the bed and sometimes upon well-placed pillows.

All movements can be encouraged prior to grafting, dressings permitting, and as soon afterwards as the surgeon will allow. Where autografts have been applied, five days usually elapse before the first dressing. Often movements can then be commenced, but only when the dressings are down, otherwise newly applied skin may be rubbed against dressings resulting in fixation and consequent destruction and loss of grafts. When lyophilized skin has been used in the form of a dressing and the area left exposed movements can start after 24 hours.

A feature of burns illness is *a mental surrender to apathy* – often aggravated by necessary isolation. Combined with this is a suppression of intellectual and aesthetic interests and a withdrawal from personal relationships. The physiotherapist's daily, or twice daily, visits give these patients a regular and closer contact with the outside world and this in turn demands of the physiotherapist a great understanding and the ability to provide mental stimulation. In some units complete isolation is maintained only during the pre-grafting period, then, after grafting, the patient is transferred to a three- or four-bedded ward where the encouragement and company of others is undoubtedly an added incentive to recovery.

The treatment of burns is extremely time-consuming for the physiotherapist. When burns are extensive it is necessary to encourage specific and general mobilization and it must be remembered that these patients tire easily and must be allowed frequent rest periods. Time must be spent in encouragement, endeavouring to give confidence to patients who, due partly to their isolation and largely to the severity of their injuries, need maximum reassurance and come to look on their physiotherapist as a source of special contact with the rest of the medical team.

AMBULATION

This varies from unit to unit. In extensive burns early ambulation is out of the question, but where leg burns are relatively minor, early ambulation with adequate support or bandaging is advocated by some, whilst others prefer the areas to be well healed before allowing the patients up and walking. The ambulation of patients with severe leg burns is obviously more delayed. In either case it is common practice to suspend the legs, well bandaged, over the side of the bed prior to weight-bearing, progressing from one minute every hour initially to two minutes every hour and so on until three or four days have elapsed when the patient is allowed onto his feet; he is then allowed to walk only for short periods and is not permitted to stand about. When sitting out the lower limbs should be elevated.

Without this gradual progression and bandage support oedema can be a complicating factor and blistering of newly grafted skin can occur due to the inadequacy of newly established circulation to the grafted area. When soundly healed it will still be necessary for patients to continue with exercises to strengthen muscles and to regain full joint movement. Crepe bandages or elastic stockings will have to be worn by those with grafted leg burns for several weeks to prevent oedema. The adapting of footwear may be necessary where there is need to compensate for contracture (e.g. tight calf contractures may need a heel raise) or to relieve specific pressure areas. This can be done with foam rubber.

Often the patient's first contact with the outside world following the burn injury is in the physiotherapy department. Here supportive therapy and great encouragement is required, because the disfigurement caused by burns is often demoralizing. Helping patients to surmount and overcome their natural self-consciousness is something in which the physiotherapist can play a very helpful role.

THE HAND

'The hand is a perfect piece of mechanism – we are constantly dependent on it.' As such it is considered necessary to dwell a little on its individual treatment.

The hands are common sites for burns not only through direct involvement, but also because they are so often used in a reflex action to protect the face. There would seem to be a higher percentage of dorsal than of palmar burns.

Once again the maintenance of a *good functional position* is essential. The wrist should be extended and the metacarpophalangeal joints flexed either by adequate positioning on pillows with foam gripping rolls in the palms, or by splinting (Plate 21/1). This functional position should be maintained of course both pre- and post-grafting and early movement must be encouraged.

Here too it should be stressed *that hands must be bandaged carefully*, so that the functional position of the fingers (with flexion at metacarpophalangeal and interphalangeal joints, with the thumb in abduction and flexion) is maintained. Any tendency there may be for bandages to be

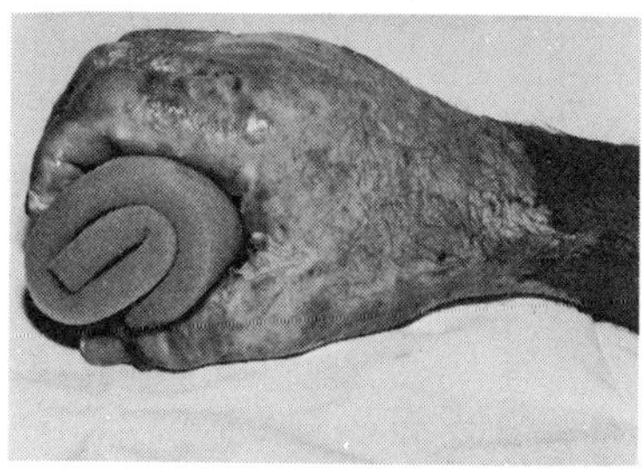

Plate 21/1 Positioning of the burnt hand (*see p. 266*)

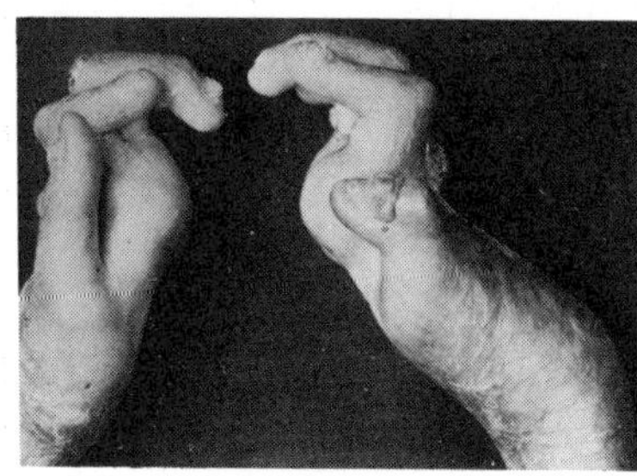

Plate 21/2 The type of deformity that can result from not maintaining good functional position (*see p. 268*)

Plate 21/3 An abdominal flap transferred via wrist to lower leg. Hand mobility must be maintained and static quadriceps and static deltoid contractions encouraged (*see p. 272*)

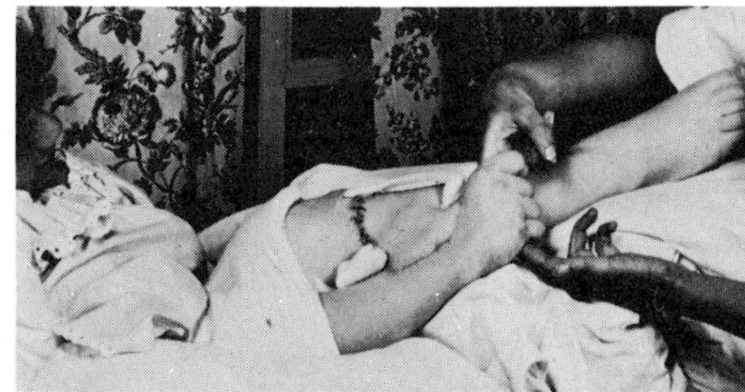

Plate 21/4 The cross-leg flap. Rolls of Sorbo rubber relieve pressure between left donor and right recipient legs (*see p. 272*)

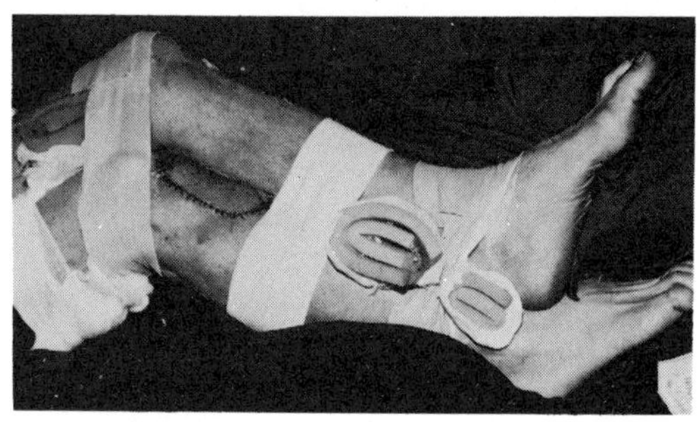

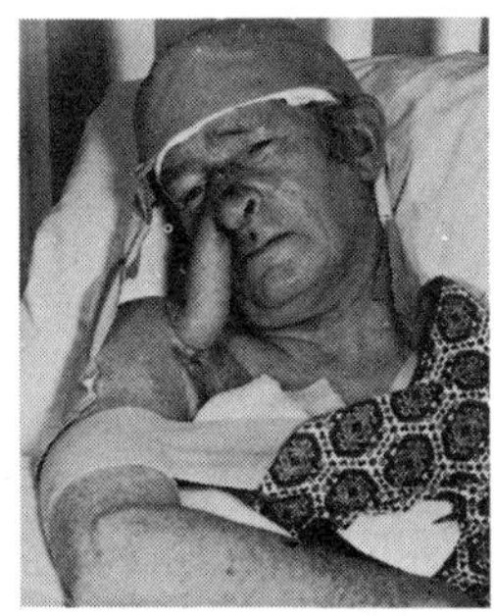

Plate 21/5 Acromio-thoracic tube pedicle raised and attached to replace a nasal defect (*see p. 272*)

applied too tightly or by the manner of their application to restrict movements of these joints, by holding them in a position of extension, must be prevented.

The shorter the time that elapses between burning and grafting, the smaller the amount of deep scar tissue likely to form. Therefore, secondary healing by granular tissue in the hand is seldom permitted. With the techniques of early excision and grafting, *movements are started* almost immediately and contracture and resultant deformities are much less likely to occur.

It was at one time categorically stated that passive movements were never used, but these should not be confused with active movements with gentle over-pressure, which often have to be employed. This, however, is something which until one has treated these cases cannot be fully appreciated. The amount of over-pressure used is not tantamount to vigorous passive movement which could only set up joint irritation and increase rather than decrease any tendency to marked joint stiffness.

All movements of the hands must be encouraged but particularly flexion of the small joints as already mentioned, and extension of the wrist and full thumb range. There is a tendency if the position is not watched, to get a flexing of the wrist and a hyperextending of the metacarpophalangeal joints, and if this is allowed to persist during healing the accompanying skin tightness will make these faulty positions difficult to correct (Plate 21/2).

One minor problem should be mentioned here and that is the difficulty that is encountered when hand burns are exposed and are too severe to allow the physiotherapist to use her hands as support or fulcra. Supported on pillows or foam rubber or when treated in a bath, encouragement can sometimes be only verbal. However, as soon as feasible, sterile gauze can be interposed between patient's and physiotherapist's hands, so that the contact thus established makes movements for the patient much easier, as will the use of plastic or rubber gloves worn by the physiotherapist when the patient has treatment in the bath or has his hand and arm in an arm bath, containing saline or Lux.

During the acute phase *movements for the unburnt areas of limbs* must be encouraged to prevent any tendency to secondary stiffness and muscle weakness such as might result in, for example, foot-drop. Patients spending prolonged periods in prone lying must of course be helped to move as much as their position will allow.

Throughout treatment co-operation of the nursing staff is essential. Their help should be sought with regard to observing and maintaining correct positioning.

When fully and firmly healed *sensory training* can play a part, but in the early stages hypersensitivity of the burnt areas discourages this, though every effort must be made to break down the patient's resistance to self-help. The holding of drinking beakers and cutlery must be encouraged as soon as feasible, and here too nursing staff help is invaluable. Those with burnt hands are often most reluctant to take the first steps towards independence.

Once the grafts are healed and the skin becomes more stable, more routine methods of treatment may be used. If the patient can come to the department *wax baths* can be given, though these must be at a lower temperature than normal, i.e. about 110°F (43°C), and excessive care must be taken in the early treatments for there is an inherent fear of being burnt again. Wax can be followed by *massage* with an hydrous ointment gently, but firmly, applied, however, an accumulation of such ointment should not be permitted and the hands should be washed with soap and water between treatments.

The use of polythene bags or gloves in the treatment of burnt hands can, with a co-operative patient, be an invaluable method. Newly burnt hands are first covered with Silver Sulphadiazine Cream, an anti-bacterial agent that can be applied painlessly to any depth of burn, and then slipped into gloves which are securely fixed at the wrist by bandage or adhesive tape, thus sealing them off. Inside these the patients find movement remarkably easy, there are no dressing restrictions, and the discomfort of the burn exposed to the air is eliminated. The physiotherapist is also able actually to see the movement achieved, as is the patient. This gives added incentive.

Advances are being made in the prevention of hypertrophic scars after burns. Originating in the USA, this method is being adopted in this country and proving most successful. This is the use of precisely measured pressure garments such as gloves and stockings made of an elasticated mesh material. The wearing of these can start one to two weeks after the burnt or grafted areas are healed. It has been found necessary to insist on their being worn 24 hours per day, except for brief periods to enable washing, etc., for six to twelve months.

These garments are often used in conjunction with Orthoplast splints – these latter maintaining pressure in axilla or neck where pressure from the elasticated mesh would be inadequate. It is the exact and even pressure of these two materials which prevents the formation of disfiguring and disabling scars.

The theory of the success of such methods is that the application of such pressure elongates the fibroblasts, thus preventing raised and bumpy scar tissue.

Watch must be retained over patients thus treated after their discharge until the pressure can safely be removed, i.e. until the hypertrophic tendencies are overcome.

SKIN GRAFTS

These are of two main types: free grafts which involve only varying thicknesses of the skin itself, and flaps and pedicles in which skin and subcutaneous tissue are transposed to make good a defect.

Free grafts

These are of two thicknesses.

WOLFE GRAFTS

These consist of full thickness skin down to, but excluding fat and usually taken from the post-auricular or supraclavicular areas to repair facial defects where skin contours need to be filled out. The donor site will not regenerate and must itself be closed by grafting.

SPLIT SKIN GRAFTS

These can vary from the very thin to three-quarter skin thickness and their donor sites heal themselves in around ten to twelve days. These grafts are cut with a knife or dermatome. Such grafts are used very largely in the surgery of repair and particularly in the grafting of burns. After cutting, they are applied to the raw areas with a backing of Tulle Gras with or without further dressings according to the wishes of the surgeon. Where the area to be repaired is small, the donor site can be selected to give a good 'match'. This means the quality and colour of the selected donor skin is taken into consideration so that these grafts match as nearly as possible the surrounding skin on the recipient site. When the area is extensive, however, grafts are taken from all available sites.

Once free grafts are in situ, blood flow into the existing capillaries occurs during the first 48 hours. Thereafter, there is a reorganization of capillaries which includes some growth.

Following free grafts, movements can be commenced after five days providing the dressings have been removed. After ten days they can be performed within the dressings. Joints not directly involved in the grafting can be moved but movement of these must once again not cause friction on newly applied skin.

When there is dryness of the grafts, once they are well established, the application – with gentle finger kneading – of olive oil or an hydrous ointment may prove beneficial. Too heavy kneading or heavy handedness must be avoided at this stage or blistering may occur – not a good psychological effect on the patient who sees this as a breakdown of soundly healed skin.

Eyelid grafts

In burns of the face, eyelids are often involved and since their contraction can lead to corneal exposure, they are of prime importance in the order of grafting. Split skin grafts are cut and held in position by stent moulds for a five-day period, and at ten days grafts may well benefit from oil massage, using light finger kneadings to maintain their pliability and aid their 'settling in'. If both eyes are involved the patient will be blindfold for the first five days and many will need all the reassurance that every member of the team can give.

Stent is a plastic resinous material, often used in dentistry. It is used

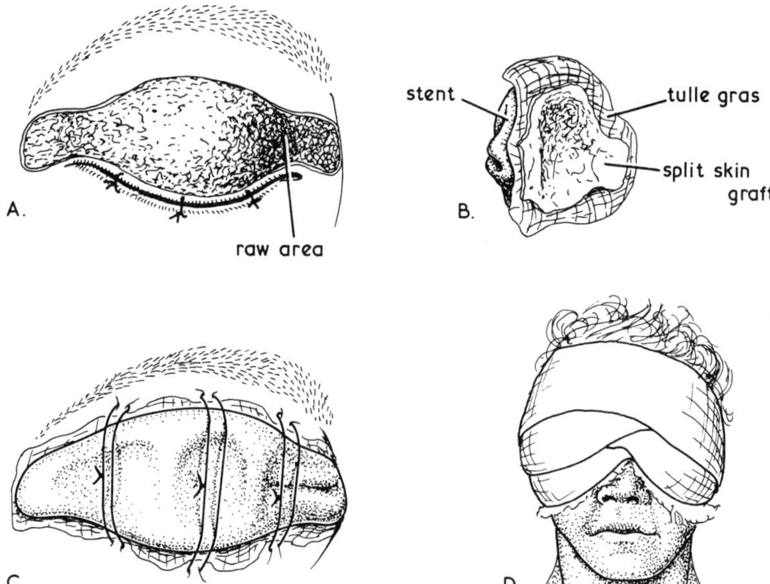

Fig. 21/3 Repair of burn of upper lid of right eye. A. Eyelids sutured together; eschar removed and raw site extended. B. Stent prepared, ready for application. C. Stent in position. D. Both eyes bandaged for 5 days

for this purpose because it is so malleable, and then sets hard, thus holding the graft in place. See Fig. 21/3.

Flaps and pedicles

From a brief summary of free grafting, we move to the surgery of repair by transplantation of skin and subcutaneous tissue. This can sometimes only be done in stages so that the viability of the graft can be maintained. The principal types of these grafts are transposition flaps, pedicle flaps and direct flaps.

TRANSPOSITION FLAPS

These are used to replace defects by transposing skin and subcutaneous tissues from an adjacent site, such as might be employed in the grafting of pressure sores. These in themselves demand little from the physiotherapist.

PEDICLE FLAPS

These are flaps raised, and sometimes tubed and used, most often, for the replacement of traumatic defects of the face and neck. Indeed, in many units these types of grafts are widely used as a means of conveying skin from one part of the body to another.

DIRECT FLAPS

These are open flaps, their undersurface remaining raw throughout their attachment period.

Pedicle and direct flaps are both means of making good one area by 'robbing' another. They can be transposed from one limb to another or can come via an intermediary, e.g. a flap or pedicle raised on the abdomen can be attached to the wrist (Plate 21/3), and after three weeks it is detached from its base and carried by the wrist to the lower leg to replace skin loss over a fractured tibia. Incidentally ununited fractures are often encouraged to heal by the fact that the compound site is given good skin cover.

Some of these flap repairs entail most acrobatic positions and often lead to discomfort in the joints involved and to muscle spasm. Such tension and consequent pain may be relieved by the application of *heat and massage* to the joints involved. Excessive care must be taken to prevent damage to the flap by heat, for the circulation is reduced and burning and destruction might therefore ensue. There is, too, an absence of skin sensation and this must be remembered for the patient will not be able to feel the heat and will, therefore, not be able to give any warning if it becomes excessive. Applied with care, however, it can be invaluable. Deep kneading can relieve spasm and discomfort in a matter of a few days. *Relevant exercises* too are given in the form of static muscle contractions and movements of joints not directly affected by the flap.

The cross-leg flap is perhaps one of the more common in use, one leg being the donor for the other. A flap is raised on the good leg and attached by its free end to the recipient site on the other, the donor site itself is then resurfaced with a split skin graft. The position is maintained for three weeks during which time the physiotherapist supervises joint care, comfort and muscle function regularly (Plate 21/4).

Nasal and chin defects are made good in several ways, but from the physiotherapy point of view, the *acromio-thoracic tube pedicle* is the important one to mention. This pedicle is raised from the upper chest wall, its lower end being swung into position to repair the nose or chin defect and it is held in position for three weeks. This will necessitate a mild side flexion and rotation of the neck (Plate 21/5).

During this period infra-red treatment and massage are given to relieve spasm and stiffness in the neck but the pedicle, of course, must be covered and protected during the application of heat.

When flaps are transposed in these stages more joints are involved and the possible final position of, for example, an arm attached to a lower leg is indeed one that calls for ingenuity in comfortable positioning and adequate physiotherapy to maintain muscle tone and movement.

GRAFTING AND PLASTIC SURGERY IN OTHER CONDITIONS

ABDOMINAL AND BREAST REDUCTIONS

When patients undergo abdominal and breast reductions, when excess tissue is removed, breathing exercises are advocated. The obese are always reluctant to move and in such cases chest complications must be avoided.

REPAIR OF SACRAL PRESSURE SORES

Sacral pressure sores are repaired by means of a local flap and those most usually treated in a plastic surgery unit are those incurred where paralysis exists. Here again the physiotherapist will be called upon to give breathing exercises and to maintain mobility by passive and active assisted movements.

Dupuytren's contracture

This is a condition frequently dealt with in plastic surgery units. It is a crippling condition in which a diseased and contracted palmar fascia causes varying degrees of deformity. In minor cases the fascia only is affected, but in severe cases the skin too is involved and in all there is a progressive pull on the fingers into the palm. In most extreme cases the skin is so contracted that in the palm creases it becomes 'soggy' and washing becomes a real problem.

Dupuytren's contracture affects men much more than women and most commonly in the 40–50 age group. It is not necessarily secondary to trauma and though it can occur unilaterally, it is much more likely to affect both hands. The little and ring fingers are much more usually involved than the thumb and index finger. Feet can be affected, but much less frequently.

Fasciectomy, or excision of the whole of the affected area of the palmar aponeurosis, is performed and this can be followed by early physiotherapy. After four to five days *gentle flexion* can be encouraged, but no extension at this stage for the palm is a poor healing area and no tension should be exerted on the stitches.

Elevation is important and every effort is made to prevent haematomas, with a firm pad bandaged into the palm, for if allowed to occur they can prevent healing and indeed cause skin loss. The palm being such a poor healing site, the wound must be allowed to become fully and soundly healed before progressing to finger extension exercises which otherwise might cause the wound edges to distract. Once the wound is healed *wax baths* and *lanolin massage* precede encouragement towards full flexion and extension. *Ultrasonics* too may play a part at this stage in softening the palmar scars.

SYNDACTYLE

This is a common congenital deformity where there is webbing between two or more digits. This can either be an extension of the normal web or can involve fusion of nerves, blood vessels and, in extreme cases, even bone.

Surgical separation is carried out early both from a functional and a cosmetic point of view. To correct this webbing, skin grafts have to be cut from a suitable area, e.g. the upper arm, and placed along the defects created by the separation. After ten days *exercises* can be given to educate the hand in its new form, particularly with regard to abduction of the fingers which has previously by nature of the webbing been inhibited.

POLLICIZATION

Loss of the thumb through trauma is a crippling condition for without a thumb the hand is at great disadvantage, and the reconstruction of the lost digit is of great importance.

This is performed either by transposition or pedicle flaps with subsequent bone graft, or by transplanting part of the index finger with its nerve and blood supply to the end of what remains of the thumb stump.

Following surgery of this kind, not only must full function of the hand be regained but the new thumb must be educated, where the latter method has been used, to work in its new role. As a finger its prime movements were those of flexion and extension and now it has to work in a position of opposition. After such operations sensory training is invaluable.

REFERENCES

Jackson, Douglas. 'Extensive Burns' in *Modern Trends in Plastic Surgery* (ed. Gibson, Thomas). Butterworth, 1964 (out of print). *Note*: 1966 edition does not contain this chapter.

Matthews, D. N. *The Surgery of Repair, Injuries and Burns*. Blackwell, 1946 (out of print).

McLaughlin, C. R. *Plastic Surgery – An Introduction for Nurses*. Faber and Faber (out of print).

Index

Moore, F. T. 'Plastic Surgery of the Hand' in *Textbook of British Surgery* (eds. Souttar, Sir Henry, and Goligher, J. C.). Heinemann, 1958, Vol. 3.

Smith, Ferris. *Plastic and Reconstructive Surgery – A Manual of Management*, Chapter III. Saunders, 1950 (out of print).

Watson, John. 'Trends in the Treatment of Burns' in *Annals of the Royal College of Surgeons of England*, **49**, 36–49, 1971.